Vestibular Disorders

VESTIBULAR DISORDERS

A Case-Study Approach

SECOND EDITION

Joseph M. Furman, MD, PhD

Professor
Departments of Otolaryngology, Neurology,
Bioengineering, and Physical Therapy
University of Pittsburgh
Pittsburgh, Pennsylvania

Stephen P. Cass, MD, MPH

Associate Professor
Department of Otolaryngology
University of Colorado Health Sciences Center
Denver, Colorado

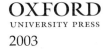
UNIVERSITY PRESS

2003

OXFORD
UNIVERSITY PRESS

Oxford   New York
Auckland   Bangkok   Buenos Aires   Cape Town   Chennai
Dar es Salaam   Delhi   Hong Kong   Istanbul   Karachi   Kolkata
Kuala Lumpur   Madrid   Melbourne   Mexico City   Mumbai
Nairobi   São Paulo   Shanghai   Taipei   Tokyo   Toronto

Published by Oxford University Press, Inc.
198 Madison Avenue, New York, New York, 10016
http://www.oup-usa.org

Oxford is a registered trademark of Oxford University Press

Library of Congress Cataloging-in-Publication Data
Furman, Joseph M., 1952-
Vestibular disorders : a case-study approach /
Joseph M. Furman, Stephen P. Cass.—2nd ed.
p. cm.
Previous ed. published under the title: Balance disorders.
Includes bibliographical references and index.
ISBN 0-19-514579-8
1. Vestibular apparatus—Diseases—Case studies.
2. Dizziness—Case studies.
3. Equilibrium (Physiology)—Case studies.
I. Cass, Stephen P., 1957-
II. Furman, Joseph M., 1952-
Balance disorders. III. Title.
RF260 .F87 2002   617.8'82—dc21   2002025789

The science of medicine is a rapidly changing field. As new research and clinical experience broaden our knowledge, changes in treatment and drug therapy do occur. The author and publisher of this work have checked with sources believed to be reliable in their efforts to provide information that is accurate and complete, and in accordance with the standards accepted at the time of publication. However, in light of the possibility of human error or changes in the practice of medicine, neither the author, nor the publisher, nor any other party who has been involved in the preparation or publication of this work warrants that the information contained herein is in every respect accurate or complete. Readers are encouraged to confirm the information contained herein with other reliable sources, and are strongly advised to check the product information sheet provided by the pharmaceutical company for each drug they plan to administer.

9 8 7 6 5 4 3 2 1

Printed in the United States of America
on acid-free paper

Preface to the Second Edition

Dizziness is one of the most common complaints that patients bring to their doctors. As many as 40% of adults experience clinically significant dizziness at some time in their lives, and nearly one in four emergency room visits includes a complaint of dizziness. Even though dizziness is common, it remains a perplexing problem for most physicians. It can be a symptom of disease in almost any organ system, and the constellation of symptoms presented by patients with dizziness often seems complex. Moreover, the same disorder may present differently, depending on the patient's personality and his or her response to disease, lifestyle, and age.

Many patients with dizziness have an abnormality related to vestibular function or to central nervous system processing of sensory information that is important for spatial orientation. The pathophysiology underlying a balance disorder can be baffling because much of vestibular physiology is grounded in physics and applied engineering, topics that are remote to most physicians. This mix of basic science and complex patient presentations makes the field of vestibular disorders challenging. Nevertheless, deducing the origin of dizziness and implementing appropriate treatment is a skill that will benefit any physician who encounters patients complaining of dizziness or disequilibrium, especially primary care physicians, otolaryngologists, neurologists, and psychiatrists.

We have chosen to use a case-study approach to outline the principles and practice of the care of patients with vestibular disorders. The use of a case-study approach is consistent with the recent evolution of problem-based learning in the medical sciences. We have tailored the case-study approach used in this book so that it can be used as part of residency training programs.

Our approach to vestibular disorders reflects the merging of ideas from the combined experience of a neurologist (Dr. Furman) and a neurotologic surgeon (Dr. Cass). We hope that this dual perspective makes this book enlightening to its readers. Each case study contains relevant material regarding history, physical examination, laboratory testing, differential diagnosis, and treatment. This material provides a springboard for discussion of either a concept in the field of vestibular disorders or the diagnosis or treatment of a particular disease state. Practical, specific treatment options are discussed throughout the book.

For our second edition, we have changed the title of the book from *Balance Disorders: A Case Study Approach* to *Vestibular Disorders: A Case-Study Approach* to reflect more accurately the focus of the diagnoses that are discussed. Each of the previous cases has been updated as much as possible based on recent advances in the field. The background material for the cases has been reorganized and now includes a chapter on the history of the dizzy patient, a chapter on the physical examination of the dizzy patient, and a chapter on psychiatric issues. The chapter on vestibular rehabilitation has been extensively revised. We have added 14 new cases, 5 of which constitute a new portion of the book concerning patients with multiple diagnoses. These cases explore the additional challenges presented by overlapping diagnostic features and conflicting treatment issues. Another new part of the book, entitled "Clinically Controversial Case Studies," includes five new cases and five previous cases, each of which addresses a disorder or a clinical issue surrounded by a particularly broad range of opinion or uncertainty.

Because of the importance of understanding the underlying physiology and pathophysiology of the conditions being discussed, Part I provides essential background information concerning vestibular physiology, history and physical examination, vestibular laboratory testing, audiology, vestibular rehabilitation, and psychiatric issues. Parts II through VI consist of case studies. In Part II, each of the six tutorial cases elucidates an essential principle or major issue in the field of balance disorders.

In Part III, 14 common disease cases review disorders that are frequently encountered. Especially common disorders are discussed in several different cases, with different specific issues addressed in each case. Part IV provides five case studies related to multiple diagnoses to illustrate the diagnostic and treatment issues that arise when a single diagnosis cannot account for the patient's ailments. Part V contains 24 case studies pertaining to unusual disorders. These cases provide the reader with an appreciation of the breadth of the field and an awareness of the rarer cause of dizziness. Part VI includes 10 case studies that address clinical controversies—8 regarding diagnosis or treatment, 1 regarding driving and dizziness, and 1 regarding malingering.

This book is not meant as a substitute for other textbooks that deal specifically with the anatomy and physiology of the vestibular system, the details of the ocular motor system, or vestibular rehabilitation. Excellent textbooks are available on each of these topics. Rather, this book spans the gap between these in-depth textbooks and the problems that arise whenever a patient presents with dizziness.

Pittsburgh, Pennsylvania   J.M.F.
Denver, Colorado   S.P.C.

Acknowledgments

We wish to acknowledge our families for their patience and support during the writing of this book. We thank Oxford University Press for publishing the second edition of this book and especially thank Ms. Fiona Stevens for her encouragement and helpful suggestions. We gratefully acknowledge Dr. Ki-Bum Sung, who provided a detailed critique of the first edition and performed extensive literature searches to assure that the second edition is up-to-date. We thank Dr. Robert Schor for help with computers, information, and media, Dr. Susan Whitney for help with the chapter entitled "Vestibular Rehabilitation," Dr. Rolf Jacob for help with the chapter entitled "Psychiatric Aspects of Vestibular Disorders," Ms. Cheryl Miller for helping us identify case material, Dr. Ja-Won Koo for helping us identify relevant literature citations, and Dr. Daniel Sklare for ideas regarding driving and dizziness. Finally, we thank Ms. Mary Grace Wojnar and Ms. Carrie Cobb for their invaluable assistance in the preparation of the manuscript.

Introduction: Guide for the Reader

The text is divided into six parts. Part I includes seven chapters that provide background information common to many of the case studies. Topics include anatomy and physiology of the vestibular system, history and physical examination of the dizzy patient, vestibular laboratory testing, audiometric testing, vestibular rehabilitation, and psychiatric issues. Parts II through VI include 59 case studies. In Part II, 6 cases illustrate major themes in the field of balance disorders; in Part III, 14 cases illustrate commonly encountered disorders; in Part IV, 5 cases illustrate how more than one disorder can be present in the same patient; in Part V, 24 cases illustrate unusual disorders, and in Part VI, 10 cases illustrate controversial disorders.

The material in this book can be approached in several ways. For individuals with minimal background in the area of vestibular disorders, Part I should be read thoroughly before beginning the case studies, which should be read in order. An alternative approach, better suited to a more knowledgeable reader, is to read Part II, the tutorial cases, first and refer to the material in Part I as needed. The reader can then study the common disease cases in Parts III and IV and the unusual disease cases in Part V. More experienced clinicians can approach the material by referring to the cases as they arise in their practice or in their own order of interest. The cases in Part VI each address a clinical controversy in vestibular disorders and should be of interest to all readers. The Appendix of Diagnoses and the Index are meant to allow the reader to find sought-after material directly. The cases also are cross-referenced extensively to alert the reader to relevant material that appears elsewhere in the text.

Contents

Part I Background for Case Studies

Chapter 1. Vestibular Anatomy and Physiology, 3

Chapter 2. History of the Dizzy Patient, 16

Chapter 3. Physical Examination of the Dizzy Patient, 21

Chapter 4. Vestibular Laboratory Testing, 30

Chapter 5. Auditory System and Testing, 41

Chapter 6. Vestibular Rehabilitation, 47

Chapter 7. Psychiatric Aspects of Vestibular Disorders, 54

Part II Tutorial Case Studies

Case 1. Unilateral Vestibular Impairment and Vestibular Compensation—
Vestibular Neuritis, 63

Case 2. Mixed Peripheral and Central Vestibular Impairment—
Cerebellopontine Angle Tumor, 72

Case 3. Impaired Vestibular Compensation—Vestibular Neuritis, 77

Case 4. Bilateral Vestibular Loss—Ototoxicity, 82

Case 5. Anxiety and Psychiatric Dizziness—Vestibulopathy,
Cause Unknown, 91

Case 6. Emergency Room Management of the Dizzy Patient—Acute
Cerebellar Infarction, 97

Part III Common Disease Case Studies

Case 7. Benign Paroxysmal Positional Vertigo—Medical Management, 105

Case 8. Migraine-Associated Dizziness, 115

Case 9. Endolymphatic Hydrops—Meniere's Disease, 121

Case 10. Disequilibrium of Aging, 128

Case 11. Labyrinthine Concussion, 133

Case 12. Vertebrobasilar Insufficiency, 139

Case 13. Benign Recurrent Vertigo of Childhood, 145

Case 14. Multisensory Disequilibrium, 149

Case 15. Recurrent Vestibulopathy, 154

Case 16. Meniere's Disease—Surgical Management, 158

Case 17. Nonspecific Vestibulopathy, 169

Case 18. Chronic Otitis Media, 174

Case 19. Cerebellar Degeneration, 180

Case 20. Multiple Sclerosis, 186

Part IV Multiple Diagnosis Case Studies

Case 21. Meniere's Disease and Migraine, 195

Case 22. Benign Paroxysmal Positional Vertigo and Anxiety Disorder, 200

Case 23. Head Trauma: Combined Central Nervous System, Labyrinthine, and Cervical Injury, 204

Case 24. Migraine-Related Dizziness and Anxiety Disorder, 208

Case 25. Meniere's Disease and Benign Paroxysmal Positional Vertigo, 213

Part V Unusual Disease Case Studies

Case 26. Mal de Débarquement Syndrome, 219

Case 27. Autoimmune Inner Ear Disease, 222

Case 28. Orthostatic Hypotension, 228

Case 29. Wallenberg's Syndrome—Posterior Inferior Cerebellar Artery Infarction, 233

Case 30. Anterior Inferior Cerebellar Artery Infarction, 237

Case 31. Benign Paroxysmal Positional Vertigo—Surgical Management, 243

Case 32. Lithium-Induced Dizziness, 249

Case 33. Syncope, 253

Case 34. Drop Attacks, 256

Case 35. Ramsay Hunt Syndrome, 260

Case 36. Convergence Spasm, 265

Case 37. Congenital Inner Ear Malformations, 269

Case 38. Ocular Tilt Reaction, 278

Case 39. Horizontal Semicircular Canal Benign Paroxysmal
Positional Vertigo, 282

Case 40. Chiari Malformation, 287

Case 41. Saccadic Fixation Instability, 293

Case 42. Congenital Nystagmus, 299

Case 43. Otosclerotic Inner Ear Syndrome, 304

Case 44. Progressive Supranuclear Palsy, 312

Case 45. Solvent Exposure, 316

Case 46. Wernicke's Encephalopathy, 321

Case 47. Vestibular Epilepsy, 326

Case 48. Prion Disease, 330

Case 49. Orthostatic Tremor, 334

Part VI Clinically Controversial Case Studies

Case 50. Acoustic Neuroma—Management, 341

Case 51. Superior Semicircular Canal Dehiscence Syndrome—
Tullio's Phenomenon, 347

Case 52. Perilymphatic Fistula, 353

Case 53. Cervicogenic Dizziness, 359

Case 54. Chronic Fatigue Syndrome, 364

Case 55. Driving and Dizziness, 368

Case 56. Malingering, 373

Case 57. Vascular Cross-Compression Syndrome of the Eighth
Cranial Nerve, 377

Case 58. Bilateral Meniere's Disease, 382

Case 59. Complementary and Alternative Therapies for Dizziness, 388

Bibliography, 393

Appendix of Diagnoses, 407

Index, 409

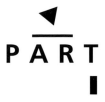

PART

I

Background for Case Studies

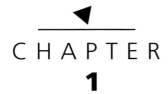

CHAPTER
1

Vestibular Anatomy and Physiology

The vestibular labyrinth contains two types of sensors, the semicircular canals and the otolith organs (Fig. 1–1). The semicircular canals sense rotational movement; the otolith organs sense linear motion and orientation with respect to gravity. There are three semicircular canals, each sensitive to rotation in a particular plane. These three planes are more or less perpendicular to one another, allowing the labyrinth to sense rotations about any spatial axis because one or more semicircular canals are stimulated by any particular rotation. For example, turning the head to the left and right stimulates predominantly the horizontal semicircular canals, whereas moving the head up and down stimulates the vertical semicircular canals. Figure 1–2 depicts the orientation of the semicircular canals in the head.

The otolith organs include the utricle and saccule. The utricle senses motion in the horizontal plane, that is, naso-occipital (forward–backward) movement, left–right movement, and combinations thereof. The saccule senses motion in the sagittal plane, such as naso-occipital movement, up–down movement, and combinations of these movements. The utricle and saccule also sense changes in orientation to gravity resulting from movements like putting the chin on the chest (pitch) and touching the ear to the shoulder (roll) . As can be seen in Figure 1–1, the cochlea is immediately adjacent to the vestibular labyrinth. Both endolymph and perilymph of the vestibular labyrinth and the cochlea are in communication with one another. The vestibular and auditory portions of the inner ear share a common blood supply as well. Because of their nearness to one another, common fluid spaces, and a shared blood supply, it is not surprising that disorders affecting the vestibular labyrinth often also affect the cochlea, so that dizziness and disequilibrium are often accompanied by hearing loss and/or tinnitus.

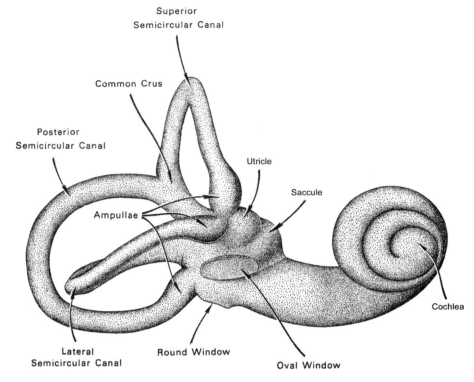

Figure 1–1 The vestibular labyrinth contains two types of sensors, the semicircular canals and the otolith organs. There are three semicircular canals: horizontal, superior (anterior), and posterior (inferior). Each semicircular canal is sensitive to rotation in the plane of the canals. The otolith organs include the utricle and saccule. The utricle senses motion both to and fro and left and right, and also senses static pitch and roll of the head, that is, movements such as putting the chin on the chest and touching the ear to the shoulder. The saccule senses up-and-down motion, to-and-fro motion, and static pitch of the head. Note the proximity of the cochlea to the vestibular labyrinth. The vestibular and auditory portions of the inner ear share a common blood supply and inner-ear fluid metabolism.

Each of the three semicircular canals contains an enlarged area known as the *ampulla*, which is important for the transduction of rotational motion into neural activity (Figs. 1–1, 1–3). Within each ampulla is a *cupula*, a gelatinous membrane that completely seals the semicircular canal. During head movement, the cupula bows like a drum head. This cupular movement, the first step in the transduction process, activates the underlying hair cells, which in turn are innervated by a semicircular canal nerve, which itself is a branch of the vestibular portion of the eighth cranial nerve.

The maculae of the vestibular labyrinth are the sensory transduction regions of the otolith organs, the utricle and saccule. The maculae are organized so that individual hair cells sense motion in a particular direction known as its *polarization vector*. The arrows shown in Figure 1–4 represent the most sensitive directions for individual hair cells on the surface of the utricular and saccular maculae. Note that for each macula there is a complete representation of directions of motion in the horizontal plane for the utricle and in the sagittal plane for the sac-

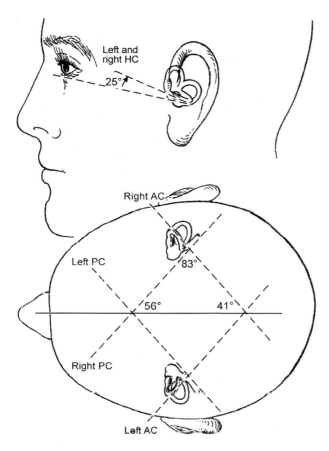

Figure 1–2 The vestibular labyrinth is oriented in the temporal bone in such a way that the lateralmost semicircular canal, which is the horizontal semicircular canal, is more or less in the head-horizontal plane. The other two semicircular canals, oriented more or less vertically and optimally, sense the oblique pitch-and-roll rotations of the head. The utricle lies more or less in the same plane as the horizontal semicircular canals, which allows it to transduce translational motion forward and backward and left and right. The saccule is oriented vertically. AC = anterior semicircular canal; HC = horizontal semicircular canal; PC = posterior semicircular canal.

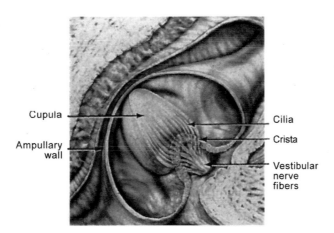

Figure 1–3 Ampulla of a semicircular canal. The ampulla of each semicircular canal is an enlarged area that is important to the transduction of rotational movement into neural activity. Within each ampulla is a cupula, a gelatinous membrane that completely seals the semicircular canal. During head movement, the cupula bows like a drum head; it does not flap like a swinging door. This cupular movement, the first step in the transduction process, activates the underlying hair cells. (*Source*: Modified with permission from Harada Y (ed): The Vestibular Organs. Amsterdam: Kugler & Guedini, 1988, p. 64.[4])

5

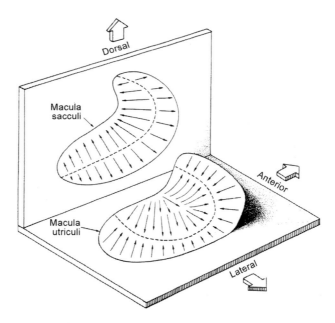

Figure 1–4 Maculae of the utricle and saccule. The maculae are the sensory transduction regions of the utricle and saccule. They are organized so that individual hair cells lie in various orientations, allowing them to optimally sense motion in a particular direction. The arrows indicate the most sensitive direction for individual hair cells on the surface of the maculae. At the center of each macula is a region called the *striola*, where the orientation of the hair cells changes abruptly. (*Source:* With permission from Baloh RW (ed): Dizziness, Hearing Loss, and Tinnitus: The Essentials of Neurotology. New York: Oxford University Press, 2001, p. 22.[5])

cule. For example, a hair cell in the utricular macula whose polarization vector points toward the left ear is stimulated by left-ear down-tilt or by linear acceleration to the right.

One component of each macula is the otolithic membrane, which contains otoconia (literally, "ear stones"), pebble-like structures composed of crystallized calcium carbonate (Figs. 1–5 and 1–6). Otoconia are constantly being formed and reabsorbed in a process involving the macular supporting cells and surrounding dark cells. This process of formation and absorption is probably important in the pathophysiology of benign paroxysmal positional vertigo (see Cases 7, 22, 25, 31, and 39).

Hair-cell stimulation results from the bending of an array of surface "hairs," or stereocilia. Bending the array toward the tallest hair (kinocilium) causes hair-cell depolarization, whereas bending the array of stereocilia away from the kinocilium causes hyperpolarization. Depolarization of the hair cells results in an increase in the firing rate of the eighth nerve afferents that innervate the hair cells, whereas hyperpolarization causes decreased activity.

Each neuron in the vestibular portion of the eighth cranial nerve has a so-called resting discharge. That is, numerous action potentials (about 90 per second) occur even with the head at rest. This is unique for sensory organs of the body. Although these neurons require an expenditure of energy even while the

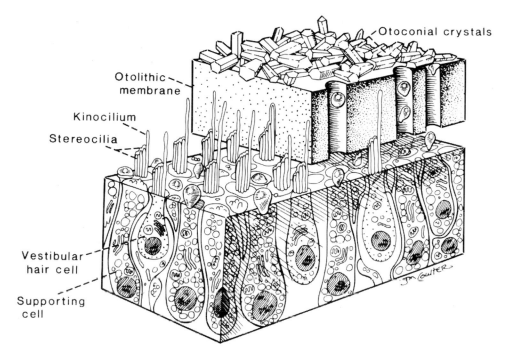

Figure 1–5 Otolithic macula. A component of each macula is an otolithic membrane containing otoconia (otoconial crystals). The otoconia add mass to the otolithic membrane. The heavy otolithic membrane deforms in response to linear motion and changes of orientation with respect to gravity. This deformation bends the hairs of the underlying hair cells. The directional sensitivity of each hair cell is determined by the location of the kinocilium with respect to the stereocilia.

head is still, their constant high-level firing rate is quite useful because such cells have a bidirectional response, that is, they can sense motion in both the excitatory and inhibitory directions, continuously monitor head motion, and are very sensitive. Vestibular neurons (Fig. 1–7) increase or decrease their firing rate as a result of depolarization or hyperpolarization, respectively, of the hair cells that they innervate.

The information regarding head movement transduced by the peripheral vestibular organs is relayed by the eighth cranial nerve, whose cell bodies lie in Scarpa's ganglion, and traverses the internal auditory canal and cerebellopontine angle before entering the brainstem at the pontomedullary junction. The vestibular nerve synapses on cells in the vestibular nuclei and other central nervous system structures such as the cerebellum. Information from the vestibular nuclei both ascends and descends in the central nervous system. Ascending pathways are important for vestibulo-ocular reflexes and for perception of vestibular sensations. Descending pathways are important for vestibulospinal reflexes.

Also included in the vestibular nerve are the vestibular efferents, neurons that project from the central nervous system to the labyrinth. Their function is uncertain, but they may be involved in modulating the sensitivity of the labyrinth.

The vestibular nucleus on either side of the brain is composed of at least four anatomic subdivisions named the *superior, medial, lateral,* and *inferior vestibular nu-*

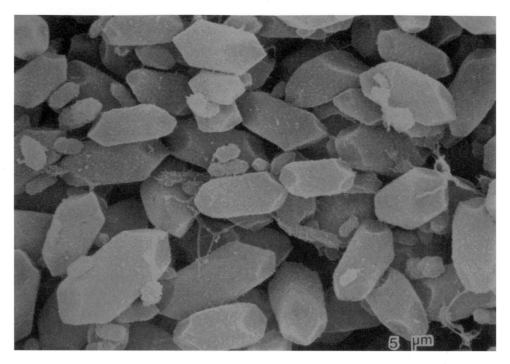

Figure 1–6 Scanning electron micrograph of otoconia, pebble-like structures composed of crystallized calcium carbonate ($CaCO_3$) that are constantly being formed and reabsorbed in a process involving the macular supporting cells and surrounding dark cells. (*Source*: With permission from Harada Y (ed): The Vestibular Organs. Amsterdam: Kugler & Guedini, 1988, p. 12.[4])

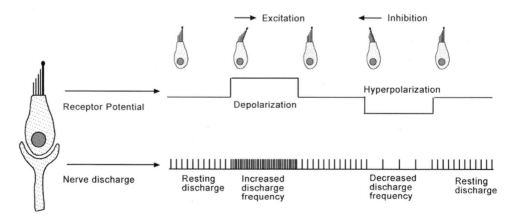

Figure 1–7 Each neuron in the vestibular portion of the eighth cranial nerve has a so-called resting discharge. That is, numerous action potentials (about 90 per second) occur even with the head at rest. Although these neurons require expenditure of energy even while the head is still, their constant high-level firing rate is useful because such cells can sense motion in both the excitatory and inhibitory directions via depolarization or hyperpolarization that increases and decreases eighth nerve firing rate, respectively. (*Source*: Adapted with permission from Kelly JP: Vestibular system. In: Kandel ER, Schwartz JH, Jessell TM (eds). Principles of Neural Science, ed 3. Norwalk, CT: Appleton & Lange, 1991, p. 506.[6])

clei. The vestibular nuclei receive inputs not only from the vestibular labyrinth but also from other sensory modalities including vision, somatic sensation, and audition. As a result of these varied sensory inputs, the name *vestibular nuclei* is somewhat misleading. These structures are, in fact, sensory integration nuclei whose output influences eye movements, truncal stability, and spatial orientation.

VESTIBULO-OCULAR REFLEX

The vestibulo-ocular reflex (VOR) is a mechanism whereby head movement automatically results in a conjugate eye movement equal and opposite to the head movement so that the eyes stay on target. For example, a leftward head movement is associated with a rightward eye movement of both eyes and vice versa. The VOR works for all types of head movements, including rotation and translation. The VOR, in its simplest form, is mediated by a three-neuron arc. For the horizontal VOR, these three neurons include the eighth cranial nerve (neuron 1), an interneuron that arises from the vestibular nucleus and terminates in the abducens nucleus (neuron 2), and the motoneuron to the eye muscles (neuron 3) (Fig. 1–8). Note that the excitation of the horizontal semicircular canal excites the contralateral abducens nucleus and thus the contralateral lateral rectus. Also stimulated, via the medial longitudinal fasciculus, which decussates (crosses), is the ipsilateral medial rectus subnucleus of the oculomotor nucleus and thus the ipsilateral medial rectus. Similar explanations can be applied to excitation of the anterior semicircular canals, for example, caused by pitching the head down, that is, chin to the chest, thereby causing upward deviation of both eyes; excitatory signals from the labyrinth cross to reach the superior rectus and inferior oblique subdivisions of the contralateral oculomotor nucleus. Because motor neurons to the superior rectus muscle decussate but those to the inferior oblique muscle do not, excitation of the anterior semicircular canals activates the ipsilateral superior rectus muscle and the contralateral inferior oblique muscle. Similarly, excitation of the posterior semicircular canals, for example by pitching the head down, causes downward deviation of both eyes; excitatory signals from the labyrinth cross to reach the contralateral rectus subnucleus and the contralateral trochlear nucleus. This neural activity causes excitation of the ipsilateral superior oblique muscle because of the crossed innervation of the superior oblique muscle by the trochlear nerve. This neural activity also causes excitation of the contralateral inferior rectus muscle because of the uncrossed innervation of the inferior rectus muscle from the oculomotor nucleus.

One remarkable feature of the VOR is that it is produced by the coordinated action of the two vestibular nuclear complexes, one on either side of the brainstem, which cooperate with one another such that when one is excited, the other is inhibited. This *push–pull* behavior is a direct result of the tonic vestibular activity in the eighth cranial nerve that allows both an increase and a decrease in neural activity during head movement. For example, when the head is turned to the left, the activity in the left eighth cranial nerve and left vestibular nuclei is increased, whereas the activity of the right eighth nerve and right vestibular nuclei is decreased (Fig. 1–9). This reciprocal effect greatly increases the sensitivity of the VOR.

Operationally, the central nervous system responds to differences in activity between the two vestibular nuclear complexes. For example, when there is no

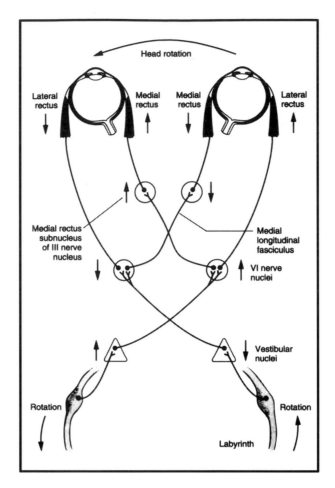

Figure 1–8 Horizontal vestibulo-ocular reflex (VOR) pathways. The VOR is mediated by a three-neuron arc that includes the eighth cranial nerve, an interneuron from the vestibular nucleus to the abducens nucleus (VI nerve), and the motoneuron to the lateral rectus muscles. To coordinate the movement of the two eyes, an interneuron connects the abducens nucleus to the oculomotor nucleus (III nerve), which contains the cell bodies of the motoneurons to the medial rectus muscle. Note that the sixth nerve nucleus contains cell bodies for the lateral rectus motoneurons as well as cell bodies for the fibers that ascend in the medial longitudinal fasciculus to innervate the motoneurons for the medial rectus muscle. The medial longitudinal fasciculus coordinates the action of the two eyes so that horizontal eye movements are conjugate. Note that a lesion of the medial longitudinal fasciculus is associated with an abnormality of adduction that manifests itself as an internuclear ophthalmoplegia. (*Source*: Adapted with permission from Furman JM: Nystagmus and the vestibular system. In: Podos SM, Yanoff M (eds). Textbook of Ophthalmology. New York: Gower Medical, 1993, p. 9.4.[7])

head movement, resting neural activity within the vestibular nuclei is symmetric. However, during movement, there is asymmetric activity in the vestibular nuclei. A left–right asymmetry in the vestibular nuclei is interpreted by the central nervous system as a head movement, even when such asymmetries are a result of pathology.

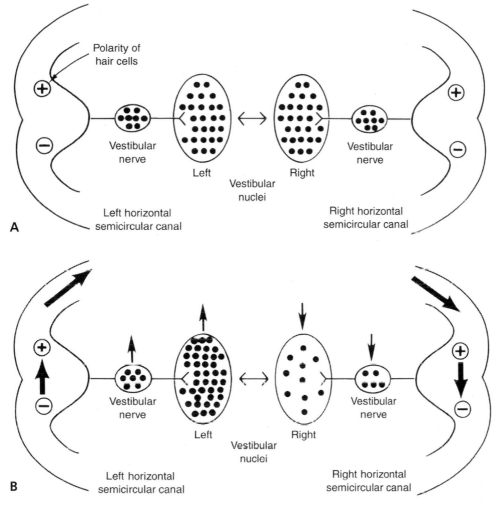

Figure 1–9 Push–pull action of the horizontal vestibulo-ocular reflex. (A) With no head movement, left and right vestibular influences are balanced. (B) With head movement to the left, endolymph flow produces an excitatory stimulus in the left horizontal semicircular canal and an inhibitory stimulus in the right horizontal semicircular canal. The excitatory stimulus increases neural activity in the vestibular nerve and vestibular nuclei, and the inhibitory stimulus decreases such activity. The brain interprets the difference in neural activity between the vestibular nuclei as a head movement to the left and generates appropriate vestibulo-ocular and postural responses.

VESTIBULOSPINAL AND NECK-RELATED REFLEXES

Information from the vestibular labyrinth descends in the nervous system to control head position, truncal stability, and limb position. The medial and lateral vestibulospinal tracts (MVST and LVST) and the reticulospinal tract (RST) carry information from the vestibular nuclei into the brainstem and spinal cord. The neck also sends neural signals to the central nervous system regarding head position. These signals, coupled with vestibular signals, provide information regarding head and trunk position. Signals from the neck can cause eye movements via the cervico-ocular reflex, which is normally almost completely inactive. Possibly, in patients with vestibular deficits, the cervico-ocular reflex becomes more active.[1,2] Another important reflex is the vestibulo-colic reflex, whereby vestibular signals are relayed to neck muscles to stabilize the head. This reflex may account for the neck stiffness experienced by many patients with vestibular asymmetries.

VESTIBULAR-AUTONOMIC PROJECTIONS

An additional projection of the vestibular system is to the autonomic nervous system, predominantly to the sympathetic nervous system and to structures that control respiration. Through these projections, patients with vestibular imbalance may experience nausea and vomiting. The physiologic necessity for the vestibuloautonomic system, especially the need for vestibular imbalance to induce nausea and vomiting, is unknown.

EFFECT OF UNILATERAL PERIPHERAL VESTIBULAR INJURY

Unilateral labyrinthine injury disrupts the reciprocal, push–pull interaction of the two labyrinths. Following the acute loss of unilateral peripheral vestibular function, there is a loss of resting neural activity in the vestibular nuclei ipsilateral to the lesion. Because the brain normally detects differences in activity between the two vestibular nuclear complexes, an acute loss of unilateral peripheral vestibular function is interpreted as a continuous rapid head movement (Fig. 1–10). The brain responds with "corrective" eye movements manifested as vestibular nystagmus.

With complete loss of unilateral vestibular function, the three semicircular canals and the two otolith organs on one side become inactive, and the resulting eye movement and body postures reflect the unopposed action of the contralateral labyrinth. In the case of eye movement, there is nystagmus. The direction of the nystagmus, which is predominantly horizontal-torsional, can be explained as follows: the remaining horizontal semicircular canal is unopposed, thus accounting for the horizontal component; the orientation of the two remaining vertical canals is such that their torsional (roll) influences add to each other but their vertical (pitch) components cancel one another. The vestibulospinal manifestation of acute unilateral peripheral vestibular loss may include head tilt. Most patients, however, do not have a static head tilt but do experience disequilibrium and postural instability that includes leaning and veering of gait to the side of the lesion.

The nystagmus, postural instability, and severe vegetative symptoms (e.g., nausea, vomiting, and diaphoresis) that are associated with acute vestibular injury gradually abate through compensatory mechanisms. This process, known as *vestibular compensation*, involves changes in the vestibular nuclei that lead to partial restoration of the lost resting neural activity within the ipsilateral vestibular nucleus, thereby reducing the asymmetry in neural activity between the left and right vestibular nuclei (Fig. 1–11A). Such changes restore the function of the vestibulo-ocular and vestibulospinal reflexes while the person is stationary.

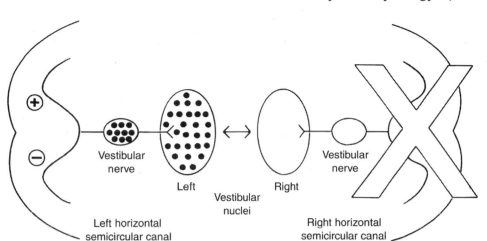

Figure 1–10 The reciprocal push–pull interaction of the two labyrinths is disrupted after acute peripheral labyrinthine injury. For example, following the acute loss of right unilateral peripheral vestibular function, there is a loss of resting neural activity in the right vestibular nerve and right vestibular nuclei. Because the brain normally detects differences in activity between the two vestibular nuclear complexes, even when stationary the imbalance in neural activity is interpreted as a rapid head movement, in this case to the left.

Vestibular compensation also improves the VOR during head movement. (Figs. 1-11B,C) The vegetative symptoms and signs resulting from stimulation of the vestibuloautonomic projections usually resolve in concert with improvement in the vestibulo-ocular and vestibulospinal reflexes.

Once the process of vestibular compensation has occurred, the neural activity in a single vestibular nerve influences the neural activity within both vestibular nuclei. Although compensation acts to rebalance brainstem vestibular activity, patients with chronic unilateral peripheral vestibular loss have a reduced VOR magnitude, abnormal timing of the VOR (see Chapter 4 regarding rotational testing), and an asymmetry of VOR during quick head movements. Occasionally, patients may overcompensate for a peripheral vestibular lesion and manifest a *recovery nystagmus*, which beats in the opposite direction from that which occurred initially. Also, such patients are susceptible to decompensation, leading to a recurrence of all or part of their acute vestibular syndrome.

The central vestibular system is profoundly influenced by the cerebellum.[3] Particular regions of the cerebellum, including the vestibulocerebellum (the flocculo-nodular lobe and the cerebellar vermis), are particularly important for control of eye movements and body position. Important and powerful connections between the vestibular nuclei and the cerebellum enable the cerebellum to influence vestibular-induced eye and trunk movements. As a result, lesions of the cerebellum are frequently associated with symptoms and signs such as gait instability and nystagmus that are indistinguishable from those seen with peripheral vestibular lesions.

The vestibular nuclear projection to the thalamus and to the cerebral cortex allows vestibular sensations to reach consciousness. However, these projections are not solely vestibular because they are mixed with somatic sensation. As a re-

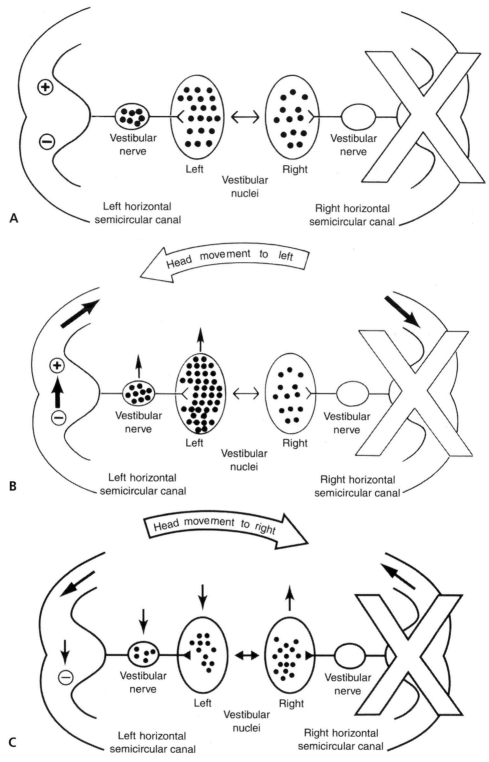

Figure 1–11 When a peripheral vestibular injury is chronic, in this case on the right, the central nervous system is able, through vestibular compensation, to partially restore the lost resting activity within the deafferented vestibular nucleus, and thus reduce the asymmetry of neural activity between the vestibular nuclei at rest (A) and partially restore the function of the vestibulo-ocular reflex (VOR). (B) Movement toward the intact ear. (C) Movement toward the lesioned ear.

sult, the distinctions that patients can make regarding other sensory systems, such as brightness, color, loudness, and pitch, are not possible for vestibular sensation. The diffuse character of the vestibulocortical projection may underlie the difficulty that patients experience when trying to describe vestibular ailments.

REFERENCES

1. Huygen PLM, Verhagen WIM, Nicolasen MGM: Cervico-ocular reflex enhancement in labyrinthine-defective and normal subjects. Exp Brain Res 87:457–464, 1991.
2. Bronstein A, Hood J: The cervico-ocular reflex in normal subjects and patients with absent vestibular function. Brain Res 373:399–408, 1986.
3. Ito M (ed): The Cerebellum and Neural Control. New York: Raven Press, 1984.
4. Harada Y (ed): The Vestibular Organs. Amsterdam: Kugler & Guedini, 1988.
5. Baloh RW, Honrubia V: Clinical Neurophysiology of the Vestibular System, ed. 3. New York: Oxford University Press, 2001.
6. Kelly JP: Vestibular system. In: Kandel ER, Schwartz JH, Jessell TM (eds). Principles of Neural Science, ed 3. Norwalk, CT: Appleton & Lange, 1991, pp 584–596.
7. Furman JM: Nystagmus and the vestibular system. In: Podos SM, Yanoff M (eds). Textbook of Ophthalmology. New York: Gower Medical, 1993, pp 9.1–9.7.

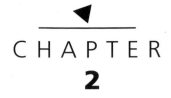

CHAPTER

2

History of the Dizzy Patient

What is meant by the term *dizziness*? What is meant by the term *vertigo*?

Dizziness means different things to different people. Thus, sensations described by a patient as *dizziness* should be further defined. Patients may use this term to mean that they feel lightheaded, have a swimming sensation in the head, and have a sense of giddiness or imbalance and unsteadiness. They may also mean that they have *vertigo*,[1] an illusory sensation of motion of either the self or the surroundings. This illusory motion can be rotational, that is, a sense of spinning or turning; translational, for example, a sense of rising; or a static reorientation of the visual world, that is, tilting of the self or the surroundings.

Why is interviewing a patient who suffers from dizziness often difficult, and what steps can be taken to yield a more satisfactory history?

Patients are often unable to describe their dizziness. This difficulty is probably related to the comparatively meager and impure neural projection from the peripheral vestibular system to the cerebral cortex. As a result, patients do not have a vocabulary for vestibular sensations, as they do for auditory and visual stimuli. Moreover, the vestibular information at cerebral levels is mixed with somatic sensation, which further degrades the specificity of vestibular complaints. Nevertheless, an attempt should be made to understand what a patient means by dizziness. Ask the patient to describe the symptoms in his or her own words, but be ready to assist the patient in learning a new vocabulary to describe the symptoms by providing descriptors such as *spinning, lightheadedness, giddiness, swimming,* and *unsteadiness when walking*. A little extra time spent in educating the patient about different subjective manifestations of dizziness can help develop a mutual understanding of what is meant by dizziness, which will improve physician–patient communication, help the physician focus on the patient's functional complaint, and save time and potential frustration later.

What categories of information should be elicited in the history of a dizzy patient?

The history should include an inquiry into (1) the characteristics of the patient's dizziness, (2) the time course and aggravating factors regarding the dizziness, (3) associated otologic symptoms, and (4) associated neurologic symptoms.

The first episode of dizziness is often vivid and is most typical of a particular disorder. Over time, either normal or maladaptive compensatory mechanisms can change the character of dizziness and obscure the diagnosis. Thus, it is often useful to begin the history by focusing on the first episode of dizziness. Once the character of the first episode is established, review the time course of the dizziness from its inception to the present. Is the dizziness episodic or constant? If the dizziness is episodic, note the duration, severity, and frequency of the episodes. If it is constant, determine whether the symptoms are getting progressively worse, slowly improving, or remaining the same.

The discovery of factors that provoke or aggravate the patient's symptoms can provide important clues to the diagnosis. Vertigo may be provoked in some people by lying down, rolling over in bed or pitching the head back to look up. In others, dizziness is associated with rising quickly from a supine or seated position. Particular environmental or social situations provoke vertigo in some individuals.

Because the hearing and vestibular apparatuses are closely linked anatomically and functionally, an inquiry into otologic symptoms is critical. Hearing loss, tinnitus, and aural fullness or pressure suggest involvement of the inner ear and may provide clues regarding which ear is involved. An inquiry into the presence of neurologic symptoms is important because of the common association of dizziness with central nervous system disorders such as cerebellopontine angle neoplasms, multiple sclerosis, migraine, and vertebrobasilar artery insufficiency. Visual symptoms can be caused by both peripheral and central vestibular abnormalities and by nonvestibular central nervous system abnormalities. Blurred vision is particularly nonspecific and can be caused by an abnormality anywhere in the vestibular, visual, or ocular motor pathways. However, blurred vision that occurs only during or immediately after head movement strongly suggests a vestibular abnormality with an impaired VOR. Double vision strongly suggests an ocular motor abnormality but can also be seen with vestibular system abnormalities, especially during or just after a head movement. Loss of vision definitely points to a visual pathway abnormality or to an alteration in level of consciousness.

Table 2–1 is a dizziness questionnaire that may be used to aid in eliciting the history. This questionnaire does not replace eliciting a history personally; rather, it focuses the patient's thinking and ensures that none of the essential elements of the history are omitted.

Which elements of the past medical history, current and previous medication use, family history, and review of systems are important in evaluating the patient with dizziness?

Table 2–1A Dizziness Questionnaire—Characteristics of Dizziness

IS YOUR DIZZINESS ASSOCIATED WITH ANY OF THE FOLLOWING SENSATIONS? PLEASE READ THE ENTIRE LIST FIRST. THEN CIRCLE <u>YES</u> OR <u>NO</u> TO DESCRIBE YOUR FEELINGS MOST ACCURATELY.

Yes No 1. Lightheadedness or swimming sensation in the head.
Yes No 2. Blacking out or loss of consciousness.
Yes No 3. Tendency to fall.
Yes No 4. Objects spinning or turning around you.
Yes No 5. Sensation that you are turning or spinning inside, with outside objects remaining stationary.
Yes No 6. Loss of balance when walking in the light: Veering to the: Right? Left?
Yes No 7. Loss of balance when walking in the dark: Veering to the: Right? Left?
Yes No 8. Headache.
Yes No 9. Nausea.
Yes No 10. Vomiting.
Yes No 11. Pressure in the head.
Yes No 12. Tingling in the fingers or toes.
Yes No 13. Tingling around the mouth.

Table 2–1B Dizziness Questionnaire—Time Course and Aggravating Factors

      1. When did your dizziness first occur? _____

      2. How often do you become dizzy? _____

      3. If dizziness occurs in attacks, how long does an attack last? _____

Yes No 4. Do you have any warning that dizziness is about to start?

Yes No 5. Does dizziness occur at any particular time of the day or night?

Yes No 6. Are you completely free of dizziness between attacks?

Yes No 7. Does change of position make you dizzy? Which movements? _____

Yes No 8. Do you become dizzy when rolling over in bed?
          To the right? _____ To the left? _____

Yes No 9. Do you know of any possible cause for your dizziness? What? _____

Yes No 10. Do you know of anything that will:

Yes No   a. Stop your dizziness or make it better? _____

          b. Make your dizziness worse? _____

Yes No 11. Do you become dizzy when you bend your head forward? _____
          Backward? _____

Yes No 12. Do you become dizzy when you cough? _____
          When you sneeze? _____
          When you have a bowel movement? _____

      13. Can any of the following make your dizziness worse or start an attack?
Yes No   Fatigue
Yes No   Exertion
Yes No   Hunger
Yes No   Menstrual period
Yes No   Stress
Yes No   Emotional upset
Yes No   Alcohol
Yes No 14. Do you have any allergies? What? _____

Table 2–1C Dizziness Questionnaire—Associated Ear Symptoms

DO YOU HAVE ANY OF THE FOLLOWING SYMPTOMS? PLEASE CIRCLE <u>YES</u> OR <u>NO</u> AND CIRCLE THE EAR INVOLVED, IF APPLICABLE.

Yes	No	1. Dizziness. Describe dizziness _____			
Yes	No	2. Difficulty in hearing?	Both Ears	Right	Left
Yes	No	3. Does your hearing change with dizziness?	Yes	No	
		If so, how? _____			
Yes	No	4. Do you have noise in your ears?	Both Ears	Right	Left
		Describe the noise: _____			
Yes	No	5. Does noise change with dizziness?	Yes	No	
		If so, how? _____			
Yes	No	6. Do you have fullness or stuffiness in your ears?	Both Ears	Right	Left
Yes	No	7. Do you have pain in your ears?	Both Ears	Right	Left
Yes	No	8. Do you have a discharge from your ears?	Both Ears	Right	Left

Table 2–1D Dizziness Questionnaire—Associated Neurologic Symptoms

HAVE YOU EXPERIENCED ANY OF THE FOLLOWING SYMPTOMS? PLEASE CIRCLE <u>YES</u> OR <u>NO</u> AND CIRCLE IF <u>CONSTANT</u> OR <u>IN EPISODES</u>.

Yes	No	1. Double vision	Constant	In Episodes
Yes	No	2. Blurred vision	Constant	In Episodes
Yes	No	3. Blindness	Constant	In Episodes
Yes	No	4. Numbness of the face or extremities	Constant	In Episodes
Yes	No	5. Weakness in the arms or legs	Constant	In Episodes
Yes	No	6. Clumsiness of the arms or legs	Constant	In Episodes
Yes	No	7. Confusion or loss of consciousness	Constant	In Episodes
Yes	No	8. Difficulty with speech	Constant	In Episodes
Yes	No	9. Difficulty with swallowing	Constant	In Episodes
Yes	No	10. Pain in the neck or shoulders	Constant	In Episodes

Table 2–1E. Dizziness Questionnaire—Past Medical History, Family History, Social History

Yes	No	1. Did you have a history of earaches or ear infections as a child?
Yes	No	2. Did you ever injure your head? When? _____
Yes	No	3. Were you ever unconscious? When? _____
Yes	No	4. Did you suffer from motion sickness before age 12? _____
Yes	No	5. Have you suffered from motion sickness in the last 10 years? _____
Yes	No	6. Do you now take any medications regularly? What? _____
Yes	No	7. Have you taken medication in the past for dizziness? Which ones? _____
Yes	No	8. Do you have a past medical history of: Diabetes? Heart disease? High blood pressure? Kidney disease? Thyroid disease? Migraine?
Yes	No	9. Do you have a family history of: Ear disease? Neurologic disease? Migraine headache?
Yes	No	10. Do you use tobacco in any form? What kind? _____ How much? _____
Yes	No	11. Does caffeine affect your dizziness? How? _____
Yes	No	12. Does alcohol affect your dizziness? How? _____

Each of the areas of the history, including the general medical history, is extremely important because all areas provide clues to the diagnosis and pertinent comorbid factors that can be helpful in planning further management of the patient. For example, the review of systems may provide clues suggesting autoimmune inner ear disease, hormonal dysfunction (reactive hypoglycemia, diabetes mellitus, thyroid dysfunction), renal disease, neurologic disease (especially multiple sclerosis and migraine), or chronic infection (human immunodeficiency virus [HIV], syphilis, Epstein-Barr virus). Patients should be asked specifically about exposure to potentially ototoxic medications (e.g., aminoglycoside antibiotics, certain chemotherapeutic agents, and loop diuretics).

REFERENCE

1. Blakely BW, Goebel J: The meaning of the word "vertigo." Otolaryngol Head Neck Surg 125:147–150, 2001.

CHAPTER 3

Physical Examination of the Dizzy Patient

COMPONENTS OF THE PHYSICAL EXAMINATION

Physical examination of the dizzy patient should include a neurologic examination, an otologic examination, and selected aspects of the neurotologic examination, that is, a subset of several special examination tools.

The neurologic examination (see Table 3–1) should include the usual subcomponents, including evaluation of mental status, the cranial nerves, the motor system, sensation, coordination, Romberg's test, and an assessment of gait including tandem walking.

The otologic examination (see Table 3–2) should include otoscopy, preferably using an operating microscope, and pneumatic otoscopy to allow an assessment of tympanic membrane mobility and sensitivity of the patient to abrupt fluctuations of external auditory canal pressure. Hearing should be assessed at the bedside; using a finger, rub a tuning fork (512 Hz). The two most commonly used tuning fork tests are Weber's test and the Rinne test.

The neurotologic examination (see Table 3–3), which provides information regarding the vestibulo-ocular and vestibulospinal systems, includes both routine and special components. The routine components include (1) a search for spontaneous nystagmus; (2) bedside (vestibulo-ocular reflex [VOR]) testing; (3) positional and positioning (Dix-Hallpike) tests to look for persistent and paroxysmal positional nystagmus, respectively; (4) postural sway while standing on a compliant (foam) surface; (5) the stepping test; and (6) several other tests used in special circumstances.

Table 3–1 Neurologic Examination

Mental status
Cranial nerves
Motor system
Sensation
Coordination
Romberg's test
Assessment of gait including tandem walking

Table 3–2 Otologic Examination

Otoscopy including pneumatic otoscopy
Bedside hearing assessment
    Finger rub
    Weber's test
    Rinne test

OCULAR MOTOR EXAMINATION

Evaluation of the ocular motor system is essential because vestibular system abnormalities, both peripheral and central, can alter eye movements in a characteristic fashion. Moreover, central nervous system lesions that produce ataxia or unsteadiness may also affect various ocular motor subsystems independent of a vestibular disorder and thus provide localizing information.

The components of the ocular motor examination include (1) an assessment of the alignment of the two eyes, (2) range of eye movement, (3) the presence of any instabilities such as nystagmus or involuntary saccades, and (4) an assessment of saccades, pursuit, and vergence. Although a complete discussion of each type of eye movement is beyond the scope of this book, elements of the ocular motor examination will be discussed in more detail below and as they arise in other case discussions. For an in-depth discussion of eye movement abnormalities, the reader is referred to Leigh and Zee's excellent work entitled *The Neurology of Eye Movements*.[1]

Misalignment of the visual axes (i.e., strabismus) may cause complaints of double vision, blurred vision, or vertiginous sensations. To assess ocular alignment, begin with a general inspection with both eyes open and viewing a single target, and look for gross misalignment of the visual axes. Ask the patient to follow a small target such as a penlight through the full range of movements including the nine cardinal positions of gaze. Look for any obvious misalignment of the eyes and ask the patient whether he or she notices any visual disturbance such as double or blurred vision in any field of gaze. The finding of an ocular misalignment may indicate a restriction or weakness of an extraocular muscle. Patients with an obvious ocular misalignment and little or no complaint of diplopia on testing usually have had strabismus since childhood. The finding of vertical misalignment suggests the presence of a skew deviation. Skew deviation has been reported mostly commonly in association with brainstem or cerebellar lesions and also can be due to injury to the otolith organs within the inner ear. Generalized limitation of range of movement may be a sign of myasthenia gravis. Limitation of voluntary vertical gaze may indicate abnormality of the midbrain including neurodegenerative disorders such as progressive supranuclear palsy, mass lesions, infarction, hemorrhage, hydrocephalus, or encephalitis.

Ocular instabilities include nystagmus and nonnystagmus movements. In nystagmus, there is a slow movement in at least one direction. With jerk nystagmus, there is a clearly defined quick and slow movement. In pendular nystagmus there is no clearly defined quick and slow movement. With the saccadic fixation instabilities, there are quick movements in both directions. Square-wave jerks are saccades away from and back to the point of fixation. Square-wave jerks are seen commonly in older individuals, and in an older person may be considered a nonspecific finding. In younger individuals, square wave jerks are considered abnormal and are most often seen with anxiety or with abnormalities of the cerebellum or brainstem. Ocular flutter and opsoclonus are rapid saccadic to-and-fro movements of the eyes without a normal intersaccadic interval. The causes of ocular flutter and opsoclonus include structural lesions of the pons or cerebellum, viral encephalitis, a paraneoplastic syndrome, or a toxic agent or medication.

Saccadic eye movements are examined by asking the patient to fixate alternately between two stationary targets. One target (e.g., the examiner's nose, finger, or pen) should be placed so that the patient can fixate upon it with the eyes in the primary position. A second target (e.g., a finger or pen) is then positioned to produce an approximate 15 degree saccade. Saccades can be tested in both the horizontal and vertical planes. The examiner should assess the velocity and accuracy of the saccades. Slowing of adducting saccades suggests brainstem dysfunction, that is, as part of internuclear ophthalmoplegia. Inaccurate saccades point to cerebellar lesions.

During vergence eye movements, the eyes move in an opposite but coordinated fashion. Both eyes move toward the nose to view nearby objects (i.e., convergence). Divergence occurs as the eyes rotate outward to view more distant objects. Vergence eye movements should be elicited by asking the patient to follow a finger or penlight as you move it toward and away from the bridge of the nose. Vergence movements are usually slow and smooth. Abnormal oscillation of the eyes during vergence, called *convergence spasm* (see Case 36), is suggestive of a functional disorder. Nystagmus that is present in primary gaze may change during vergence. For example, congenital nystagmus is typically dampened by convergence, and central vestibular nystagmus may be exaggerated or change direction during convergence.

BEDSIDE ASSESSMENT OF HEARING

Weber's test is performed by placing the vibrating tuning fork on the vertex of the head (forehead) and noting whether the sound is heard in the midline (*Weber midline*) or in one ear or the other (*Weber right* or *Weber left*). With unilateral disease, Weber's test usually lateralizes away from the ear with a sensorineural hearing loss or toward the ear with a conductive hearing loss.

The Rinne test can be performed by first placing the stem of the vibrating tuning fork on the subject's mastoid bone (the bony prominence behind the pinna) and then placing the tines of the vibrating tuning fork near the external auditory canal without touching the patient. If the sound is perceived as louder during air conduction, which is normal, the result is called *Rinne positive*. If the sound is perceived as louder during bone conduction, the result is called *Rinne negative*.

Weber's test and the Rinne test are generally used together to help indicate whether an asymmetry of hearing is present and whether the hearing loss is conductive or sensorineural. Used in conjunction, these tests provide valuable information about the relative hearing between the patient's two ears and whether a hearing loss is primarily sensorineural or conductive.

NEUROTOLOGIC EXAMINATION

All patients should undergo a routine neurotologic examination (see Table 3–3). A search for spontaneous nystagmus should include the observation of a patient's eyes open in the dark using infrared glasses (Fig. 3–1) or with reduced visual fixation using Frenzel's glasses. Nystagmus that increases in intensity or is seen only with infrared or Frenzel glasses suggests a peripheral vestibular system imbalance. Post-head-shaking nystagmus is observed using infrared glasses following about 15 seconds of brisk to-and-fro passive horizontal head rotation.[2,3] With asymmetric central vestibular function, patients may manifest a transitory nys-

Table 3–3 Neurotologic Examination

ROUTINE TESTS

Search for Spontaneous Nystagmus
    Eyes open in the dark; requires use of infrared/Frenzel's glasses
    Post-Head-Shaking Nystagmus

Bedside Vestibulo-Ocular Reflex (VOR) Tests
    Head thrust test
    VOR ophthalmoscopy
    Illegible E test

Positional Testing

Dix-Hallpike Test

Stability on a Foam Pad

Stepping Test

SPECIAL TESTS

Cervical-Ocular Testing (Head-Fixed, Body-Turned Maneuvers)

Head Roll Test for Horizontal Semicircular Canal Benign Paroxysmal Positional Vertigo

Hyperventilation

Tragal compression and Pneumatic Otoscopy while Observing Eye Movements

Valsalva Maneuver

Pastpointing

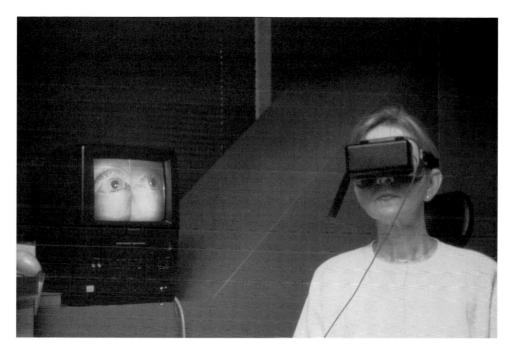

Figure 3–1 Infrared video goggles. The patient's eyes are illuminated by invisible infrared light sources behind opaque goggles. Infrared goggles eliminate visual fixation while allowing the examiner to observe vestibular nystagmus.

tagmus. Unfortunately, post-head-shaking nystagmus is not a specific test for vestibular abnormalities; that is, it has a relatively high false-positive rate.

Bedside VOR testing can be accomplished in three ways: (1) observing eye movements following abrupt head movements, that is, the head thrust test[4]; (2) head shaking while observing the fundus of one eye with an ophthalmoscope while the other eye is occluded[5]; and (3) assessing visual acuity during head shaking.[6]

To perform the head thrust test, grasp the patient's head, rotate it slowly 30 degrees to the right or left, and then briskly return the head to the center. Normally, the amount of eye movement required to refixate a visual target immediately upon cessation of an abrupt 30 degree passive horizontal head rotation is negligible. Unilateral vestibular loss results in an asymmetry of eye movement seen following the head thrust, that is, a refixation saccade. Bilateral vestibular loss leads to a refixation saccade following head thrusts to both the right and the left.

To best accomplish head shaking during ophthalmoscopy, the patient should be asked to make high-frequency head rotations of very small amplitude. Normally, the fundus appears fixed in space. If the fundus appears to move, either an uncompensated vestibular loss or a bilateral vestibulopathy with decreased gain of the VOR is suggested.

The assessment of visual acuity during head shaking, also known as the *illegible E test*, can uncover an abnormal VOR. Loss of more than two lines of acuity on a Snellen chart usually indicates an abnormally low VOR magnitude. Un-

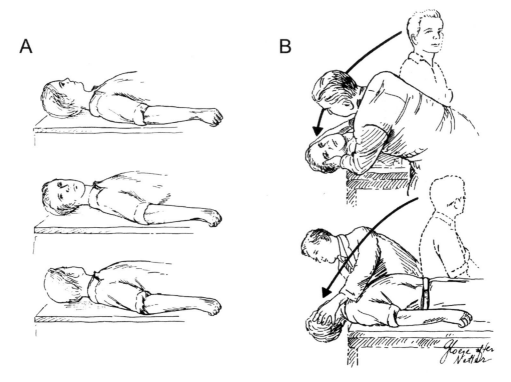

Figure 3–2 Techniques for performing positional and positioning testing. (A) Head positions for observing persistent positional nystagmus. (B) The Dix-Hallpike test for diagnosing benign paroxysmal positional vertigo. In the sitting position, the patient's head is turned 45 degrees to the right or left. Next, the patient is taken rapidly from the sitting to the supine position. The head is then gently moved to the final head-hanging position. (*Source*: With permission from Baloh RW: Dizziness, Hearing Loss, and Tinnitus: The Essentials of Neurotology. Philadelphia: FA Davis, 1984, p. 81.[12])

fortunately, this type of testing is inexact because the head movement delivered to each patient differs. Nonetheless, this bedside maneuver can provide useful information, especially when used to detect a change in vestibular function by serial testing of the same patient over time.

Positional testing is performed by observing the patient's eyes using infrared or Frenzel glasses while the patient assumes the supine, head left, left lateral, head right, and right lateral positions (Fig. 3–2A). The significance of persistent positional nystagmus is uncertain. However, a direction-fixed positional nystagmus (a nystagmus that beats in the same direction in all positions) is more likely to be related to a peripheral vestibular abnormality. A direction-changing positional nystagmus (a nystagmus whose direction changes when the patient changes from one ear down to the other ear down) can be caused by either peripheral or central vestibular lesions.

Paroxysmal positioning testing, that is, the Dix-Hallpike test, is used in diagnosing benign paroxysmal positional vertigo, which is discussed in Cases 7, 22, 25, 31, and 39. The Dix-Hallpike test is performed by first turning the patient's head 45 degrees either to the right or to the left and then rapidly bringing the pa-

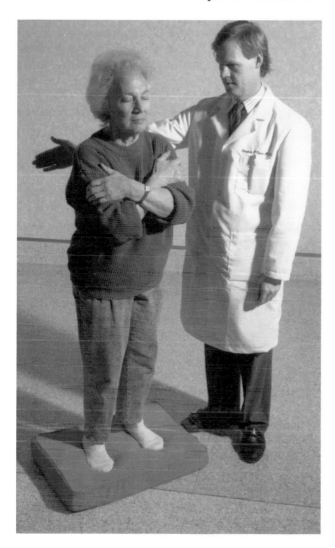

Figure 3–3 Clinical foam posturography. The patient stands on a dense foam pad with the arms folded on the chest and with the eyes open, then closed.

tient from the seated to the supine position (Fig. 3–2B). The patient's eye movements should be observed once they reach the supine head-turned position, if possible using infrared or Frenzel's glasses. The onset of geotropic vertical and torsional nystagmus that follows a short delay and is transitory (typically lasting less than 30 seconds) and associated with a perception of vertigo is diagnostic of benign paroxysmal positional vertigo.

Romberg's test for the patient with dizziness and dysequilibrium should be modified to include the use of a compliant surface such as a foam wheelchair pad[7,8] (Fig. 3–3). Because movement at the ankle is greatly diminished while standing on foam, the somatosensory system provides an erroneous estimate of postural sway. Thus, if a patient stands on foam with the eyes closed, only the vestibular system remains to provide accurate information regarding orientation.

The stepping test is performed by asking patients to march in place with their eyes closed[9] (Fig. 3–4). This test should be performed using a standard number of steps such as 60 and a threshold of normality such as a rotational deviation

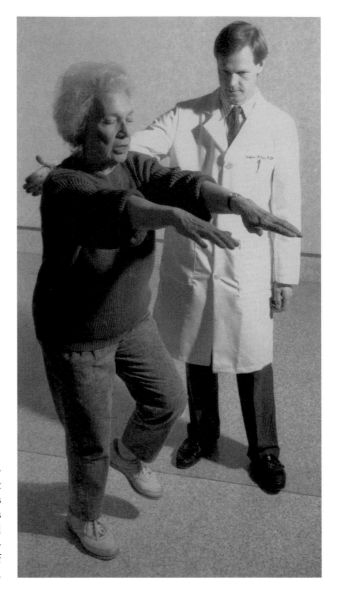

Figure 3–4 Unterberger (Fukuda) stepping test. The patient marches in place with the eyes closed. Typically, the patient is asked to march 60 steps and the angle of deviation is observed. Less than 45 degrees of deviation is considered normal.

greater than 45 degrees. Forward movement is not pathologic.[10,11] Excessive rotation suggests the presence of a vestibulospinal imbalance but is not localizing.

Several examination tools may be used in special circumstances. Head-fixed, body-turned maneuvers are performed to assess the cervico-ocular reflex by keeping the head fixed with the eyes open in the dark, thereby eliminating visual and vestibular inputs (see Case 53). Nystagmus seen during head-fixed, body-turned maneuvers suggests an abnormal cervico-ocular reflex and is called *cervical nystagmus*. This test can be performed in both the seated and recumbent positions.

Other bedside neurotologic tests include an assessment of eye movements following hyperventilation, during tragal stimulation, and during the Valsalva maneuver. These tests will be described in other cases as they arise. Pastpointing is performed by asking the patient to extend his or her arm and point to the ceiling. Then, with the eyes closed, the patient is asked to touch the examiner's finger. If the patient moves in such a way that he or she would miss the examiner's finger, the examiner moves under the patient's finger and the test is abnormal. Pastpointing should not be confused with dysmetria. Pastpointing indicates a vestibular system imbalance.

REFERENCES

1. Leigh RJ, Zee DS: The Neurology of Eye Movements, ed 3. New York: Oxford University Press, 1999.
2. Kamei T, Kornhuber H: Spontaneous and head-shaking nystagmus in normals and in patients with central lesions. Can J Otolaryngol 3:372–380, 1974.
3. Hain TC, Fetter M, Zee DS: Head-shaking nystagmus in patients with unilateral peripheral vestibular lesions. Am J Otolaryngol 8:36–47, 1987.
4. Halmagyi G, Curthoys I: A clinical sign of canal paresis. Arch Neurol 45:737–739, 1988.
5. Zee D: Ophthalmoscopy in examination of patients with vestibular disorders. Ann Neurol 3(4):373–374, 1978.
6. Longridge NS, Mallinson AI: A discussion of the dynamic illegible "E" test. A new method of screening for aminoglycoside vestibulotoxicity. Otolaryngol Head Neck Surg 92:671 677, 1984.
7. Shumway-Cook A, Horak FB: Assessing the influence of sensory interaction of balance. Phys Ther 66:1548–1550, 1986.
8. Weber PC, Cass SP: Clinical assessment of postural stability. Am J Otol 14(6):566–569, 1993.
9. Fukuda T: The stepping test. Acta Otolaryngol 50:95–108, 1959.
10. Zilstorff-Pedersen K, Peitersen E: Vestibulospinal reflexes. Arch Otolaryngol 77:237 245, 1963.
11. Peitersen E: Vestibulospinal reflexes. Arch Otolaryngol 79:481–486, 1976.
12. Baloh RW: Dizziness, Hearing Loss, and Tinnitus: The Essentials of Neurotology. Philadelphia: FA Davis, 1984.

CHAPTER
4

Vestibular Laboratory Testing

Vestibular laboratory testing of the dizzy patient should be reserved for those in whom such testing may be useful in establishing a diagnosis. Laboratory testing is most useful when a thorough history has been obtained and a physical examination has been performed to guide both the selection of appropriate tests and the interpretation of those tests. Vestibular laboratory testing may be helpful in distinguishing between a peripheral and a central vestibular abnormality. Also, for disorders thought to be peripheral, vestibular laboratory testing may enable lateralization of the abnormality, which is often helpful when designing and monitoring therapy. Vestibular laboratory testing is also useful in allowing documentation of an abnormality suspected as the result of a bedside evaluation. This is particularly helpful when patients are being evaluated by several physicians and may also be useful for medical/legal situations.

In patients who are undergoing treatment either specifically for a balance disorder or for another condition that requires potentially ototoxic medication, vestibular laboratory testing may be useful because it allows patients to be evaluated during their course of treatment. Certain tests, such as rotational testing and posturography, lend themselves more to serial evaluation than does caloric testing.

Vestibular laboratory tests can be divided into vestibulo-ocular and vestibulospinal tests. Each type of testing relies on a measure of motor response or output resulting from vestibular sensory input. Because of this reliance on measuring a motor output, either eye movements or postural sway, currently available vestibular laboratory tests provide only an indirect measure of vestibular end-organ function.

Vestibulo-ocular testing is well-established and relies on the vestibulo-ocular reflex (VOR). To properly evaluate the VOR, it is necessary first to assess the neural motor output, that is, the ocular motor system, independent of the vestibular system. Because eye movement abnormalities, if undetected, could lead to the erroneous conclusion that an abnormality is a result of a vestibular system lesion, an ocular motor screening battery is performed to identify difficulties with the neural control of eye movements. VOR tests, which include caloric, positional, and rotational testing, are described in the remainder of this chapter.

The vestibulospinal reflexes are not as well understood as the VOR, and to date, vestibulospinal testing consists mostly of using a moving posture platform to record sway. As with testing the VOR, vestibulospinal testing requires an assessment of the neural motor output (i.e., postural sway, independent of the vestibular system) before assessment of the vestibular effects on posture. The neural motor output (i.e., the postural motor control system) is evaluated by exposing patients to both translation and rotation of the platform while postural responses are recorded. The vestibulospinal system is then studied by altering vision and somatic sensation so that patients must rely on vestibular sensation to maintain balance.

OCULAR MOTOR TESTING

Ocular motor testing is designed to uncover abnormalities in ocular motor control in both the rapid and slow eye-movement systems. Ocular motor testing consists of (1) a search for nystagmus with and without visual fixation, (2) a search for gaze nystagmus with both horizontal and vertical gaze deviation, (3) an assessment of saccadic eye movements, (4) a recording of ocular pursuit, and (5) a recording of optokinetic nystagmus.

Videoculography and electro-oculography are the most commonly used methods for recording eye movements. The physiologic basis for electro-oculography is the corneal-retinal dipole potential. This is created by the metabolic activity of the retina, which causes the eye to act as a dipole oriented more or less outward along the visual axis. Videoculography uses computerized digital image processing and is rapidly replacing electro-oculography.

By convention, for horizontal recordings, upward deflections of the chart recorder pen denote rightward eye movement and downward deflections denote leftward eye movement. For vertical recordings, upward deflections denote upward eye movement and downward deflections denote downward eye movements. An example of nystagmus recorded with electro-oculography is shown in Figure 4–1.

POSITIONAL TESTING

Positional testing is performed by placing the patient in the following positions—supine, head left while supine, left lateral, head right while supine, and right lateral—while recording eye movements in the dark. Positional testing is designed to search for *static* positional nystagmus. Static positional nystagmus is not paroxysmal since it is present as soon as the patient assumes the provocative position and persists as long as the patient stays in that position. Static positional nystagmus is a nonspecific, nonlocalizing sign.

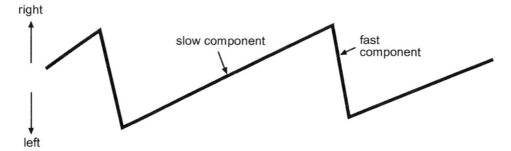

Figure 4–1 Shown diagrammatically are the two components of nystagmus: slow and fast. By convention, for horizontal eye movements, upward deflections on the eye movement record correspond to rightward eye movements, and downward deflections on the record correspond to leftward eye movements. Note that the velocity of the slow component is lower than the velocity of the fast component, as evidenced by the slope of the lines representing these components of nystagmus.

Paroxysmal positional nystagmus, that is, nystagmus induced by the Dix-Hallpike maneuver, may have the typical characteristics of benign paroxysmal positional nystagmus; that is, it (1) appears predominantly torsional and upbeating (that is, beating toward the forehead), (2) has a brief latency of 5 to 10 seconds prior to its appearance, (3) lasts for 15 to 45 seconds, (4) is typically associated with vertigo, and (5) diminishes or disappears with repeated provocation. Because electro-oculography and commercially available videoculography systems are insensitive to torsional eye movements and vertical electro-oculography is plagued by artifacts and a high signal-to-noise ratio, typical benign paroxysmal positional nystagmus, which is largely torsional, is difficult to record in the vestibular laboratory. Although there are benign variants of typical benign paroxysmal positional vertigo, if a nystagmus is recorded during the Dix-Hallpike maneuver that does not conform in every respect to the typical pattern seen with benign paroxysmal positional nystagmus, it should be considered the result of a central nervous system abnormality until proven otherwise.

CALORIC TESTING

Caloric irrigation of the labyrinth is the mainstay of vestibular laboratory testing and forms the basis for so-called electronystagmography. The basis for caloric testing is the establishment of a thermal gradient across the horizontal semicircular canal. By positioning the patient in such a way that the horizontal semicircular canal lies in the vertical plane, for example, 30 degrees of head flexion from the supine, a convection current is developed that is thought to induce a change in activity in the vestibular nerve. Although research from microgravity (outer space) experiments has indicated that the thermal stimulus, independent of the convection current, actually generates a portion of the caloric response, the convection current theory still accounts for the majority of the caloric response (Fig. 4–2).

The caloric stimulus to the labyrinth can be delivered into the external auditory canal using either water or air. Water irrigation can use either direct irriga-

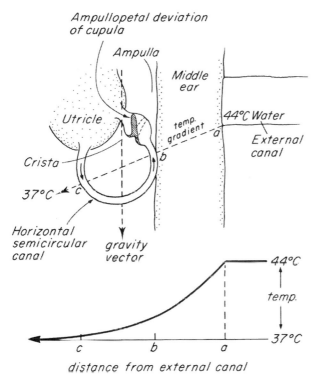

Ampullopetal deviation of cupula

Ampulla

Middle ear

Utricle

temp. gradient

44°C Water

External canal

Crista

37°C

Horizontal semicircular canal

gravity vector

44°C

temp.

37°C

distance from external canal

c   b   a

Figure 4–2 Caloric testing. The physiologic basis for caloric testing is the establishment of a thermal gradient across the horizontal semicircular canal and placement of the horizontal canal in the vertical plane such that a convection current is developed. (*Source*: Adapted with permission from Baloh RW, Honrubia V (eds): Clinical Neurophysiology of the Vestibular System, ed 2. Philadelphia: FA Davis, 1999, p. 159.[5])

tion of the external auditory canal or a small distensible balloon that is filled with cold or warm water from a reservoir. This so-called closed-loop irrigation has many advantages: the stimulus can be reproduced; caloric testing can be performed despite perforations in the tympanic membrane; and testing is well tolerated even by children.

Nystagmus responses induced by caloric irrigation are analyzed by measuring the velocity of the slow component of the nystagmus, whose magnitude reflects the intensity of the vestibular response (Fig. 4–3) Many studies have shown that the peak slow component velocity attained following caloric irrigation is the best determinant of the intensity of a particular response.[1]

To compare the responsiveness of one ear to that of the other ear, established practice is to use Jongkees' formula to compute a percent *reduced vestibular response*. Quite simply, the peak slow component velocities are summed for each ear and then subtracted from the sum of responses to irrigation of the opposite ear. The difference is normalized by dividing by the sum of the four responses and then multiplying by 100 to develop a measure of reduced vestibular response in percent. Each vestibular laboratory should establish its own normative values. For many laboratories, a reduced vestibular response of less than 25 is considered within normal limits. A unilateral caloric reduction almost always signifies a *peripheral* vestibular lesion, which by definition includes a lesion localized to the vestibular end organ, the vestibular nerve, or the vestibular nerve root entry zone. Typically, the side of the reduced vestibular response is the lesion side. Rarely, however, the lesion side may have a hyperactive rather than a hypoactive response as the result of an excitatory rather than a ablative lesion. In such cases, the lesion side may actually be contralateral to the side of the caloric reduction.

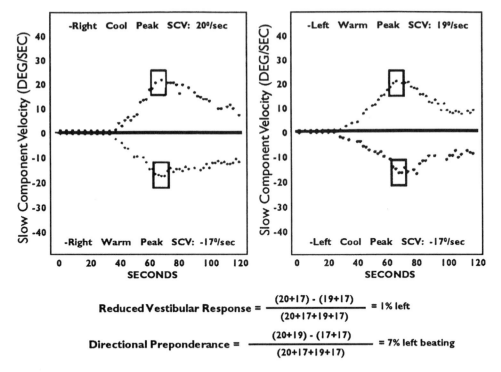

$$\text{Reduced Vestibular Response} = \frac{(20+17) - (19+17)}{(20+17+19+17)} = 1\% \text{ left}$$

$$\text{Directional Preponderance} = \frac{(20+19) - (17+17)}{(20+17+19+17)} = 7\% \text{ left beating}$$

Figure 4–3 Slow-component velocity response to caloric irrigations. Note that the peak slow-component velocity is bracketed and that the reduced vestibular response and directional preponderance values from Jongkees' formula are normal. (*Source*: Furman JM, Cass SP: Laboratory Testing. I. Electronystagmography and Rotational Testing. In Baloh RW, and Halmagyi M (eds): Disorders of the Vestibular System. New York: Oxford University Press, 1996, p. 201.[6])

When responses in an ear to warm and cool irrigation are absent, most laboratories use ice-water irrigation to provoke a response. Like any alerting stimulus, ice-water irrigation may unmask a latent spontaneous nystagmus. Thus, caloric responses induced by ice-water irrigation should be recorded with the patient both supine (head up 30 degrees) and prone (head down 30 degrees) in order to invert the orientation of the horizontal semicircular canal. Only if the direction of the caloric nystagmus reverses is it certain that the ear truly has a caloric response.

In patients with bilateral vestibular loss, caloric responses are reduced or absent in both ears. Some patients require ice-water irrigation of both ears (sequentially) to ascertain the overall level of unresponsiveness. However, some patients may have reduced or even absent caloric responses and preserved rotational responses. This apparent contradiction can be explained by understanding that caloric stimulation is a nonphysiologic but useful laboratory curiosity, whereas rotation is the natural stimulus of the labyrinth. Also, because thermal stimulation is gradual, caloric stimulation is comparable to a very low frequency rotational stimulus with an equivalent frequency of about 0.003 Hz.[2] Thus, some patients may respond minimally to caloric testing because of its very low equivalent frequency, yet still have robust responses during rotational testing, which uses much higher frequencies.[3]

Rarely, patients may exhibit increased caloric responses. As in the case of increased gain on rotational testing (see below), increased responses usually signify cerebellar disease. Also available from the caloric response is a measure of so-called directional preponderance, which expresses numerically whether the amount of right-beating nystagmus exceeds the amount of left-beating nystagmus or vice versa. Unlike the measure of reduced vestibular response, the directional preponderance of caloric testing is a nonspecific and nonlocalizing sign of vestibular dysfunction. Moreover, the measure is more variable than the reduced vestibular response. Most laboratories use a value of 30% directional preponderance as a threshold of normality.

The great advantage of caloric testing is that it provides lateralizing information that is not available from any other vestibular laboratory test. Disadvantages of the caloric test include its variability, its propensity for inducing nausea and occasional vomiting, and the unwillingness of most patients to undergo repeated caloric testing even when such testing would be helpful for management.

ROTATIONAL TESTING

Rotational testing relies on natural stimulation of the labyrinth, namely, angular acceleration. Rotational testing typically uses so-called earth-vertical axis rotation, in which a subject sits on a computer-controlled turntable and is turned left and right in a prescribed fashion (Fig. 1 4). Assessment of the VOR independent of vision is accomplished by rotating the patient with the eyes open in the dark. Rotational testing can also be used to assess visual–vestibular interaction by rotating patients in various visual conditions.

Unlike caloric testing, rotational testing stimulates both labyrinths simultaneously; one is inhibited while the other is excited. Many different types of rotation can be used for rotational testing. The most common types are sinusoids, that is, sinusoidal harmonic acceleration. With this type of stimulus, subjects are rotated first to the right and then to the left, then right, then left, and so on in a smooth, sinusoidally varying pattern of velocity and acceleration. Patients may also be rotated at a constant velocity followed by an abrupt deceleration to a stop.

To analyze the nystagmus induced by rotational testing, it is necessary to identify the slow components, because these reflect the influence of vestibular stimulation. The slow components induced by rotational stimulation are pieced together to generate a so-called cumulative slow-component eye position. This response measure is typically differentiated mathematically to yield the slow-component eye velocity, which can be compared with the turntable velocity to establish the response parameters of gain, phase, and symmetry (directional preponderance).

The gain of the nystagmus response to sinusoidal earth-vertical axis rotation is, by definition, the ratio of the magnitude of the response to the magnitude of the stimulus. The estimate of gain is obtained by using a computer to fit the best sinusoid through the slow-component eye velocity and then by dividing the magnitude of that best fit by the peak velocity of the sinusoidal rotational stimulus.

Reduced gain indicates decreased vestibular sensitivity. Unilateral vestibular loss may or may not reduce gain below normal. Thus, reduced gain usually indicates bilateral vestibular loss. Rarely, gain can be abnormally large, usually as a result of a cerebellar lesion.

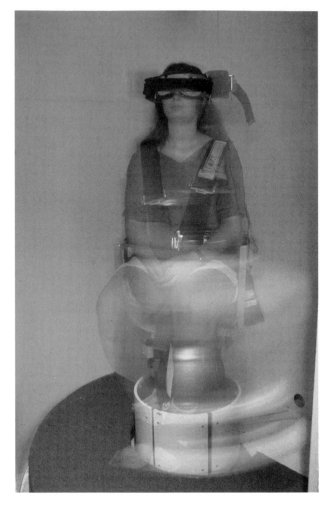

Figure 4–4 Earth-vertical axis rotational testing is usually performed using a test chair located inside an enclosure with a computer-controlled turntable. Testing of the vestibulo-ocular reflex (VOR) is performed with the eyes open in darkness or occluded with opaque goggles.

The phase of the response to sinusoidal earth-vertical axis rotation is also determined following generation of the best-fit sinusoid through the slow-component eye velocity response. Phase represents the timing relationship between the eye velocity response and turntable velocity. Phase is a highly sensitive but nonspecific measure of vestibular system function. Phase commonly changes with peripheral vestibular injury, and the changes are often permanent. Another measure, comparable to phase, can be obtained from constant velocity rather than sinusoidal rotations. That measure, the so-called time constant of the VOR, is a measure of how rapidly the vestibular nystagmus decays following an abrupt stop of the rotational chair. Like phase, the VOR time constant is a sensitive but nonspecific measure of vestibular system abnormality.

Many patients, especially those who are symptomatic at the time of testing, display an asymmetric response, that is, a directional preponderance (Fig. 4–5). Despite a symmetric stimulus with equal rotations to the right and to the left, patients with a directional preponderance display an excessive amount of either right-beating or left-beating nystagmus. Such an asymmetry of response can manifest simply as a shift in the average velocity of the response, or the slow-component velocity may have a nonsinusoidal shape with a higher velocity in

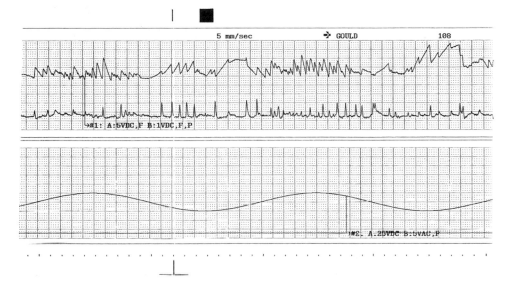

Figure 4–5 A recording of horizontal (top trace) and vertical (middle trace) eye position during earth-vertical axis rotation. The recording uses the standard convention of upward pen deflection indicating a rightward or an upward movement. The record shows a horizontal nystagmus in the horizontal recording and eye-blink artifacts in the vertical recording. The lowest trace indicates turntable velocity, which in this case is varying sinusoidally at 0.05 Hz. Note that in this patient, who is abnormal, there is much more right-bearing nystagmus than left-beating nystagmus.

one direction or the other. A rotational response asymmetry indicates an ongoing vestibulo-ocular imbalance but does not provide localizing information.

Another type of rotational testing, visual–vestibular interaction, which is usually reserved for detailed testing of patients suspected of having a central vestibular lesion, is performed by asking patients to look at a small target that rotates with them or by having them view earth-fixed full-field stripes or dots while undergoing earth-vertical axis rotation. In this way, vision is used to either reduce or augment the vestibular response, respectively. Visual–vestibular interaction testing is particularly useful when assessing central vestibular abnormalities because appropriately combining visual and vestibular information depends upon the normal functioning of brainstem and cerebellar structures. Typically, patients are rotated at a single sinusoidal frequency (1) in the dark, (2) with a fixation target, and (3) with earth-fixed stripes. A sinusoidal optokinetic stimulus while the patient is stationary may be used as a pure visual stimulus. The responses to these visual, vestibular, and combined visual–vestibular stimuli are recorded and analyzed in a manner similar to the response to sinusoidal rotational acceleration in the dark, that is, to yield gain and phase.

Rotational testing has several advantages: (1) the stimulus can be controlled precisely; (2) rotation consists of the natural stimulation of the labyrinth, that is, angular acceleration; (3) rotation is rarely bothersome; (4) rotation can be used for serial evaluations; and (5) in special circumstances, visual–vestibular interaction can be assessed. Testing can be performed at several rotational frequencies and amplitudes, allowing flexibility in the design of the stimulus so that patients with particular types of abnormalities, such as bilateral vestibular loss, can be evaluated more thoroughly. In particular, higher frequencies and amplitudes of rotation can be used to determine the degree, if any, of remaining vestibular function in patients who have suffered bilateral vestibular loss either from ototoxic medication or from an underlying disease state.[4] The great disadvantage of rotational testing is that it does not provide lateralizing information since both labyrinths are stimulated simultaneously. Thus, rotational testing is best used as an adjunct to caloric testing.

POSTUROGRAPHY

Posturography is now performed in many vestibular laboratories using the commercially available EquiTest device. Testing is divided into two broad types, which have been named *motor control* (formerly *movement coordination*) testing and *sensory organization* testing. Motor control testing employs repeated translations and rotations of the support surface that are designed to assess a patient's ability to maintain balance.

The sensory organization test is designed to manipulate vision and somatic sensation, which constitute two of the three sensory modalities important in maintaining upright balance. Using a technique called *sway referencing*, the platform and/or the visual surroundings are rotated in the same way that the patient is swaying, thereby distorting these sensory inputs. Sway referencing the platform and visual surroundings in various combinations can force patients to rely primarily on their vestibular system to maintain upright balance. Thus, the sensory organization portion of the posturography evaluation includes six conditions, illustrated in Figure 4–6.

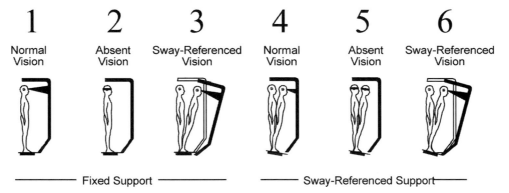

1	2	3	4	5	6
Normal Vision	Absent Vision	Sway-Referenced Vision	Normal Vision	Absent Vision	Sway-Referenced Vision

———— Fixed Support ————   ———— Sway-Referenced Support————

Figure 4–6 The sensory organization portion of computerized dynamic posturography includes six paradigms: (*1*) eyes open, platform stable; (*2*) eyes closed, platform stable; (*3*) eyes open with visual surroundings moving and platform stable; (*4*) eyes open, platform moving; (*5*) eyes closed, platform moving; and (*6*) both visual surroundings and platform moving. The movements of the visual surroundings, the platform, or both are designed to parallel movements of the patient's center of mass, the so-called sway referencing, thereby providing distorted visual or proprioceptive input. The fifth and sixth conditions, wherein the patient's eyes are closed or the patient is viewing moving visual surroundings while the floor moves, require the patient to rely on the vestibulospinal system to maintain balance. (*Source:* With permission from NeuroCom International Inc., Clackamas, Oregon.)

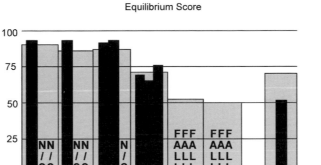

Figure 4–7. Computer analysis of postural sway provided by the EquiTest device for a patient who was able to stand during the first four sensory conditions but unable to stand on the fifth and sixth conditions. This patient has a vestibular pattern on posturography, suggesting an ongoing vestibulospinal abnormality.

Figure 4–7 shows an example of the computer analysis of postural sway provided by the EquiTest device. This patient was able to stand during the first four sensory conditions but was unable to stand during the fifth and sixth conditions; the patient lost balance and put tension on the safety harness. This patient therefore has a vestibular pattern on posturography suggesting an ongoing vestibulospinal abnormality. Another pattern of abnormality, shown in Figure 4–8, is called a *surface-dependent pattern* and suggests a combined visual and vestibular abnormality regarding postural control. Only when provided with reliable proprioceptive input can such an individual stand.

An advantage of dynamic posturography is that it evaluates upright balance and thus provides a functional evaluation that depends on vestibulospinal function. In this regard, dynamic posturography provides information distinctly dif-

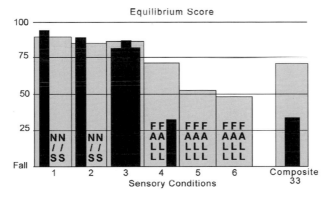

Figure 4–8 Computer analysis of postural sway provided by the EquiTest device for a patient who was able to stand during the first three sensory conditions but unable to stand on the fourth, fifth, and sixth conditions. This patient has a surface-dependent pattern on posturography, suggesting a combined visual/vestibular abnormality regarding postural control. Such an individual can stand only with reliable proprioceptive input.

ferent from that provided by caloric and rotational testing, which assess vestibulo-ocular responses. Dynamic posturography is noninvasive and has been shown to be repeatable. Although a lack of patient cooperation and effort will lead to abnormal responses, only with great sophistication can particular patterns of abnormalities be spuriously produced.

A disadvantage of dynamic posturography is that the results are nonspecific and nonlocalizing and may indicate vestibular disease even when not present.

REFERENCES

1. Jacobson GP, Newman CW: Handbook of Balance Function Testing. St. Louis: Mosby Year Book, 1993.
2. Hamid M, Hughes G, Kinney S: Criteria for diagnosing bilateral vestibular dysfunction. In: Graham MD, Kemink JL (eds). The Vestibular System: Neurophysiologic and Clinical Research. New York: Raven Press, 1987, pp 115–118.
3. Furman JM, Kamerer DB: Rotational responses in patients with bilateral caloric reduction. Acta Otolaryngol (Stockh) 108:355–361, 1989.
4. Baloh RW, Honrubia V, Yee RD, Hess K: Changes in the human vestibulo-ocular reflex after loss of peripheral sensitivity. Ann Neurol 16:222–228, 1984.
5. Baloh RW, Honrubia V: Clinical Neurophysiology of the Vestibular System, ed 2. Philadelphia: FA Davis, 1999.
6. Furman JM, Cass SP: Laboratory testing. I. Electronystagmography and rotational testing. In: Baloh RW, Halmagyi M (eds). Disorders of the Vestibular System. Oxford University Press, New York, 1996, pp 191–210.

CHAPTER
5

Auditory System and Testing

The cochlea, the human organ of hearing, consists of a membranous structure called the *cochlear duct*, which is approximately 33 mm in length and twisted into a spiral with two and three-quarter turns (Fig. 5–1). The cochlear duct is supported by a bony skeleton consisting of a central modiolus and a surrounding otic capsule. The afferent auditory neuronal cell bodies form the spiral ganglion, which is located inside the modiolus of the cochlea. The spiral arrangement of the cochlear duct results in a spiral arrangement of neurons within the spiral ganglion. The auditory nerve, which is a component of the eighth cranial nerve, carries approximately 30,000 primary afferent neurons and about 1000 efferent nerve fibers, whose function is unknown. Because the vestibular and auditory apparatus share common inner ear fluids, nerves, blood supply, and location within the temporal bone, disorders that affect the peripheral vestibular apparatus often affect hearing. Vertigo associated with a unilateral hearing loss suggests a peripheral vestibular abnormality on the side with the hearing loss. Thus, it is important to assess hearing in the evaluation of the dizzy patient because hearing loss may help to localize a vestibular system disorder to the labyrinth and also may help to lateralize the problem to a particular ear.

Many vertigo syndromes have characteristic associated audiologic findings that can help establish a specific diagnosis. For example, a fluctuating low-frequency sensorineural hearing loss is characteristic of endolymphatic hydrops, that is, Meniere's disease. Acute vestibular neuritis is characterized by the absence of auditory symptoms and normal hearing. Compression of the vestibular-cochlear nerve within the internal auditory canal or cerebellopontine angle by a neoplasm can produce symptoms of unsteadiness and disequilibrium as well as a sensorineural hearing loss, which typically presents at high frequencies and is

41

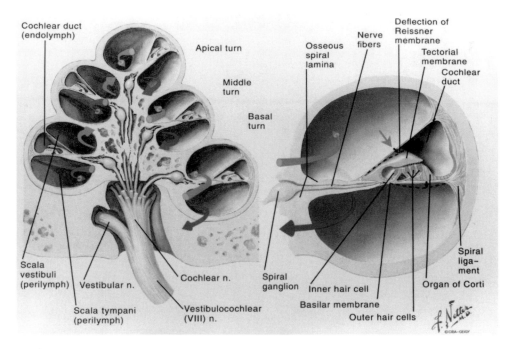

Figure 5–1 Two views of the anatomy of the cochlea. The left panel shows the three turns of the cochlear duct. The cochlear nerve enters the center of the cochlea from the internal auditory canal. The right panel shows one turn of the cochlea in greater detail. The organ of Corti contains the hair cells involved in transduction of sound to neural activity. (*Source*: With permission from Silverstein, H, Wolfson, RJ, Rosenberg, S: Diagnosis and management of hearing loss. Clin Symp 44(3):5, 1992.[10])

slowly progressive. Such lesions also cause diminished word recognition. Otosclerosis, which may cause dizziness, produces a characteristic conductive hearing loss.

LABORATORY ASSESSMENT OF HEARING

Audiogram and Word Recognition Test

The mainstay of hearing assessment consists of two psychophysical tests: the pure-tone audiogram and the word recognition test.[1,2] The pure-tone audiogram summarizes hearing thresholds compared to those of normal persons at standardized pure-tone frequencies that range from 250 to 8000 Hz. These hearing thresholds are plotted in a graphic format, wherein the abscissa (horizontal axis) is frequency and the ordinate (vertical axis) is hearing threshold in decibels (dB) referenced to the sound pressure level of normal hearing at each test frequency (Fig. 5–2). The word recognition test measures the ability of a patient to repeat correctly words represented at 30 to 40 dB louder than the patient's hearing threshold. The percentage of words correctly recognized is reported for each ear separately.

Normally, hearing thresholds are symmetric in the two ears. When one ear is found to have significantly worse hearing than the other ear, further evaluation of the auditory system is warranted, especially to rule out eighth nerve or

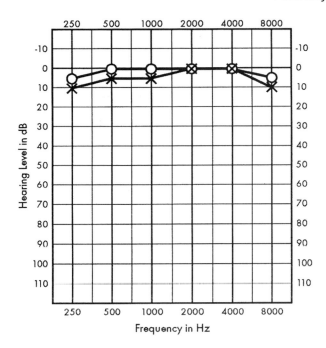

Word Recognition Score			Right	Left
Right : 100% Left : 100%	Air	unmasked masked	o——o △——△	×——× ப——ப
	Bone	unmasked masked	◄---◄ Ɛ---[	>--->]---]

Figure 5–2 Audiogram.

cerebellopontine angle lesions. Although there are no strict guidelines as to when to pursue further evaluation of asymmetric hearing loss, a significant hearing difference is considered to be 10 dB or more at two adjacent test frequencies or a 15% or greater difference in word recognition scores. It is recommended that whenever a significant hearing asymmetry is present that cannot be explained by other clinical circumstances, such as unilateral noise-induced hearing loss, either brainstem auditory-evoked potential testing (see later) or brain imaging be performed to rule out a structural lesion of the auditory system.[3]

Tympanometry and Acoustic Reflex Testing

Tympanometry and acoustic reflex testing are commonly used audiologic screening tests.[4] Tympanometry assesses the compliance (acoustic resistance) of the tympanic membrane and middle ear ossicles and is largely used to help diagnose middle ear infection. Tympanometry is also used as part of the electronystagmographic perilymphatic fistula test. This test consists of changing external auditory canal pressure while recording eye movements. Patients with a perilymphatic fistula may develop nystagmus or eye deviation in response to pressure changes. Acoustic reflex testing assesses the integrity of the stapedius reflex by exposing the ear to loud sound and then assessing changes in acoustic resistance; thus, it provides information about the afferent sensory (auditory) and efferent motor (facial nerve) limbs of this reflex. Historically, acoustic reflex testing has been used as part of a *site-of-lesion* test battery. However, more advanced audiologic tests (see below), such as brainstem auditory-evoked potential testing and electrocochleography, have superseded acoustic reflex testing and other previously used site-of-lesion tests for localizing disorders of the auditory system.

Brainstem Auditory-Evoked Potential Testing

Brainstem auditory-evoked potential testing is an electrophysiologic test used to evaluate the integrity of the auditory pathway from the cochlea through several brainstem auditory relay centers.[5] In the brainstem auditory-evoked potential testing procedure, auditory clicks or brief tone bursts are delivered through headphones to evoke a highly synchronous and repeatable neural response. This response is measured using surface electrodes and standard signal averaging techniques. The evoked neural potentials that occur early, that is, within 1 to 12 milliseconds, reflect cochlear nerve and brainstem activity and are collectively called *brainstem auditory-evoked potentials* or the *auditory brainstem response*. The brainstem auditory-evoked potential is characterized by a series of five vertex-positive waves (I to V) that are thought to correspond to relay centers within the auditory pathway: wave I—cochlear nerve at the level of the spiral ganglion; wave II—cochlear nerve/brainstem junction; wave III—cochlear nucleus; wave IV—

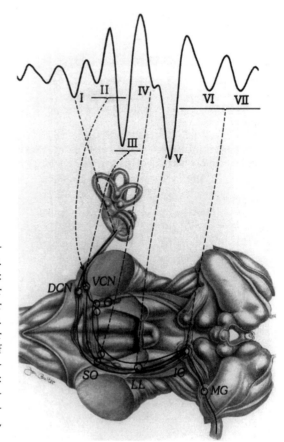

Figure 5–3 Neural generators of brainstem auditory-evoked potentials. VCN: ventral cochlear nucleus; DCN: dorsal cochlear nucleus; SO: superior olive; LL: lateral lemniscus; IC: inferior colliculus; MG: medial geniculate. (*Source*: With permission from Moller AR, Jannetta PJ: Neural generators of the brainstem auditory evoked potentials. In: Nodar RH, Barber C (eds): Evoked Potentials II: The Second International Evoked Potentials Symposium. Boston: Butterworths, 1984, p. 144.[11])

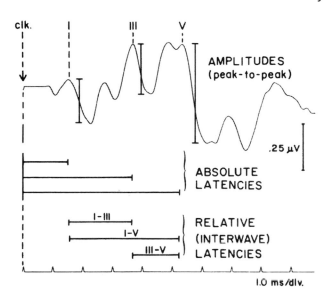

Figure 5–4 Analysis of brainstem auditory-evoked potentials (BAEP). Latency measurements are used more commonly than amplitude measurements. Absolute latencies, relative latencies, and interaural latencies (not shown) can be used in the analysis and interpretation of BAEP.

superior olive complex; wave V—lateral lemniscus; and waves VI and VII—inferior colliculus (Fig. 5–3). The interpretation of the brainstem auditory-evoked potential is based on the qualitative morphology of the waveforms and the quantitative latency and amplitude of each wave.

Brainstem auditory-evoked potential testing can be used for site-of-lesion testing since the latencies of waves I to V can be compared between the two ears and to normative data[6,7] (Fig. 5–4). These measurements can be used to determine whether abnormal wave latencies exist and the likely anatomic site of such delays. Disruption of auditory neural transduction may be caused by neoplasia, by compression or invasion of the eighth cranial nerve or brainstem, or by demyelination anywhere along the central auditory pathway. Auditory system abnormalities may be associated with concomitant vestibular abnormalities caused by the close anatomic relationship between the vestibular nerve and the auditory nerve and between the vestibular nuclei and the cochlear nuclei. Thus, brainstem auditory-evoked potential testing, which provides information regarding the integrity of central auditory pathways, also provides information regarding central vestibular pathways. Brainstem auditory-evoked potential testing can also be used for determining auditory thresholds in patients who cannot otherwise cooperate, such as adults with altered mental status and infants.

Electrocochleography

Electrocochleography is a modification of the brainstem auditory-evoked potential test in which wave I is amplified to reveal both the *action potential* of the cochlear nerve, also called N1, and another wave preceding the action potential referred to as the *summating potential.* Normally, the ratio of the summating potential to the action potential is less than 1:3. However, when endolymphatic hydrops is present, the summating potential increases relative to the action potential (Fig. 5–5). When the ratio of summating potential to action potential amplitude exceeds 0.5, it is considered abnormal and indicative of endolymphatic hydrops.

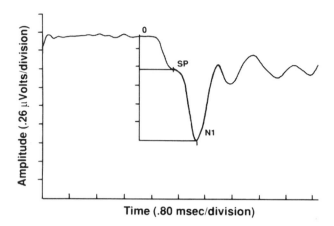

Figure 5–5 The SP/AP ratio is calculated by measuring the amplitudes of the summating potential (SP) and action potential (AP, labelled N1 in the figure) from baseline (0). (*Source*: With permission from Campbell K, Harker AL, Abbas PJ: Interpretation of electrocochleography in Meniere's disease and normal subjects. Ann Otol Rhinolaryngol 101: 497, 1992.[12])

The association of an elevated summating potential/action potential ratio with endolymphatic hydrops has been substantiated both experimentally and clinically.[8,9] Thus, electrocochleography can be helpful in diagnosing endolymphatic hydrops as the underlying cause of a balance disorder.

Electrocochleography is particularly useful in patients whose symptoms are not characteristic of a particular disorder. Also, in cases in which both ears appear to be affected, electrocochleography may be helpful in localizing underlying endolymphatic hydrops to an actively pathological ear.

REFERENCES

1. Katz J (ed): Handbook of Clinical Audiology. Baltimore: Williams & Wilkins, 1994.
2. Rintelmann WF (ed): Hearing Assessment. Perspectives in Audiology Series. Austin: Pro-Ed, 1991.
3. Selesnick SH, Jackler RK: A typical hearing loss in acoustic neuroma patients. Laryngoscope 103:437–446, 1993.
4. Sheehy JL, Hughes RL: The ABC's of impedance audiometry. Laryngoscope 134(11):1935–1949, 1974.
5. Moller AR: Audiotory neurophysiology. J Clin Neurophysiol 11(3):284–308, 1994.
6. Selters WA, Brackmann DE: Acoustic tumor detection with brain stem electric response audiometry. Arch Otolaryngol 103:181–187, 1977.
7. Wilson DF, Hodgson RS, Gustafson MF, Hogue S, Mills L: The sensitivity of audiotory brainstem response testing in small acoustic neuromas. Laryngoscope 102:961–964, 1992.
8. Ferraro JA, Arenberg K, Hassanein S: Electrocochleography and symptoms of inner ear dysfunction. Arch Otolaryngol 111:71–74, 1985.
9. Arenberg IK, Ackley RS, Ferraro J, Muchnik C: EcoG results in perilymphatic fistula: Clinical and experimental studies. Otolaryngol Head Neck Surg 99(5):435–443, 1988.
10. Silverstein H, Wolfson RJ, Rosenberg S: Diagnosis and management of hearing loss. Clin Symp 44(3):5, 1992.
11. Moller AR, Janetta PJ: Neural generators of the brainstem auditory evoked potentials. In: Nodar RH, Barber C (eds). Evoked Potentials II: The Second International Evoked Potentials Symposia. Boston: Butterworths, 1984, pp 137–144.
12. Campbell K, Harker AL, Abbas PJ: Interpretation of electrocochleography in Meniere's disease and normal subjects. Ann Otol Rhinol Laryngol 101:497, 1992.

CHAPTER
6

Vestibular Rehabilitation

Physical therapy evaluation and treatment have become an important resource in the management of the dizzy patient. In the 1940s, Cawthorne,[1] Cooksey,[2] and later, Dix and Hood[3] recognized that patients who actively moved their heads recovered more quickly and completely from acute peripheral vestibular lesions than those who did not. These early clinical observations led to numerous experimental and clinical studies that have supported the concept that vestibular exercises promote functional balance recovery and compensation following vestibular system injury. More recently, the writings of Shumway-Cook and Horak[4] and Herdman[5] have focused the expertise of therapists on the problem of functional recovery following vestibular system injury. Attention to the specific problems of each patient has improved the quality of such intervention. The formerly common practice of dispensing a generic list of head movement exercises has evolved into a referral for a comprehensive sensory and motor evaluation by a skilled therapist with specialized training in balance disorders who then develops a treatment plan for a program of vestibular rehabilitation. There is evidence that a customized exercise program improves function faster than a generic treatment program.[6,7] The goal of vestibular rehabilitation is to develop a specific program of movements directed at improving a patient's functional balance deficits, decreasing the risk of falling, decreasing dizziness, increasing activity level, and improving functional abilities in general.

Who is a candidate for vestibular rehabilitation? Patients who typically respond favorably to vestibular rehabilitation include those with nonfluctuating peripheral vestibular loss, chronic uncompensated peripheral vestibulopathy, multisensory disequilibrium, drug-induced vestibulopathy, head trauma, migraine-related vestibulopathy, cervical dizziness, stroke (anterior inferior and posterior inferior cerebellar arteries), panic/anxiety disorders, and the vestibular imbalance that follows a destructive surgical procedure. Patients with episodic vertigo who have otherwise normal balance (e.g., many patients with Meniere's disease) are not candidates for therapy because exercises do not influence the frequency or severity of episodes. Patients with benign paroxysmal positional vertigo do not typically require vestibular rehabilitation unless their evaluation uncovers evidence for an ongoing vestibulo-ocular or vestibulospinal imbalance. However, there is recent evidence that persons with benign paroxysmal positional vertigo may experience balance dysfunction for at lease 1 month after resolution of their benign paroxysmal positional vertigo.[8] Therapy is thus indicated in selected patients, especially those at risk for falling.

Despite the fact that some disorders are easier to treat than others and that some disorders have poorer prognoses than others, vestibular rehabilitation has few contraindications. The therapist should be informed of the patient's medical problems and diagnoses, results of vestibular testing, medications, and contraindicated exercises such as vigorous neck exercises in patients with vertebral vascular disease. Patients should be reassured that they must often be willing to "feel worse before they begin to feel better." There is no age limit for a trial of vestibular rehabilitation.

THEORETIC BASIS FOR PHYSICAL THERAPY

Although considered primarily reflexive, vestibular responses are actually quite malleable. The ability to alter the vestibulo-ocular reflex (VOR) forms one of the theoretic bases for vestibular rehabilitation. Physiologic alterations of the VOR can be brought about by (1) changing the magnitude of the VOR using an altered visual environment such as that produced by magnifying or miniaturizing lenses[9]; (2) changing the timing of the VOR using repeated rotations[10,11]; and (3) altering vestibulo-ocular responses by imagining an earth-fixed or a head-fixed visual target.[12] This capacity for vestibulo-ocular responses to change, depending on the demands of the situation, provides the therapist with a modifiable substrate.

As discussed in Chapter 1, following a peripheral vestibular injury, the vestibular system is known to alter its properties to produce a more functional response. Unilateral vestibular injury is known to be followed immediately by an acute vestibular syndrome. However, in a matter of hours or days, depending on the patient's age and central nervous system status, the symptoms of acute vestibular loss abate so that the patient can perform the activities of daily living. This process of central nervous system compensation for unilateral peripheral injury occurs by mechanisms as yet unknown. However, certain types of movement and exposure to visual surroundings enhance this compensation process, especially for dynamic relexes.[13] Also, certain pharmaceutic agents (e.g., meclizine) may slow this process.[14] Neurophysiologically, the response to unilateral peripheral vestibular injury undoubtedly includes changes in the neural activity in the vestibular nuclei. The crossed pathways of the vestibular commissures may be important for the compensatory process.[15] After compensation, if a subsequent injury occurs to the contralateral vestibular system, some individuals appear to have only an acute vestibular injury on the newly affected side. Bilateral peripheral vestibular injury is a more challenging problem than unilateral vestibular injury. Proprioceptive and visual influences may assume a more important role in stabilization of the eyes and the body following severe bilateral vestibular deficits. The therapist can exploit this process during vestibular rehabilitation.[7]

TECHNIQUE OF VESTIBULAR REHABILITATION

A thorough discussion of the technique of vestibular rehabilitation is beyond the scope of this book. However, a brief overview follows. For an in-depth discussion of this topic, the reader is referred to the excellent textbook by Herdman entitled *Vestibular Rehabilitation*.[5]

VESTIBULAR REHABILITATION ASSESSMENT

A thorough evaluation of each patient by the therapist on an individualized basis precedes the development of a treatment plan for vestibular rehabilitation. This evaluation begins by reviewing material supplied by the referring physician, which typically includes the diagnosis/differential diagnosis and past medical history including medications, recently prescribed medications, and laboratory test results. Even though a diagnostic evaluation by the referring physician has already been undertaken, the therapist personally evaluates the patient's vestibular, proprioceptive, and visual systems from his or her own perspective to uncover any deficits that may be affecting the patient's balance. The patient's height, weight, cognitive function, attentional capacity, vision, strength, posture, coordination, presence of joint pain, and range of motion can all affect balance and are thus evaluated as well. Because some patients are able to balance without difficulty if they are in an environment with little extraneous movement but have marked problems in more dynamic environments that contain extraneous movement, the patient should be evaluated in different settings if possible. The therapist must obtain a history of the patient's problem, with an emphasis on his or her functional deficits. This may include a Dizziness Handicap Inventory[16] to assess the patient's perception of handicap at each visit. The Dizziness Handicap Inventory attempts to quantify the effects of dizziness on a patient's function, physical status, and emotional well-being. The activities-specific balance confidence scale, another self-report measure, can be used to quantify balance confidence with each visit.[17]

The therapist then elicits a detailed social history to determine whether or not the patient is living in a safe environment. The therapist may make recommendations that attempt to improve the level of safety in the patient's home environment. For example, it may be suggested that a patient use a night light in the bedroom, remove throw rugs, or install handrails. It is also helpful to know whether any family members can assist the patient in a home exercise program. Then the therapist performs a physical examination to assess the patient's ability to perform functional movements with the eyes open, eyes closed, and at various speeds. Transitional movements that are tested include rolling, sitting, reaching, standing, and the Dix-Hallpike test (see Chapter 3 and Case 7). Then the therapist assesses head and eye movements. This assessment parallels that of the physical examination performed by the physician. However, the patient's symptoms, such as dizziness and blurred vision, are especially important during these movements. The therapist then assesses sensation and the patient's ability to sit, stand,

Table 6–1 Functional Balance Assessment

Test	Type of Data	Scale
Dynamic Gait Index[18]	Ordinal	0–24 (24 is the best score)
Timed "Up & Go"[19]	Ratio	0 to as much time as required (lower scores are best)
Clinical Test of Sensory Integration and Balance (CTSIB)[20]	Ratio if timed	0–30 seconds (30 seconds is best)
Berg Balance Scale[21]	Ordinal	0–56 (56 is the best score)
Modified Gait Abnormality Rating Scale[22]	Ordinal	
Physical Performance Test[23]	Ordinal	0–36 points (36 is the best score)
Functional reach[24]	Length	0 inches to as long as the person can reach (higher scores best)
Gait speed[25]	Velocity	0 to whatever speed is achieved (higher scores are best)
Five times sit to stand test[26]	Time	0 to as long as is required (shorter is best)

and walk in different situations. *Static* balance measures include Romberg testing, single leg stance, and tandem Romberg testing. Following the elicitation of a history and the performance of a physical examination, the therapist may perform a functional balance assessment (Table 6–1). The functional balance assessment is a tool box that the physical therapist uses to determine function in persons with vestibular disorders or those who are at risk of falling. All of the tools except the Physical Performance Test, the five times sit to stand, and the modified Gait Abnormality Scale have been validated with persons with vestibular disorders. Use of the tools permits subjective and objective comparisons of the patient's perceived status and assists in determining if the patient is improving.

VESTIBULAR REHABILITATION TREATMENT

Herdman[5] recommends that therapists identify the specific problems and functional limitations of each patient so that a list of vestibular rehabilitation goals can be constructed. Once these goals are established, the therapist has numerous movements from which to choose to develop a program for each patient. Many of these movements can be performed by the patient at home. They are designed to potentiate compensation for peripheral vestibular lesions and to help patients learn how to substitute other sensory inputs, such as vision and somatosensory inputs, for vestibular sensation. Substitution of other sensory modalities is especially important in patients with bilateral vestibular deficits.

Herdman[5] states that "The goals of physical therapy intervention are to improve the patient's mobility, overall general physical condition and activity level, functional balance, safety for gait and gait-related activities, and the magnitude of the patient's symptoms." Because many patients' symptoms worsen in the early stages of vestibular rehabilitation, vestibular suppressants may be prescribed when therapy begins. Subsequently, these medications, which may actually impair vestibular compensation, should be discontinued.

Table 6–2 Balance and Gait Exercises

1. Perform the following exercises while standing. Stand near a kitchen counter, but hold on only if needed.
   a. Walk sideways 15 ft. Repeat in both left and right directions _____ times, twice a day.
   b. Walk backward 15 ft. Repeat _____ times, twice a day.
2. Perform the following exercises while standing. Stand with a wall behind you. Have a family member stand nearby if needed. Stand on a pillow or couch cushion for _____ seconds.
   a. Do this with your eyes open. Repeat _____ times, twice a day.
   b. Do this with your eyes closed. Repeat _____ times, twice a day.
   c. Stand on one leg with your eyes closed. Repeat _____ times, twice a day.
3. Walk down a corridor and practice moving your head left and right. Keep your head turned in either direction for about three steps. Walk _____ ft. Repeat _____ times, twice a day. Also repeat by moving your head up and down.
4. Set up an obstacle course. Use chairs, pillows, and furniture as obstacles. Place smaller objects on the floor that you must step over. Change the course each time so that you do not get used to the same routine.

   You can incorporate stair climbing, sitting to standing, or picking up and carrying objects during the obstacle course. Set a timer or clock yourself to see how quickly you can finish.

   To add difficulty, have a family member give commands (e.g., "Turn left now") or throw a ball toward you unexpectedly.
5. Walk around a darkened room (preferably carpeted) in your house for _____ minutes.
6. Go grocery shopping as tolerated.
7. Do your walking program at a shopping mall one or two times a week.

Source: Adapted from Herdman SJ (ed): *Vestibular Rehabilitation.* Philadelphia: FA Davis, 2000, p. 404.[5]

Table 6–2 lists balance and gait exercises used at the University of Pittsburgh Medical Center. Table 6–3 lists the general principles for helping patients make progress in their rehabilitation.

Patients with bilateral vestibular reduction generally have a more serious balance problem and a worse prognosis than those with unilateral vestibular loss. Many of the principles that underlie the vestibular rehabilitation of patients with unilateral vestibular loss also apply to patients with bilateral vestibular loss, but there are several special considerations: recovery is slower; sensory substitution is the primary means of rehabilitation; exercises may be needed chronically; visual input (proper lighting) is critical; and a cane or walker may provide a great deal of help, especially early in the rehabilitation process.[5] After assessment and development of a treatment plan, patients are typically seen in follow-up every 1 to 2 weeks, for a total of six visits, so that progress can be monitored and the

Table 6–3 General Principles for Progression in Vestibular Rehabilitation

Slow to fast movement
Wide to narrow base of support
Reaching inside to outside the base of support
Eyes open to eyes closed
Stable support surface to compliant support surface
Vary environmental constraints
Eye movement with no head movement to eye movement with coordinated head movement
Walking with head stable on trunk to walking with head moving on trunk

Table 6–4 Factors That Affect the Outcome of Vestibular Rehabilitation

Abnormalities of strength or range of motion
Age
Combined central and peripheral vestibular disorders
Duration and chronicity of illness
Medical comorbidities such as diabetes, kidney disease, or liver disease
Migraine
Neck dysfunction
Ongoing litigation
Peripheral neuropathy
Preexisting eye movement disorders such as strabismus or amblyopia
Preexisting or associated psychiatric disorders
Preexisting orthopedic conditions

treatment program modified as needed. Factors that affect the outcome of vestibular rehabilitation are listed in Table 6–4. Note that the patients least likely to benefit include those with fluctuating conditions, those with pure central nervous
system disorders, those with mixed central and peripheral disorders, and those
involved in litigation.

REFERENCES

1. Cawthorne TE: Vestibular injuries. Proc R Soc Med 39:270–273, 1945.
2. Cooksey FS: Rehabilitation in vestibular injuries. Proc R Soc Med 39:275, 1945.
3. Dix MR, Hood JD: Vestibular habituation: Its clinical significance and relationship to vestibular neuronitis. Laryngoscope 80:226–232, 1970.
4. Shumway-Cook A, Horak FB: Rehabilitation strategies for patients with vestibular deficits. In: Arenberg IK (ed). Dizziness and Balance Disorders. New York: Kugler, 1993, pp 667–691.
5. Herdman SJ (ed): Vestibular Rehabilitation. Second Edition, Philadelphia: FA Davis, 2000.
6. Shepard NT, Telian SA. Programmatic vestibular rehabilitation. Otolaryngol Head Neck Surg 112:173–182, 1995.
7. Krebs DE, Gill-Body KM, Riley PO, Parker SW. Double-blind, placebo-controlled trial of rehabil- itation for bilateral vestibular hypofunction: Preliminary report. Otolaryngol Head Neck Surg 109(4):735–741, 1993.
8. Di Girolamo S, Paludetti G, Briglia G, Cosenza A, Santarelli R, Di Nardo W. Postural control in benign paroxysmal positional vertigo before and after recovery. Acta Otolaryngol 118(3):289–293, 1998.
9. Melvill Jones, G: Adaptive modulation of VOR parameters by vision. In: Berthoz, A, Melvill Jones G (eds). Adaptive Mechanisms in Gaze Control: Reviews in Oculomotor Research. Amsterdam: Elsevier, 1985, pp 21–50.
10. Schmid R, Jeannerod M: Vestibular habituation: An adaptive process? In: Berthoz A, Melvill Jones G (eds). Adaptive Mechanisms in Gaze Control. Amsterdam: Elsevier, 1985, pp 113–122.
11. Baloh RW, Henn V, Jager J: Habituation of the human vestibulo-ocular reflex by low frequency harmonic acceleration. Am J Otolaryngol 3:235, 1982.
12. Melvill Jones G, Berthoz A: Mental control of the adaptive process. In: Berthoz, A, and Melvill Jones G (eds). Adaptive Mechanisms in Gaze Control. Amsterdam: Elsevier, 1985, pp 203–212.
13. Igarashi M: Physical exercise and acceleration of vestibular compensation. In: Lacour M et al (eds). Vestibular Compensation. Amsterdam: Elsevier, 1989, pp 131–144.
14. Peppard SB: Effect of drug therapy on compensation from vestibular injury. Laryngoscope 96:878–898, 1986.
15. Bienhold H, Flohr H: Role of commissural connexions between vestibular nuclei in compensation following unilateral labyrinthectomy. J Physiol 284:178, 1978.

16. Jacobson GP, Newman CW: The development of the Dizziness Handicap Inventory. Arch Oto-laryngol Head Neck Surg 116:424–427, 1990.
17. Powell LE, Myers AM: The activities-specific balance confidence (abc scale). J Gerontol Med Sci 50(1):M28–M34, 1995.
18. Shumway-Cook A, Woollacott M: Motor Control: Theory and Practical Applications. Baltimore: Williams & Wilkins, 1995.
19. Podsiadlo D, Richardson S: The timed "up & go": A test of basic functional mobility for frail elderly persons. JAGS 39:142–148, 1991.
20. Shumway-Cook A, Horak FB: Assessing influence of sensory interaction on balance. Phys Ther. 66:1548–1550, 1986.
21. Berg KO, Wood-Dauphinee SL, Williams JI, Maki B: Measuring balance in the elderly: Validation of an instrument. Can J Public Health 83:S7–S11, 1992.
22. VanSwearingen JM, Paschal KA, Bonino P, Yang JF. The modified Gait Abnormality Rating Scale for recognizing the risk of recurrent falls in community-dwelling elderly adults. Phys Ther 76(9):994–1002, 1996.
23. Reuben DB, Siu AL: An objective measure of physical function of elderly outpatients. JAGS 38:1105–1112, 1990.
24. Duncan P, Weiner D, Chandler J, Studenski S: Functional reach: A new clinical measure of balance. J Gerontol 45:M192–M197, 1990.
25. Cerny K: Clinical method of quantitative gait analysis. Phys Ther 63:1125–1126, 1983.
26. Nevitt MC, Cummings SR, Kidd S, Black D: Risk factors for recurrent nonsyncopal falls. A prospective study. JAMA 261(18):2663–2668, 1989.

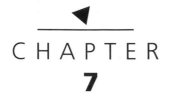
Psychiatric Aspects of Vestibular Disorders

It is common practice to assign a single diagnosis to a patient with dizziness. This strategy is usually appropriate, though in some cases two or more neurotologic disorders may present simultaneously. For dizzy patients with psychiatric disorders, it is generally inappropriate to assign a single diagnosis, that is, to consider a patient's dizziness as arising from either a neurotologic disorder or a psychiatric disorder. The "either-or, but not both" approach usually leads to suboptimal care. Typically, neurotologic disorders and psychiatric disorders coexist and interact. It is common practice to regard a patient's description of his or her dizziness as an indication of the origin of the problem. That is, spinning of the outside world has been thought to indicate a vestibular disorder, whereas spinning in the head has been thought to indicate a psychiatric disorder. Unfortunately, such inferences are not uniformly accurate. Thus, when evaluating a patient with dizziness, it is best to regard psychiatric symptoms as a comorbidity rather than a complete explanation for all of the patient's symptoms.

OVERLAP BETWEEN VESTIBULAR DISORDERS AND PSYCHIATRIC DISORDERS

The interrelationship between vestibular disorders and psychiatric disorders is complex. This chapter aims to provide a brief background to this topic. Figure 7–1 provides a framework for classifying patients with a chief complaint of dizziness. The central area indicates patients with well-defined neurotologic syndromes such as benign paroxysmal positional vertigo, Meniere's disease, and vestibular neuritis. The area, just above it represents patients who have a balance system disorder that cannot be assigned a specific diagnosis. Rather, such patients

Normal Vestibular Function

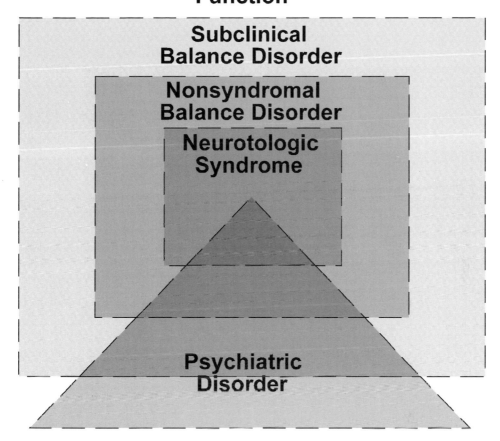

Figure 7–1. Framework for a taxonomy of dizziness. This Venn-type diagram illustrates the overlap between neurotologic and psychiatric etiologies for dizziness. Note that dizzy patients can manifest a neurotologic (balance) disorder, a psychiatric disorder, or both. Moreover, because of the difficulty in establishing a neurotologic diagnosis definitively, there are subgroups of patients with subclinical balance disorders, nonsyndromal balance disorders, and those with a well-defined neurotologic syndrome. A contemporaneous psychiatric disorder can be seen with all groups.

have examination or laboratory abnormalities that suggest a balance system disorder, but the etiology is uncertain. Diagnostic labels given to such patients include *vestibulopathy of unknown cause*. The area above this one represents that group of dizzy patients whose symptoms are highly suggestive of a balance disorder but who have no objective findings to substantiate even a provisional neurotologic diagnosis. The top area represents dizzy patients with normal vestibular function such as individuals with orthostatic hypotension.

Patients with dizziness, with or without a vestibular abnormality, may also manifest psychiatric disorders such as anxiety. Thus, superimposed on the areas that classify vestibular disorders is the broad category of psychiatric disorders. That is, as illustrated diagrammatically in Figure 7–1, a patient may have a psychiatric disorder that coexists with any of the four categories of dizziness. Thus, the presence of a psychiatric disorder does not rule out a balance disorder. In fact, as noted below, some psychiatric disorders are clearly associated with a higher likelihood of an associated vestibular disorder. So, patients with dizziness may have a balance disorder, a psychiatric disorder, both, or neither. This scheme helps to clarify how patients with both a vestibular disorder and a psychiatric disorder can be categorized. However, this scheme does not provide any details regarding the type or manner of interaction between the two types of disorders.

INTERACTION BETWEEN VESTIBULAR DISORDERS AND PSYCHIATRIC DISORDERS

Figure 7–2 presents a framework for understanding the interface between psychiatric disorders and vestibular disorders. The categories illustrated in this figure can be used to classify dizzy patients who present with psychiatric disorders in isolation or in association with a vestibular disorder. Category A represents individuals whose dizziness can be explained by their psychiatric disorder alone, that is, patients with psychiatric dizziness.[1] The term *psychiatric dizziness* should be reserved for those patients in whom the dizziness (*1*) is part of a recognized psychiatric syndrome (e.g., the dizziness during a panic attack or the abnormal

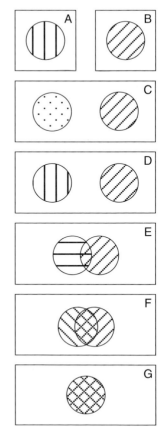

Figure 7–2. Framework for the interface between balance disorders and psychiatric disorders. This interface is depicted as several levels of interaction ranging from non-coexistent disorders to a complete overlap in pathophysiology. (A) Psychiatric disorder without a balance disorder. (B) Balance disorder without a psychiatric disorder. (C) Co-occurrence of a psychiatric disorder that does not provoke dizziness and a balance disorder with no functional overlap. (D) Co-occurrence of psychiatric dizziness and a balance disorder with no functional overlap. (E) Psychiatric overlay. (F) Behavioral/psychological mediation. (G) Neurological linkage.

gait of conversion hysteria) and (2) cannot be explained by vestibular dysfunction. Thus, dizziness occurring during a panic attack should be labeled *psychiatric dizziness,* whereas dizziness between panic attacks should not. Category B represents individuals with a balance disorder alone, that is, without an associated psychiatric disorder.

Categories C and D represent individuals with no functional overlap between a vestibular disorder and a psychiatric disorder, that is, nonfunctionally related, independently occurring disorders.

Category E represents individuals with *psychiatric overlay,* in which a patient's personality or psychiatric disorder influences his or her perception of the dizziness and the way the patient presents to and interacts with the medical profession. This category includes the role of *coping behaviors,* which may influence both physiologic and psychological aspects of the patient's problem.

Category F represents a complex blend of mutual influences of psychiatric disorders and vestibular disorders on one another. This category, termed *psychological/behavioral mediation,* implies a causal relationship between vestibular disorders and psychiatric disorders. That is, a vestibular disorder may cause, trigger, or exacerbate a psychiatric abnormality (somatopsychic mechanism) or a psychiatric disorder may cause, trigger, or exacerbate a vestibular abnormality (psychosomatic mechanism).

Category G represents individuals in whom a vestibular disorder and a psychiatric disorder are manifestations of a common underlying disorder. This circumstance, called *linkage,* may pertain to some patients with anxiety disorders. The linkage concept is that vestibular disorders and psychiatric disorders may be two different manifestations of a common underlying central nervous system abnormality. Balaban and Thayer[2] have postulated that the linkage between vestibular disorders and anxiety disorders may be based upon shared brain pathways that mediate autonomic responses. Central nervous system structures that may be critical for this linkage include the parabrachial nucleus and its connections with other structures. The vestibular disorder–anxiety disorder linkage also may be based on the effects of neurotransmitters, such as the monoamines noradrenaline and serotonin.

SOMATOPSYCHIC MECHANISMS

Somatopsychic mechanisms refer to psychological, psychiatric, and behavioral consequences of vestibular dysfunction. One possible consequence of vestibular dysfunction is anxiety. Anxiety has two components, somatic symptoms and cognitive symptoms. Somatic anxiety includes heart palpitations, nausea, diaphoresis, feeling hot or cold, shortness of breath, chest discomfort, dizziness, numbness or tingling, and feeling detached. Cognitive anxiety includes anxious thoughts such as "What if I have a life-threatening illness?" There are several different types of anxiety disorders. The Diagnostic Manual of the American Psychiatric Association (DSM-IV)[3] lists 11 different anxiety disorders; two of these are Panic Disorder without Agoraphobia and Panic Disorder with Agoraphobia. These disorders seem to have a particularly strong association with vestibular disorders.[4] The anxiety associated with vestibular dysfunction also has two components, one related to the somatic component and the other associated with the cognitive component.

Dizziness is often situation-specific. For example, rolling over in bed can trigger benign paroxysmal positional vertigo. Similarly, because the balance system receives input from three sensory systems, that is, the visual system, the somatosensory system, and the vestibular system, situations that are characterized by inconsistencies among visual, vestibular, and somatosensory signals can lead to dizziness even in normal individuals. Such situations may be particularly bothersome to patients with vestibular disorders. Such patients may show unusual sensitivity to, or need for, visual and/or somatosensory information to maintain balance. This heightened awareness of nonvestibular sensation is called *space and motion sensitivity*.[5] A subgroup of these patients experience space and motion discomfort, that is, these sensory stimuli are unpleasant. A subgroup of these individuals may actually avoid environments with inadequate or misleading balance information such as shopping malls or grocery stores. It is tempting to label patients who avoid such environments as having *psychogenic* dizziness. In fact, such patients are likely to have vestibular dysfunction.[4] Space and motion sensitivity, and space and motion discomfort, may help explain why some patients with vestibular disorders avoid certain environments. In some patients with vestibular disorders, space and motion discomfort may interfere with social, occupational, or academic functioning.

Other psychiatric disorders that can be induced or exacerbated by vestibular dysfunction include depression and social withdrawal. Depressed patients pay attention to depressing things. Thus, a depressed patient with dizziness may focus selectively on those symptoms that remain even after partially successful treatment has been instituted. Dizziness and imbalance also can cause social withdrawal since patients may be afraid of appearing drunk. Social withdrawal can also be a result of a patient adopting the *sick role*, that is, behaving as one would expect someone to act if he or she were sick.

Some patients with dizziness become angry with the health care delivery system. Jacob et al.[6] suggest that dizzy patients may trigger a *clinician's dismissive behaviors*, which include a failure on the part of the physician to recognize that there is a problem, a physician minimizing the impact of the problem, the patient's perception that the time spent by the physician is inadequate, and offense to the patient when the physician suggests that the patient's problem might be "mental."

Not every patient with dizziness develops a psychiatric disorder. Why? Possibly, preexisting anxiety, somatization, that is, the tendency to report and be preoccupied with medical symptoms from varied organ systems, perfectionist traits, and obsessive-compulsive personality disorder predispose patients to develop a psychiatric problem as a result of dizziness.[6]

PSYCHOSOMATIC MECHANISMS

Psychosomatic mechanisms refer to the alteration in vestibular function that may result from psychiatric conditions. For example, the gain of the VOR decreases with somnolence and increases with arousal. Therefore, increased anxiety may affect vestibular function. Similarly, hyperventilation may affect vestibular responses.[7] Psychosomatic mechanisms also may be important in patients who have compensated for a peripheral vestibular disorder and then have become symptomatic because of a psychiatric-induced reemergence of vestibular symptoms.

TREATMENT IMPLICATIONS

What are the treatment implications for patients with combined vestibular and psychiatric disorders? Such patients should be treated for both their vestibular and psychiatric disorders. Treatment considerations include pharmacotherapy, behavioral therapy, and vestibular rehabilitation.[8] The presence of a vestibular disorder should not preclude the appropriate psychiatric treatment. Similarly, the presence of a psychiatric disorder should not preclude appropriate treatment for a patient's balance disorder. In some patients, the same treatment may be helpful for both disorders.

REFERENCES

1. Furman JM, Jacob RG: Psychiatric dizziness. Neurology 48:1161–1166, 1997.
2. Balaban CD, Thayer JF: Neurological bases for balance-anxiety links. J Anxiety Disorders 15:53–79, 2001.
3. American Psychiatric Association: Diagnostic and Statistical Manual of Mental Disorders, ed 4. Washington, DC: American Psychiatric Association, 1994.
4. Jacob RG, Furman JM, Durrant JD, Turner SM: Panic, agoraphobia, and vestibular dysfunction. Am J Psychiatry 153:503–512, 1996.
5. Jacob RG, Woody SR, Clark DB, Lilienfeld SO, Hirsch BE, Kucera GD, Furman JM, Durrant JD: Discomfort with space and motion: A possible marker of vestibular dysfunction assessed by the Situational Characteristics Questionnaire. J Psycopathol Behav Assess 15:299–324, 1993.
6. Jacob RG, Furman JM, Cass SP: Psychological sequelae of vestibule disorders. In: Luxon LM, Martini A, Furman JM, Stephens D (eds). Textbook of Audiological Medicine London: Martin Dunitz, Ltd. (in press).
7. Theunissen EJ, Huygen PL, Folgering HT: Vestibular hyperactivity and hyperventilation. Clin Otolaryngol 111:161–169, 1986.
8. Jacob RG, Whitney SW, Detweiler-Shostak G, Furman JM: Vestibular rehabilitation for patients with agoraphobia and vestibular dysfunction: A pilot study. J Anxiety Disorders 15(1-2).131–146, 2001.

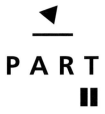

PART

II

Tutorial Case Studies

Unilateral Vestibular Impairment and Vestibular Compensation— Vestibular Neuritis

HISTORY

A 25-year-old woman who worked as a registered nurse presented with the chief complaint of acute vertigo that began 3 days before evaluation. The patient's vertigo was associated with nausea and vomiting for several hours. Following this episode, the patient had disequilibrium, gait instability, and a complaint of poor vision for 2 days. She had no associated complaints of hearing loss or tinnitus and no fullness or stuffiness in the ears. There were no complaints of changes in strength or sensation. The patient had experienced a flu-like illness that had begun approximately 2 weeks before the onset of the vertigo. At the time of evaluation, she noticed imbalance in the dark and spatial disorientation, especially after large head movements. She had no significant past medical history, and the family history was noncontributory.

Question 1: Based on the patient's history, what is the most likely diagnosis?

Answer 1: This patient's history is consistent with an acute vestibular syndrome characterized by vertigo, nausea, vomiting, blurred vision, and disequilibrium. The absence of auditory symptoms and the prior flu-like illness suggest the possibility of vestibular neuritis. Other, less likely conditions include endolymphatic hydrops and a demyelinating disorder. The absence of other otologic symptoms argues against endolymphatic hydrops (see Cases 9, 16, 21, 25). The absence of nonvestibular neurologic symptoms and the absence of previous neurologic deficits make a demyelinating lesion very unlikely. A demyelinating lesion would have to be located precisely at the root entry zone of the eighth nerve to present in this way (see Case 20).

PHYSICAL EXAMINATION

Neurologic examination revealed a left-beating horizontal-torsional nystagmus on leftward gaze with the upper poles of the eyes beating to the left. The remainder of the cranial nerve examination was normal. Strength, sensation, and coordination were normal. The patient had a negative Romberg's test. Gait was wide-based, and the patient could not tandem walk. The otologic examination was normal. The neurotologic examination was abnormal. Behind infrared glasses, the patient's nystagmus increased in intensity; it was now observed in the primary position, and both the frequency and amplitude of the nystagmus were higher. The head thrust test was abnormal, with refixation saccades noted following head rotation from left to right. The patient was unable to stand on a compliant foam surface with her eyes closed without losing her balance. Past-pointing was present with arm deviation to the right. On the stepping test, the patient rotated almost 180 degrees to the right.

Question 2: What is the pathophysiology of the patient's symptoms and signs?

Answer 2: The patient is suffering from an acute vestibular syndrome almost certainly caused by an acute, profound imbalance between the afferent activity from the left and right labyrinths. Because a large difference in neural activity normally occurs only during large head movements, the central nervous system interprets an acute loss of vestibular activity on one side as the head rotating briskly toward the intact ear. Patients thus experience vertigo. Vegetative symptoms of nausea, vomiting, and diaphoresis result from activity in the pathways from the vestibular system to the autonomic nervous system.

Question 3: What is the significance of the patient's nystagmus being horizontal-torsional?

Answer 3: The patient's nystagmus is caused by the imbalance in afferent activity from the left and right labyrinths and is probably a result of imbalanced semicircular canal activity rather than imbalance of otolith activity. Because of the orientation of the three semicircular canal pairs, the afferent activity from the intact ear, if unopposed by activity in the affected ear, combines to produce a slow component of nystagmus whose direction has specific characteristics. The unopposed left (lesioned) ear, horizontal semicircular canal activity drives the eyes horizontally toward the right, and the combined activity of the two left vertical semicircular canals, that is, the left superior and left posterior semicircular canals, causes a slow torsional movement of the eyes, with the upper poles moving toward the right. No vertical component is produced because the left superior semicircular canal tends to drive the eyes up, while the left posterior semicircular canal tends to drive the eyes down, thereby canceling the vertical influences. Thus, the predominantly horizontal-torsional nystagmus suggests a net effect of three unopposed semicircular canals of the patient's left ear combining to produce a nystagmus whose slow component has a horizontal direction toward the lesioned ear and whose quick component (for which the nystagmus direction is named) beats horizontally toward the intact ear.

Question 4: Why did the patient's nystagmus increase during gaze toward the right and decrease during gaze toward the left?

Answer 4: The alterations in the patient's nystagmus as a function of eye position in the orbit are typical of most types of nystagmus wherein the intensity of

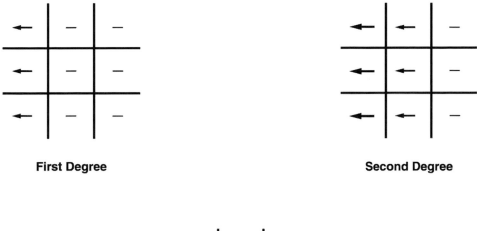

First Degree   **Second Degree**

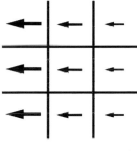

Third Degree

Figure Case 1–1 Alexander's system of grading vestibular nystagmus. Note that only the horizontal components of the nystagmus are illustrated. The length of the arrows signifies the intensity of the nystagmus.

the nystagmus, including its frequency and amplitude, increases when a patient looks in the direction of the quick component. This phenomenon, whereby the magnitude of the nystagmus changes as a function of eye position, is known as *Alexander's law* and is illustrated in Figure Case 1–1. The physiologic basis for Alexander's law may relate to an alteration in the *neural integrator* leading to a combined effect of a vestibular nystagmus and a gaze-evoked nystagmus. For example, when a patient with a right-beating nystagmus looks to the right, both the gaze-evoked nystagmus and the vestibular imbalance cause leftward eye movement, thereby increasing the magnitude of the nystagmus. However, on left gaze, the vestibular imbalance and the gaze-evoked nystagmus oppose one another, thereby decreasing the intensity of the nystagmus.

Vestibular nystagmus, which is undirectional, is sometimes graded in severity based upon its presence in different horizontal gaze positions. Specifically, Alexander's system,[1] which was originally applied to patients observed during visual fixation, includes *first-degree, second-degree,* and *third-degree vestibular nystagmus.* In third-degree nystagmus, the nystagmus is undirectional and can be observed regardless of horizontal gaze position, but the intensity of the nystagmus is maximizal with gaze in the direction of the quick component of nystagmus and is minimal, but still observable, when horizontal gaze is directed away from the

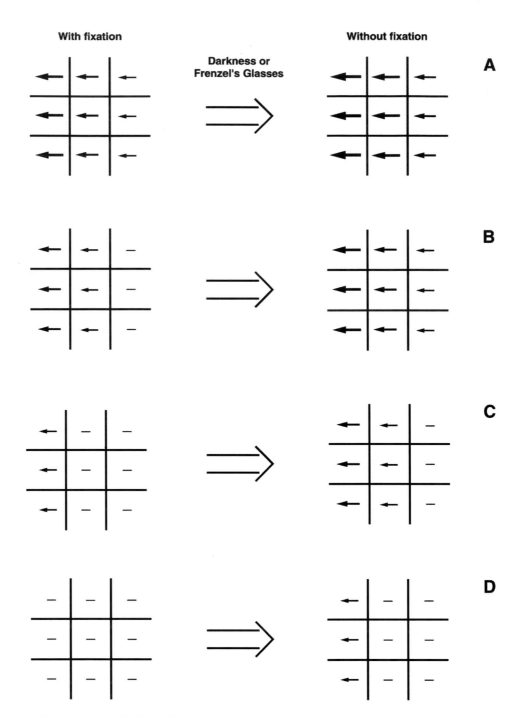

Figure Case 1–2 The influence of loss of visual fixation on vestibular nystagmus. Note that in its mildest form, a latent vestibular nystagmus will be absent in a lighted room but present in darkness on lateral gaze.

quick component. In second-degree nystagmus, the nystagmus is observed only when the patient gazes straight ahead or in the direction of the quick component. In first-degree nystagmus, the nystagmus can be observed only with gaze in the direction of the quick component. This patient had a first-degree vestibular nystagmus since left-beating nystagmus was observed only with leftward gaze.

Question 5: Why is the patient's nystagmus increased in magnitude when she is wearing infrared glasses?

Answer 5: Vestibular nystagmus, whether physiologic or pathologic, can be significantly inhibited by visual fixation when vision and visual fixation and visual tracking mechanisms are intact. Infrared or Frenzel glasses allow the patient's eyes to be observed while they significantly reduce visual fixation. An increase in a patient's nystagmus on wearing infrared or Frenzel glasses supports the idea that the patient's nystagmus originates from a vestibular imbalance, usually peripheral. Figure Case 1–2 illustrates the influence of loss of visual fixation on the various grades of severity of vestibular nystagmus. Note that in its mildest form, a vestibular nystagmus may be absent with visual fixation and observed only with loss of visual fixation with lateral gaze to the right or to the left, depending on the direction of the nystagmus. In clinical parlance, a horizontal-torsional nystagmus that increases in magnitude with loss of visual fixation is called *vestibular nystagmus*.

LABORATORY TESTING

Videonystagmography: Ocular motor testing was normal. Testing confirmed the presence of a left-beating spontaneous vestibular nystagmus that increased with loss of visual fixation. Caloric testing revealed absent responses in the right ear, including absent responses to ice-water irrigation.

Audiometric testing was normal.

An MRI scan of the brain was normal.

Question 6: How do results of laboratory testing influence the diagnostic considerations for this case?

Answer 6: The most significant finding on vestibular laboratory testing is the reduced vestibular response in the right ear on caloric testing. Although a unilateral caloric weakness was suspected from the clinical evaluation, laboratory testing provides objective evidence of a severe loss of sensitivity in the right labyrinth, confirming the clinical suspicion.

The normal audiometric test suggests that the patient is suffering from a pure vestibular syndrome such as vestibular neuritis as opposed to a more generalized *labyrinthitis*, which is commonly associated with a high-frequency hearing loss, or from endolymphatic hydrops, which is often associated with a low-tone sensorineural hearing loss.

DIAGNOSIS/DIFFERENTIAL DIAGNOSIS

As noted, this patient is almost certainly suffering from vestibular neuritis[2–4] (Fig. Case 1–3). Other names for this condition include *vestibular neurolabyrinthitis*,

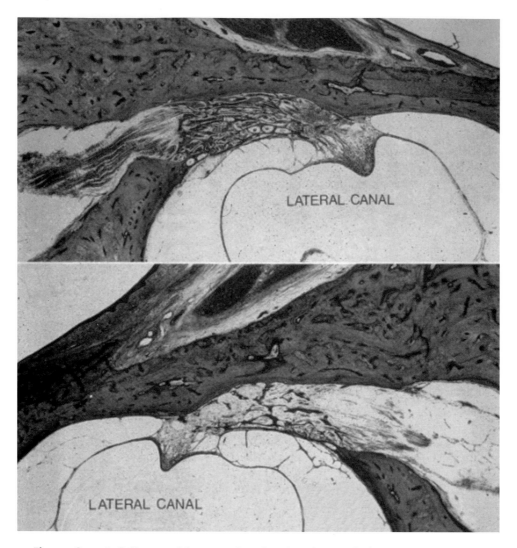

Figure Case 1–3 Temporal bone section showing the vestibular nerve innervating the lateral semicircular canal. The upper panel shows a normal nerve. The lower panel shows atrophy of the vestibular nerve thought to be the result of a viral vestibular neuritis. (*Source:* With permission from Schuknecht HR, Kitamura K: Vestibular neuritis. Ann Otol Rhinol Laryngol (suppl) 78(90):1–19, 1981.[3])

vestibular labyrinthitis, vestibular neuronitis, and *acute vestibulopathy of uncertain etiology.* These terms are used interchangeably. It should be realized that a *peripheral* vestibular lesion could actually be affecting the hair cells, the eighth nerve afferents, or the eighth nerve root entry zone. From the vestibular signs and symptoms alone, a distinction cannot be made among these three localizations. Postmortem temporal bone histopathology suggests that Scarpa's ganglion is affected primarily.[5] Figure Case 1–3 illustrates atrophy of the vestibular nerve thought to be the result of a viral vestibular neuritis. Vestibular neuritis appears to have a predilection for the superior division of the vestibular nerve.[6,7] Other entities that should be considered include labyrinthine infarction (see Case 30). It would be rare for a mass lesion such as an acoustic neuroma to present solely with an acute vestibular syndrome without hearing loss, tinnitus, or other neurologic signs or symptoms (see Cases 2, 50).

The patient was given a diagnosis of vestibular neuritis.

TREATMENT/MANAGEMENT

A short (10- to 14-day) course of corticosteroids, for example prednisone, 1 mg/kg per day, decreases the duration of vestibular symptoms and may also reduce the chance of future recurrent episodes of acute vertigo.[8] Corticosteroids also have been shown experimentally to speed vestibular compensation. Antiviral agents such as acyclovir may be considered since viral reactivation is thought to be involved in the pathogenesis of the condition; however, there are no data to conclusively support its use in this setting.[9] This patient was treated with a 2 week course of corticosteroids. Vestibular suppressants and antinausea agents were also prescribed on an as-needed basis for symptomatic relief (see Case 17).

FOLLOW-UP

The patient was seen in follow-up 1 month after the initial presentation. At that time, she was very much improved and experienced symptoms only during rapid head movement, which caused transitory dizziness and lightheadedness, and during walking in dimly lit or dark environments. The patient also noted some difficulty with driving, especially immediately after rapid head movements just before changing lanes.

Physical examination at the 1-month follow-up visit revealed no nystagmus with visual fixation. However, behind infrared glasses, a low-amplitude, left-beating horizontal-torsional nystagmus was observed. The head thrust test was unchanged, that is, still abnormal. The patient's gait had a normal base, but there was some difficulty during tandem walking. The patient was able to stand on a compliant foam pad even with her eyes closed with minimal difficulty. Her rotation on the stepping test improved, rotating only 45 degress right, and past-pointing was absent.

The patient was referred for a course of vestibular rehabilitation (see Chapter 6).[10]

Question 7: By what process did this patient's symptoms and signs almost completely resolve?

Answer 7: Despite the fact that the patient's vestibular loss in the right ear almost certainly persists, vestibular *compensation* (see Chapter 1), a process that involves rebalancing of the activity in central vestibular structures, has occurred. Through this mechanism, vestibulo-ocular, vestibulospinal, perceptual, and autonomic symptoms and signs improve substantially, athough some symptoms (as noted above in this patient) are likely to persist. Vestibular compensation occurs automatically in individuals with a normal central nervous system, normal vision and proprioception, and adequate physical activity. This patient's recovery is typical even for individuals who have suffered complete unilateral peripheral vestibular loss. The process of vestibular compensation is thought to involve brainstem and cerebellar structures, so that resting activity in the left and right vestibular nuclei becomes more or less balanced despite unilaterally reduced or absent vestibular nerve activity.

SUMMARY

A 25-year-old woman presented with the acute onset of a vestibular syndrome indicative of an acute unilateral peripheral vestibular loss. The patient's history suggested a viral/postviral affliction of the vestibular labyrinth or nerve. Examination revealed horizontal-torsional spontaneous vestibular nystagmus, poor tandem walking, and an inability to stand on a compliant foam surface with the eyes closed. Laboratory testing revealed a right reduced vestibular response. The patient was treated with a 2-week course of corticosteroids. Vestibular suppressant agents and antinausea agents were used only on an as-needed basis. Through the process of vestibular compensation, the patient's symptoms decreased dramatically. At the 1 month follow-up evaluation, nystagmus was present only while the patient was wearing infrared glasses, and she could tandem walk and stand on a compliant surface.

TEACHING POINTS

1. **An acute unilateral vestibular syndrome is characterized by vertigo, nausea, vomiting, blurred vision, and disequilibrium.** These symptoms and signs result from an imbalance between the afferent activity from the left and right labyrinths. The central nervous system interprets this imbalance as a brisk continuous head rotation toward the intact ear.
2. **Vegetative symptoms of nausea, vomiting, and diaphoresis are caused by activity in the pathways from the vestibular system to the autonomic nervous system.**
3. **The direction of acute vestibular nystagmus is typically horizontal-torsional.** This direction of nystagmus results primarily from the unopposed horizontal semicircular canal afferent activity from the intact side that produces a horizontal direction of nystagmus. The afferent activity from the two intact vertical semicircular canals sum with one another such that torsionally the upper pole of the eye drifts (torts or rolls) toward the lesioned ear. The vertical eye movement drives of the two vertical semicircular canals cancel one another. The net effect of the three unopposed semicircular canals of the intact ear thus combines to produce a predominantly horizontal-torsional nystagmus whose slow component is toward the lesioned ear and whose quick component (for which the nystagmus direction is named) beats toward the intact ear.
4. **Alexander's law, wherein the intensity of nystagmus (including its frequency and amplitude) increases when a patient looks in the direction of the quick component, is typical of most types of nystagmus.** The physiologic basis for Alexander's law may be related to changes in the *neural integrator* leading to gaze-evoked nystagmus.

5. **Visual fixation inhibits vestibular nystagmus when vision and visual fixation/visual tracking mechanisms are intact.** Infrared or Frenzel glasses allow the patient's eyes to be observed while visual fixation is significantly reduced. Thus, an increase in a patient's nystagmus when wearing infrared or Frenzel glasses supports the idea that the patient's nystagmus originates from a vestibular imbalance. In clinical parlance, a horizontal-torsional nystagmus that increases in magnitude with loss of visual fixation is called *vestibular nystagmus.*

6. **Vestibular compensation rebalances the neural activity in central vestibular structures.** This process causes a reduction of the symptoms and signs of an acute vestibular syndrome. Through compensation, vestibulo-ocular, vestibulospinal, perceptual, and autonomic symptoms and signs of the acute vestibular syndrome largely resolve. Vestibular compensation occurs automatically in individuals with a normal central nervous system, normal vision and proprioception, and adequate physical activity. The process of vestibular compensation is thought to involve brainstem and cerebellar structures, so that resting activity in the left and right vestibular nuclei becomes more or less balanced despite unilaterally reduced or absent vestibular nerve activity. *Vestibular neuritis* **is the diagnostic designation given to an acute vestibular syndrome, without obvious cause, that occurs without auditory or neurologic signs or symptoms.** The underlying pathogenesis is thought to involve viral activation within the vestibular nerve. Other conditions that can cause an acute vestibular syndrome include endolymphatic hydrops, a demyelinating disorder, and infarction involving the labyrinth or brainstem/cerebellum.

7. **Treatment of vestibular neuritis with a short (10- to 14-day) course of corticosteroids may decrease the duration of vestibular symptoms and may improve long-term recovery.**

REFERENCES

1. Leigh RJ, Zee DS: Neurology of Eye Movements, ed 3. New York: Oxford University Press, 1999.
2. Dix MR, Hallpike CS: The pathology, symptomotology and diagnosis of certain common disorders of the vestibular system. Proc R Soc Med 45:341–354, 1952.
3. Coats AC: Vestibular neuronitis. Acta Laryngol (suppl) 251:5–28, 1969.
4. Schuknecht HF, Kitamura K: Vestibular neuritis. Ann Otol Rhinol Laryngol (suppl) 78(90):1–19, 1981.
5. Baloh RW, Lopez I, Ishiyama A, Wackym PA, Honrubia V: Vestibular neuritis: Clinical–pathologic correlation. Otolaryngol Head Neck Surg 114:586–592, 1996.
6. Fetter M, Dichgan J: Vestibular neuritis spares the inferior division of the vestibular nerve. Brain 119:755–763, 1996.
7. Gacek RR, Gacek MR: Vestibular neuronitis. Am J Otol 20:553–554, 1999.
8. Ariyasu L, Byl FM, Sprague MS, Adour KK: The beneficial effect of methylprednisolone in acute vestibular vertigo. Arch Otolaryngol Head Neck Surg 116:700–703, 1990.
9. Flohr H, Luneburg U: Effects of ACTH on vestibular compensation. Brain Res 248:169–173, 1982.
10. Strupp M, Arbusow V, Maag KP, Gall C, Brandt T: Vestibular exercises improve central vestibulospinal compensation after vestibular neuritis. Neurology 51(3):838–844, 1998.

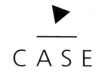

Mixed Peripheral and Central Vestibular Impairment— Cerebellopontine Angle Tumor

HISTORY

A 65-year-old man had a chief complaint of dizziness that had been worsening during the past 6 months. The patient's major symptom was disequilibrium without vertigo, which was present daily, occurred with head movement, and was particularly bothersome when walking. He noted veering of his gait both to the right and to the left. There also was a complaint of tinnitus in the left ear that was worsening gradually. He had no significant past medical history, and the family history was noncontributory.

Question 1: Based on the patient's history, what diagnoses should be considered?

Answer 1: The patient's history is consistent with both vestibular and auditory abnormalities. Moreover, disequilibrium without vertigo and the gradually worsening course suggest the possibility of a central vestibular abnormality. Diagnostic considerations that can account for both the patient's tinnitus and the imbalance include a cerebellopontine angle mass or, less likely, a peripheral otologic condition. The differential diagnosis for the patient's balance symptoms independent of tinnitus is quite broad.

PHYSICAL EXAMINATION

Neurologic examination indicated a Bruns' nystagmus, that is, a coarse, gaze-evoked nystagmus during leftward horizontal gaze and a fine vestibular (horizontal-torsional) nystagmus on rightward gaze. With infrared glasses, the patient was noted to have a primary-position, right-beating, horizontal-torsional nystagmus of small amplitude. There was no alteration of strength or sensation or incoordination of the limbs. The patient had an ataxic gait. Romberg's test was negative. Bedside evaluation of the patient's hearing indicated that Weber's test lateralized to the right and the Rinne test was positive bilaterally, indicating a sensorineural hearing loss on the left.

Question 2: What is the mechanism of this patient's nystagmus?

Answer 2: Bruns' nystagmus is a combination of a gaze-evoked nystagmus in one direction and a vestibular nystagmus that beats in the opposite direction. The gaze-evoked nystagmus is based on a cerebellar lesion ipsilateral to the direction of the gaze-evoked nystagmus. The vestibular nystagmus is based on a vestibular lesion contralateral to the direction of the vestibular nystagmus. In this patient's case, the gaze-evoked nystagmus is left-beating on left gaze and suggests a left-sided cerebellar lesion. The vestibular nystagmus is right-beating on right gaze and suggests a left-sided vestibular lesion. Thus, this patient is likely to have a left-sided cerebellar lesion and a left-sided vestibular lesion.[1,2] Right-beating vestibular nystagmus observed in the primary position with infrared glasses can often be seen only on right lateral gaze when the patient is examined in the light (see Case 1 for a discussion of Alexander's law).

Question 3: Based on the patient's history and physical examination, what is the most likely abnormality and what diagnostic test(s) should be performed?

Answer 3: This patient is likely to have a left cerebellopontine angle neoplasm. Diagnostic considerations include a large acoustic neuroma or meningioma; an aneurysm acting as a mass lesion; one of a number of uncommon posterior fossa neoplasms, such as an epidermoid tumor, chordoma, or lipoma; or, rarely, a metastatic tumor. The patient should undergo MRI of the brain, with special attention to the cerebellopontine angle. Auditory and vestibular testing would also be helpful to delineate the patient's functional abnormalities.

LABORATORY TESTING

Videonystagmography: Ocular motor testing revealed overshoot saccades to the left, an asymmetric impairment of ocular pursuit with difficulty pursuing targets moving to the left, and normal optokinetic nystagmus. A right-beating spontaneous vestibular nystagmus was seen in the dark. Caloric testing revealed a reduced vestibular response of moderate degree on the left. Rotational testing revealed asymmetric responses with more right-beating nystagmus than left-beating nystagmus.

Posturography testing indicated excessive sway on conditions 5 and 6, that is, a vestibular pattern.

Audiometric testing revealed a moderate to severe sensorineural hearing loss on the left with a word recognition score of 30%. Hearing was normal on the right.

An MRI scan of the brain revealed a 4-cm mass in the left cerebellopontine angle that filled the porus of the left internal auditory canal. There was a shift of the cerebellum and brainstem caused by mass effect of the tumor (Fig. Case 2–1).

Question 4: What additional information was provided by the laboratory testing?

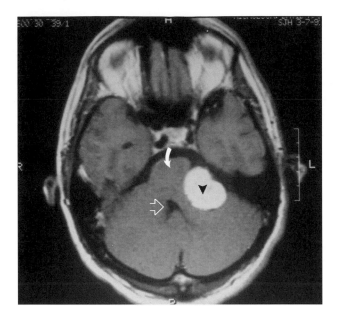

Figure Case 2–1 Axial magnetic resonance imaging of the brain demonstrating a 4-cm cerebellopontine angle neoplasm consistent with an acoustic neuroma. Note the compression and shift of the brainstem and distortion of the fourth ventricle. Arrowhead = neoplasm; curved arrow = brainstem; open arrow = fourth ventricle.

Answer 4: The MRI scan confirms the clinical suspicion of a cerebellopontine angle tumor. The scan is most suggestive of an acoustic neuroma. Audiometric testing suggests that the patient has little functional hearing remaining in the left ear. Vestibular laboratory testing confirms the presence of both peripheral vestibular and central nervous system abnormalities. The patient's caloric reduction suggests impairment of afferent vestibular activity. The abnormal saccades and pursuit suggest impairment of cerebellar/brainstem function. The patient's spontaneous nystagmus and directional preponderance on rotational testing indicate an ongoing vestibulo-ocular asymmetry. Posturography suggests that some of the patient's imbalance is a result of vestibular dysfunction.

DIAGNOSIS/DIFFERENTIAL DIAGNOSIS

This patient's history, physical examination, and laboratory studies indicate a cerebellopontine angle lesion with a mixed central and peripheral vestibular disorder.

Question 5: In what way do combined peripheral and central vestibular abnormalities interact to cause a synergistic adverse effect on a patient's balance?

Answer 5: As noted in Case 1, patients with a normal central nervous system can compensate for a peripheral vestibular lesion and become nearly symptom free. Vestibular compensation requires changes in vestibular processing in the brainstem and cerebellum, particularly the vestibulocerebellum (see Chapter 1). This patient's cerebellopontine angle lesion has caused a left–right vestibular asymmetry and, as evidenced by the patient's neurologic signs, has impaired the function of some of the central nervous system structures important for vestibular compensation. Thus, despite a vestibular loss that is gradual rather than acute and partial rather than complete, this patient has symptoms of dizziness and imbalance suggesting that vestibular compensation has not occurred.

Question 6: What are the causes of combined peripheral and central vestibular dysfunction?

Answer 6: The causes of combined peripheral and central vestibular lesions include large cerebellopontine angle lesions,[3] as in this case; anterior inferior cerebellar artery territory infarction (see Case 30); trauma (see Cases 11 and 23); and multisystem degenerations (see Case 14), for example, Friedreich's ataxia. Also, some patients with peripheral vestibular lesions have preexisting central nervous system abnormalities that prevent normal compensation from occurring (see Case 3).

TREATMENT/MANAGEMENT

The patient was treated surgically using a translabyrinthine approach. The diagnosis of an acoustic neuroma was confirmed on pathologic analysis. Complete tumor resection was accomplished with preservation of all cranial nerves except the eighth nerve, which was resected with the tumor.

Postoperatively, the patient had no complications and was referred for vestibular rehabilitation therapy (see Chapter 6).

FOLLOW-UP

The patient recovered uneventfully from the surgery. Three months after surgery, he reported tiring easily and continued to have mild to moderate unsteadiness and disequilibrium. He was reassured and encouraged to keep up with his home vestibular rehabilitation program and to avoid vestibular suppressant medications.

SUMMARY

A 65-year-old man presented with a gradual onset of imbalance and unilateral hearing loss over 6 months. Physical examination suggested a mixed central and peripheral vestibular lesion. MRI scanning confirmed the presence of a cerebellopontine angle tumor. Vestibular studies documented both peripheral and central vestibular abnormalities and abnormalities of ocular motor control. The patient demonstrated impaired compensation for his peripheral vestibular abnormality. Treatment consisted of surgical resection of the tumor. Follow-up evaluation showed mild to moderate residual unsteadiness, but the patient reported no significant disability caused by his balance dysfunction.

TEACHING POINTS

1. **A cerebellopontine angle lesion should be suspected in the setting of dizziness associated with unilateral or asymmetric hearing loss or tinnitus.** Diagnostic considerations should include a large acoustic neuroma or meningioma involving the posterior fossa. Several uncommon tumors may also affect the posterior fossa, including epidermoid tumor, chordoma, lipoma, or (rarely) metastatic tumor. A vertebrobasilar aneurysm acting as a mass lesion may also present with similar symptoms. The patient should undergo MRI of the brain, with special attention to the cerebellopontine angle.

2. **Large cerebellopontine angle tumors may produce a combination of peripheral and central vestibular abnormalities.** Both vestibular nerve and cerebellar function may be impaired. These impairments may be manifested by abnormal ocular motor tests, spontaneous nystagmus, a reduced vestibular response on caloric testing, a directional preponderance on rotational testing, and abnormal posturography.

3. **Combined peripheral and central vestibular abnormalities interact to cause a synergistic adverse effect on a patient's balance.** With a normal central nervous system, patients can compensate for a peripheral vestibular lesion and become nearly symptom free. However, if central nervous system abnormalities involve the structures that are critical for vestibular compensation, a peripheral vestibular lesion may produce persistent symptoms resulting from impaired compensation. Combined peripheral and central vestibular dysfunction may be caused by large cerebellopontine angle lesions, anterior inferior cerebellar artery territory infarction, trauma, and multisystem degenerations. Also, some patients with peripheral vestibular lesions have preexisting central nervous system abnormalities that prevent normal vestibular compensation from occurring.

4. **Bruns' nystagmus represents a manifestation of a combined peripheral and central vestibular abnormality.** It is a combination of a gaze-evoked nystagmus in one direction, presumably based on an ipsilateral cerebellar lesion, and a vestibular nystagmus in the opposite direction. Bruns' nystagmus is highly suggestive of a cerebellopontine angle tumor.

REFERENCES

1. Lundborg T: Diagnostic problems concerning acoustic tumors. Acta Otolaryngol (suppl) 99:1–111, 1950.
2. Nedzelski JM: Cerebellopontine angle tumors: Bilateral flocculus compression as cause of associated oculomotor abnormalities. Laryngoscope 93:1251–1260, 1983.
3. Baguley DM, Beynon GJ, Grey PL, Hardy DG, Moffat DA: Audio-vestibular findings in meningioma of the cerebellopontine angle: A retrospective review. J Laryngol Otol 111:1022–1026, 1997.

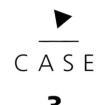

C A S E

3

Impaired Vestibular Compensation— Vestibular Neuritis

HISTORY

A 65-year-old man presented with a complaint of 6 months of dizziness and disequilibrium. His symptoms were characterized by nearly constant imbalance when walking or standing and lightheadedness even when seated. Rapid head movement exacerbated the patient's dizziness, which was associated with blurred vision. He did not complain of recent vertigo or any positional symptoms. Specifically, there were no complaints of dizziness when rolling over in bed. The patient noted no recent change in hearing or any tinnitus or aural fullness. He was essentially asymptomatic when lying still.

The patient dated his symptoms to an acute episode of vertigo associated with nausea, vomiting, and severe disequilibrium lasting for several hours 6 months before evaluation. He had not complained of dizziness before that episode. He was evaluated by his primary care physician and was believed to have a peripheral vestibular ailment. The patient was treated with meclizine, 25 mg orally, three times daily. This provided some relief but was not entirely successful in alleviating his symptoms. The patient had to decrease his activity level to such a degree that he no longer drove an automobile or took his morning walk and discontinued gardening. Despite these changes in his activities, he continued to experience daily dizziness, and his physician increased the dosage of his meclizine to 25 mg, four times daily. Other than dizziness, the patient had no significant past medical history. The family history was noncontributory.

Question 1: Based on the patient's history, what is the most likely diagnosis? Why is the patient experiencing dizziness?

Answer 1: This patient's most likely diagnosis is vestibular neuritis (see Case 1). Acute vertigo unaccompanied by associated hearing loss, tinnitus, and aural fullness is unlikely to be caused by Meniere's disease. Other possibilities include an ischemic insult to the vestibular labyrinth or nerve or some other nonspecific vestibulopathy. In any case, the patient's history is consistent with an acute peripheral vestibular ailment 6 months before evaluation.

The patient's persistent dizziness suggests that he has not compensated for his presumed peripheral vestibular loss. His continued symptoms of instability during standing and walking suggest an ongoing vestibulospinal abnormality. The patient's blurred vision immediately following head movement suggests a vestibulo-ocular abnormality. Meclizine does not appear to be a successful treatment. Possibly, this medication is actually worsening the patient's symptoms by suppressing needed vestibular input and interfering with vestibular compensation.

PHYSICAL EXAMINATION

General examination revealed an elderly-appearing man who made minimal spontaneous head movements. Neurologic examination revealed a few beats of right-beating nystagmus on right-lateral gaze that were unsustained. Otherwise, the patient's cranial nerve examination was normal. There were no changes in strength or sensation. There was no incoordination. The patient's gait was slow, with a short stride length. His head was held rigidly during walking. The patient could tandem walk only with assistance. Romberg's test was negative. Otologic examination was normal. A low-amplitude right-beating nystagmus was seen in the primary position with infrared glasses.

The head thrust test was normal. Dix-Hallpike maneuvers were negative. The patient could not stand on a compliant foam surface with the eyes open or closed. Pastpointing was absent. On the stepping test, the patient's stepping was tentative and wide-based, and she rotated almost 180 degrees to the left.

Question 2: What additional information regarding the cause of this patient's dizziness was provided by the physical examination?

Answer 2: The patient's examination suggests that he is avoiding vestibular stimulation by severely limiting head movement. Moreover, the patient's nystagmus, although minimal, suggests an ongoing vestibulo-ocular asymmetry and a vestibular compensation abnormality. It is likely that the patient has not compensated for his presumed peripheral vestibular deficit. One reason for the patient's failure to compensate may be inadequate vestibular stimulation because he limits head movement so severely.

LABORATORY TESTING

Videonystagmography: Ocular motor function was normal. A very-low-amplitude right-beating nystagmus was seen with the eyes open in the dark while seated and during positional testing. This nystagmus increased with rightward gaze. Caloric testing revealed a 50% reduced vestibular response on the left.

Rotational testing revealed responses of normal amplitude and timing. However, there was a right-directional preponderance.

Posturography indicated a *surface dependence* pattern wherein the patient had excessive postural sway whenever he was standing on a *sway-referenced* platform regardless of the visual condition, that is, on conditions 4, 5, and 6. He was able to maintain his balance only when the support surface was fixed.

Audiometric testing showed a mild high-frequency sensorineural hearing loss that was symmetric in both ears. Word recognition scores were 100% bilaterally.

An MRI scan of the brain was normal.

Question 3: What additional information does laboratory testing provide?

Answer 3: Laboratory testing indicates that the patient has both a unilateral peripheral vestibular reduction and an ongoing vestibulo-ocular and vestibulospinal asymmetry. Moreover, the patient's posturography abnormalities suggest that he has become dependent on a rigid surface for maintaining balance. Taken together, the findings suggest impaired vestibular compensation for a unilateral peripheral vestibular insult despite the passage of 6 months since the patient's acute vestibular syndrome.

Question 4: What are the causes of impaired vestibular compensation for peripheral vestibular injury? Which of these causes may be underlying this patient's persistent symptoms?

Answer 4: Vestibular compensation depends upon consistent peripheral vestibular activity, even if reduced or only from one labyrinth, in combination with other sensory inputs such as that from vision and somatosensation, and normal function of central vestibular structures.[1-3] Thus, failure to compensate for a peripheral vestibular lesion can be based on fluctuating or aberrant peripheral vestibular activity, a central nervous system abnormality that impairs vestibular compensation, clinical or subclinical involvement of the contralateral ear, multiple sensory deficits, or a sedentary lifestyle. Impaired vestibular compensation can be a result of both structural abnormalities of the brain[4] and dysfunction caused by certain drugs such as benzodiazepines (Table Case 3-1)

This patient's failure to compensate for a peripheral vestibular lesion is probably the result of a combination of a sedentary lifestyle and overmedication with vestibular suppressants that together caused inadequate vestibular stimulation and impaired vestibular compensation. The absence of vertigo and the constancy of symptoms do not suggest fluctuating or aberrant vestibular input from the in-

Table Case 3-1 Causes of Impaired Compensation

Fluctuating vestibular function
Aberrant vestibular function
Subclinical involvement of the contralateral labyrinth
Central nervous system
  Structural
  Medication-induced
Sedentary lifestyle
Multisensory impairment
  Visual dysfunction
  Somatosensory dysfunction

volved ear, although this cannot be ruled out entirely. Also, there is nothing to suggest abnormalities in other sensory systems.

DIAGNOSIS/DIFFERENTIAL DIAGNOSIS

This patient's history, physical examination, and laboratory studies suggest left-sided vestibular neuritis and impaired compensation, that is, the patient has failed to undergo normal vestibular compensation for his peripheral vestibular ailment.

TREATMENT/MANAGEMENT

This patient was treated by gradually discontinuing meclizine. Additionally, he was scheduled for a course of vestibular rehabilitation therapy in the hope of potentiating compensation for his peripheral vestibular deficit. Physical therapy was recommended with the intent of reducing the patient's symptoms of dizziness and improving his balance by expediting vestibular compensation and reducing his dependence upon somatosensation, that is, eliminating his *surface dependence.*

SUMMARY

A 65-year-old man presented with a history of an episode of acute vertigo, nausea, and vomiting 6 months prior to evaluation. The patient's symptoms evolved into constant disequilibrium. Physical examination suggested an ongoing vestibular imbalance. This was confirmed by laboratory testing, which indicated a reduced vestibular response and both vestibulo-ocular and vestibulospinal abnormalities. The patient was believed to have a peripheral vestibular ailment with poor compensation centrally. His vestibular suppressant medication was discontinued, and she was enrolled in a course of vestibular rehabilitation therapy.

TEACHING POINTS

1. **Persistent dizziness that continues following an acute peripheral vestibular ailment may be the result of impaired vestibular compensation.** Typical symptoms of impaired compensation include instability during standing and walking and blurred vision associated with quick head movements.
2. **Patients with impaired vestibular compensation for a peripheral vestibular injury often avoid vestibular stimulation by severely limiting head movements.** Gait is often slow, with a short stride length, and the head is held rigidly during walking. Although limiting head movements reduces vestibular stimulation and thus the sensation of dizziness, this strategy is maladaptive because vestibular stimulation is necessary to stimulate the process of vestibular compensation.
3. **Failure to compensate for a peripheral vestibular lesion can be the result of one or more factors.** These include fluctuating or aberrant peripheral vestibular activity; a central nervous system abnormality; clin-

ical or subclinical involvement of the contralateral ear; the presence of other sensory deficits, especially involving vision and somatosensation; or a sedentary lifestyle. Central nervous system abnormalities that impair vestibular compensation include both structural abnormalities and dysfunction caused by certain drugs such as benzodiazepines.

4. **Vestibular laboratory test results that are consistent with impaired vestibular compensation include the presence of a spontaneous nystagmus, directional preponderance on rotational testing, and abnormal platform posturography testing. Treatment of patients with impaired vestibular compensation includes tapering vestibular suppressant medications and instituting a course of rehabilitation therapy.**

REFERENCES

1. Hart C, McKinley P, Peterson B: Compensation following acute unilateral total loss of peripheral vestibular function. In: Graham M, Kemink J (eds). The Vestibular System: Neurophysiologic and Clinical Research. New York: Raven Press, 1987, pp 187–192.
2. Lacour M, Toupet M, Denise P, Christen Y (eds): Vestibular Compensation: Facts, Theories and Clinical Perspectives. Proceedings of the International Symposium. Paris: Elsevier, 1988.
3. Smith P, Curthoys I: Mechanisms of recovery following unilateral labyrinthectomy: A review. Brain Res Rev 14:155–180, 1989.
4. Furman JM, Balaban CD, Pollack IF: Vestibular compensation following cerebellar infarction. Neurology 48:916–920, 1997.

Bilateral Vestibular Loss—Ototoxicity

HISTORY

A 59-year-old woman who did not work outside the home presented with a complaint of dizziness, difficulty with vision, and instability while walking, especially in dimly lit environments or when the floor was uneven. The patient's complaints were constant during the previous 6 months. She was asymptomatic when sitting or lying still. Visual complaints were most noticeable when she was moving her head rapidly or riding in a motor vehicle, during which she experienced jumbling of the visual surroundings. Meclizine provided no relief of the patient's symptoms but was still being used occasionally. There was no complaint of hearing loss, tinnitus, or aural fullness. The patient also had no complaints of double vision, loss of vision, weakness, loss of sensation, or incoordination aside from difficulty walking.

Question 1: Based on this portion of the patient's history, what are the diagnostic considerations?

Answer 1: Constant imbalance, absence of vertigo, and absence of associated complaints of hearing loss or tinnitus all point away from a unilateral peripheral vestibular ailment. The patient may be suffering from a central nervous system abnormality affecting the balance system, such as a cerebellar abnormality. However, the fact that the patient's ambulation is worse in dimly lit environments suggests a vestibular component. Also, the patient's poor vision when the head is moving, particularly in motor vehicles, suggests an impaired VOR.

ADDITIONAL HISTORY

Upon further questioning, the patient related that she had noted the onset of her symptoms approximately 1 week after discharge from the hospital where she had been admitted because of complicated cholecystitis. During that hospitalization, she had been treated with intravenous gentamicin for 2 weeks. The patient stated that, to the best of her knowledge, the gentamicin was given at an appropriate dose, with drug levels ascertained regularly. The patient also indicated that she had a past history of Sjogren's syndrome, which had been in remission for approximately 2 years. There was no significant family history.

PHYSICAL EXAMINATION

Neurologic examination revealed full extraocular movements without nystagmus. The remainder of the neurologic examination was normal, except that the patient had gait ataxia with a widened base. Romberg's test was negative. Otoscopic examination was normal. Decreased audibility to finger rub was noted in both ears. The patient's visual symptoms could be reproduced by applying a gentle vibratory motion with the index finger to the head just lateral to the outer canthus of the eye while the opposite eye was occluded. On neurotologic examination, there was no nystagmus behind infrared glasses. On head thrust testing, refixation saccades were noted with head movement both to the right and to the left. During ophthalmoscopy, the patient was asked to move her head back and forth at a high frequency with very small excursions. The optic disc was noted to move with the patient's head movements rather than remain stable in space. The dynamic visual acuity test was abnormal in that the patient's visual acuity decreased by three lines on a Snellen chart during passive head movement. The patient was unable to stand on a compliant foam surface with her eyes closed without falling.

Question 2: Based upon the additional historical information and the physical examination, what is the patient's likely diagnosis?

Answer 2: This patient is probably suffering from bilateral vestibular loss as a result of aminoglycoside ototoxicity, which causes hair cell damage (Fig. Case 4–1). The patient is manifesting Dandy's syndrome, that is, the combination of oscillopsia (jumbling of the visual surround) and gait ataxia caused by the bilateral loss of vestibular function.[1] Dandy popularized vestibular nerve section as a treatment for Meniere's disease in 1928.[2] Many of Dandy's patients underwent bilateral vestibular nerve sections that resulted in oscillopsia and gait ataxia, a symptom complex that now bears his name. Abnormal head thrust test bilaterally, motion of the fundus during head movement, and abnormal reduction in visual acuity with head movement indicate a reduced VOR. The past history of Sjogren's syndrome is of uncertain significance. Because Sjogren's syndrome is an autoimmune disorder that may be associated with vestibular loss (see Case 27), the patient may have had a combination of autoimmune inner ear disease and ototoxicity. By some unknown mechanism, the patient may have been more susceptible to ototoxicity because of her Sjogren's syndrome.

Question 3: What are the causes of bilateral vestibular loss? What laboratory tests should be requested?

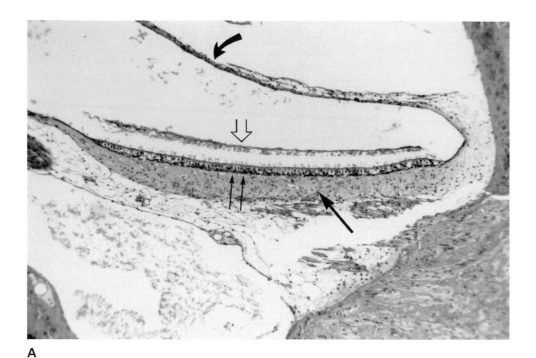

A

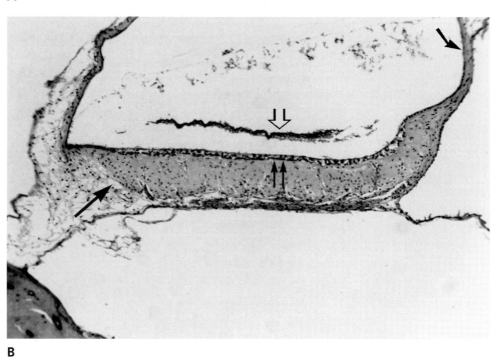

B

Figure Case 4–1 Histopathology of aminoglycoside ototoxicity. (A) Normal utricular macula. (B) Utricular macula following aminoglycoside-induced ototoxicity. Note the flattening of the sensory epithelium and loss of stereocilia, denoting destruction of the utricular hair cells. Thick straight arrow = utricular macula; double arrows = sensory epithelium (hair cells) with stereocilia extending from their upper surface (panel A); open arrowhead = otolithic membrane; curved arrow = endolymphatic membrane surrounding the utricle.

Table Case 4–1 Commonly
Used Ototoxic Medications

Aminoglycoside antibiotics
    Streptomycin
    Gentamicin
    Tobramycin
Chemotherapeutic/anticancer agents
    Cisplatinum
Diuretics
    Furosemide
    Ethacrynic acid
Erythromycin
Salicylates

Answer 3: Bilateral vestibular loss is most commonly a result of ototoxicity from aminoglycosides, including gentamicin, tobramycin, and streptomycin.[3] Commonly used medications that are ototoxic are listed in Table Case 4–1. Other pharmaceutical agents, such as cisplatinum, can cause bilateral vestibular loss. Diagnostic considerations for bilateral vestibular loss besides ototoxicity include bilateral Meniere's disease, otosclerosis, Paget's disease, a history of meningitis, multiple cranial neuropathies, congenital abnormalities, neurofibromatosis type II (bilateral acoustic neuroma), autoimmune inner ear disease (Case 27), syphilis and vestibular loss in association with neurodegenerative syndromes that cause deafness (e.g., Friedreich's ataxia), and idiopathic causes.[4] Thus, further laboratory testing should include rheumatologic parameters, such as an erythrocyte sedimentation rate and antinuclear antibody measurement, as well as a serum fluorescent treponemal antibody absorption test (FTA-ABS). Audiometry should be performed to determine whether or not there is a hearing loss associated with the patient's vestibular loss. Quantitative vestibular laboratory testing, including rotational testing, should be requested to confirm the extent of vestibular loss.

In the case of bilateral vestibular loss in the presence of bilateral hearing loss, the patient should have an MRI scan to rule out the unlikely occurrence of bilateral mass lesions such as acoustic neuroma or cerebellopontine angle tumors.

LABORATORY TESTING

Videonystagmography: Ocular motor testing was normal. There was no static positional nystagmus. Caloric testing revealed absent responses in both ears even to ice-water irrigation.

Rotational testing revealed markedly reduced responses such that no eye movements were generated at frequencies below 0.5 Hz and there were only a few beats of nystagmus following deceleration from a constant velocity rotation of 90 degrees per second.

Posturography indicated excessive sway on conditions 5 and 6, that is, a vestibular pattern. Audiometric testing indicated a bilateral asymmetric sensorineural hearing loss (Fig. Case 4–2).

The left ear had primarily a high-frequency hearing loss. The right ear had a flat hearing loss. An MRI scan of the brain was normal.

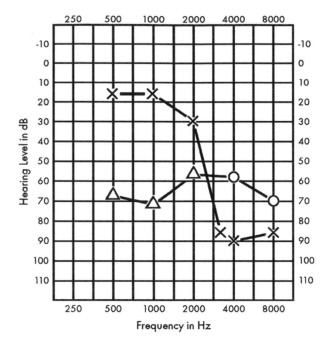

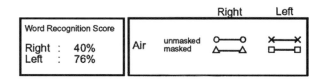

Figure Case 4–2 Audiogram.

The patient had a normal erythrocyte sedimentation rate and negative antinuclear antibody and FTA-ABS measurements.

Question 4: What information does vestibular laboratory testing provide for diagnosis and treatment?

Answer 4: The patient's laboratory test indicates bilateral vestibular loss confirmed by both caloric and rotational testing. Posturography supports the diagnosis by indicating an inability to control upright balance when forced to rely on vestibular information. Regarding treatment, this patient will require therapy to potentiate nonvestibular sensory inputs.

Question 5: What is the value of assessing hearing in the evaluation of the dizzy patient?

Answer 5: Because the vestibular and auditory periphery share common inner-ear fluid homeostasis, blood supply, nerves, and location within the temporal bone (see Chapter 1), disorders that affect the peripheral vestibular apparatus often affect hearing as well. An evaluation of hearing can help to localize a vestibular system disorder to the periphery and often can help to lateralize an abnormality. In addition, certain vertigo syndromes have characteristic types of associated hearing loss, for example, endolymphatic hydrops, which is frequently associated with a low-tone sensorineural hearing loss with good word recognition, whereas vestibular neuritis is characterized by normal hearing. Compression of the eighth cranial nerve bundles within the internal auditory canal and/or cerebellopontine angle by a tumor can also produce symptoms of unsteadiness and disequilibrium as well as hearing loss. In this situation, the hearing loss is usually primarily in the high frequencies, and word recognition is relatively poor.

DIAGNOSIS/DIFFERENTIAL DIAGNOSIS

This patient is manifesting bilateral vestibular loss as a result of aminoglycoside ototoxicity.

TREATMENT/MANAGEMENT

Question 6: Prevention is the best management for ototoxicity. What factors should alert the physician to the possible occurrence of ototoxicity?

Answer 6: The major risk factors for the occurrence of bilateral vestibulopathy when using ototoxic drugs include impaired renal function, age greater than 65, prior use of ototoxic drugs, high serum levels of ototoxic drugs, preexisting sensorineural hearing loss, and a medical course greater than 14 days. Some patients may have a genetic predisposition to aminoglycoside ototoxicity,[5] but there is currently no clinically available test for this condition. Symptoms of bilateral vestibular loss can be progressive and also delayed from weeks to months even after the drug has been stopped.[3]

Question 7: Based on the patient's diagnosis and laboratory test findings, what are the appropriate strategies for managing her disequilibrium?

Answer 7: This patient is suffering from bilateral vestibular loss. Treatment should include discontinuation of all vestibular-suppressant medications. Also, the patient should be referred for a course of vestibular rehabilitation therapy to encourage the use of sensory input other than that from the vestibular system, such as from vision and proprioception. A properly fitted cane can provide increased proprioceptive input. The patient should also be cautioned to remove all loose rugs from the home, install night lights, and install hand rails on stairways and in the bathroom.

Question 8: Aside from discontinuing vestibular suppressants and encouraging the use of alternative sensory inputs, what other modalities are available to patients with bilateral vestibular loss to develop spatial orientation and stable vision while the head is moving?

Answer 8: Possible strategies for patients with bilateral vestibular loss are listed in Table Case 4–2. The use of nonvestibular sensory inputs such as vision and proprioception is the primary means of partially overcoming the effects of bilateral vestibular loss. During head movements, stabilization of vision can be achieved, in part, by alterations of patterns of head movement such that the head is moved more slowly. Some patients can learn to *preprogram* slow compensatory eye movements in anticipation of head movements. Also, the cervico-ocular re-

Table Case 4–2 Strategies for Patients with Bilateral Vestibular Loss

Sensory substitution
Altered patterns of head motion
Preprogramming of slow eye movements in anticipation of head movements
Potentiation of the cervico-ocular reflex
Saccidic substitution
Perceptual adjustments to decrease oscillopsia

flex can be potentiated in such patients[6,7] (see Case 53). Saccadic eye movements can be substituted for slow eye movements. There can be a perceptual adjustment to decrease the effect of oscillopsia.[8] These behavioral adjustments may occur spontaneously to a greater or lesser extent in an individual patient. However, by working with a physical therapist, patients with bilateral vestibular loss can be helped to achieve optimal ocular motor and balance function while decreasing symptoms[9] (see Chapter 6).

The patient was treated with discontinuation of vestibular-suppressant medications and a course of vestibular rehabilitation therapy. The therapist provided the patient with a cane.

FOLLOW-UP

The patient improved somewhat, especially in regard to her symptoms of dizziness while still. Unfortunately, although improved, the patient still had oscillopsia and gait instability in poorly lighted environments and poor balance when walking on uneven flooring.

SUMMARY

A 59-year-old woman presented with oscillopsia and ataxia that began following treatment with an aminoglycoside antibiotic for cholecystitis. The patient had a past history of Sjogren's syndrome that may have predisposed the patient to ototoxicity. Laboratory testing confirmed the presence of bilateral vestibular loss and did not reveal any evidence of autoimmune disease. The patient was treated with discontinuation of vestibular-suppressant medications, a cane, and a course of vestibular rehabilitation therapy designed to train the patient to use other sensory modalities and to adopt other behaviors to substitute for her vestibular function. Following treatment, the patient had decreased symptoms and was functionally improved but still impaired.

TEACHING POINTS

1. **The combination of oscillopsia and ataxia (Dandy's syndrome) is pathognomonic for bilateral vestibular loss.**
2. **Bilateral vestibular loss most commonly occurs as a result of aminoglycoside-induced ototoxicity.** Other pharmaceutical agents such as cisplatinum can also cause bilateral vestibular loss. Bilateral vestibular

loss may also be caused by bilateral Meniere's disease, autoimmune inner ear disease, otosyphilis, or bilateral acoustic neuromas or may be idiopathic.

3. **Laboratory testing of patients with bilateral vestibular loss is helpful.** Testing should include rheumatologic parameters, such as an erythrocyte sedimentation rate and antinuclear antibody and serum FTA-ABS measurements. Audiometry should be performed to evaluate the pattern of any associated hearing loss. Quantitative vestibular laboratory testing should be requested to confirm the extent of vestibular loss. Rotational testing is particularly helpful in this regard. An MRI scan should be performed if bilateral acoustic neuromas are suspected.

4. **Hearing assessment is a fundamental part of the evaluation of the dizzy patient.** Because the vestibular and auditory periphery share common inner-ear fluid homeostasis, blood supply, nerves, and location within the temporal bone, disorders that affect the peripheral vestibular apparatus often affect hearing as well. An evaluation of hearing can help to localize a vestibular system disorder to the periphery and can often help to lateralize an abnormality.

5. **The type of hearing loss can help to diagnose vestibulopathy.** Several vertigo syndromes have characteristic types of associated hearing loss. For example, endolymphatic hydrops is frequently associated with a low-tone sensorineural hearing loss with good word recognition, whereas vestibular neuritis is characterized by normal hearing. Compression of the eighth cranial nerve bundles within the internal auditory canal and/or cerebellopontine angle by a tumor can produce a hearing loss that is usually worse in the high frequencies, with impaired word recognition.

6. **Prevention is the best management for ototoxicity.** The major risk factors for the occurrence of bilateral vestibulopathy when using aminoglycoside antibiotics include impaired renal function, age greater than 65, prior use of ototoxic drugs, high serum levels of ototoxic drugs, preexisting sensorineural hearing loss, and drug exposure longer than 14 days. Symptoms of bilateral vestibular loss can be progressive and can be delayed for weeks to months following discontinuation of an aminoglycoside antibiotic.

7. **Treatment for bilateral vestibular loss should include discontinuation of all vestibular-suppressant medications and referral for a course of vestibular rehabilitation therapy.** Patients should be taught how to use sensory input other than that from the vestibular system, such as from vision and proprioception. A properly fitted cane can provide increased proprioceptive input. The patient should also be cautioned to remove all loose rugs from the home, install night lights, and install hand rails on stairways and in the bathroom. If possible, the patient should not receive further ototoxic medications.

REFERENCES

1. "JC": Living without a balancing mechanism. N Engl J Med 246:458–460, 1952.
2. Dandy WE: Meniere's disease: Its diagnosis and methods of treatment. Arch Surg 16:1127, 1928.

3. Rybak LP, Matz GJ: Auditory and vestibular effects of toxins. Manifestations of systemic disease. In: Cummings W (ed). Otolaryngology—Head and Neck Surgery, Vol 4. St Louis: CV Mosby, 1986, pp 3161–3172.

4. Baloh RW, Jacobson K, Honrubia V: Idiopathic bilateral vestibulopathy. Neurology 39:272–275, 1989.

5. Casano RA, Johnson DF, Bykhovskaya Y, Torricelli F, Bigozzi M, Fischel-Ghodsian N: Inherited susceptibility to aminoglycoside ototoxicity: Genetic heterogeneity and clinical implications. Am J Otol 20:151, 1999.

6. Kasai T, Zee DS: Eye–head coordination in labyrinthine-defective human beings. Brain Res 144:123–141, 1978.

7. Bronstein AM, Hood JD: The cervico-ocular reflex in normal subjects and patients with absent vestibular function. Brain Res 373:399–408, 1986.

8. Wist ER, Brandt T, Krafczyk S: Oscillopsia and retinal slip. Brain 106:153–168, 1983.

9. Herdman SJ (ed): Vestibular Rehabilitation, ed 2. Philadelphia: FA Davis, 2000.

C A S E

5

Anxiety and Psychiatric Dizziness—Vestibulopathy, Cause Unknown

HISTORY

A 43-year-old woman who worked as an accountant presented with the chief complaint of dizziness for the last several years. Her symptoms were described as a sense of lightheadedness and disequilibrium without true vertigo. Lightheadedness was constantly present at a low level. The patient suffered periodic exacerbations. She was particularly bothered by rapid head movements and by certain environments, such as shopping malls, grocery stores, and driving on winding roads. Additionally, she occasionally experienced tingling of the fingers and toes associated with her dizziness. She also related that she avoided heights. There was no positional sensitivity, hearing loss, or tinnitus. She had had a history of panic attacks in her 20s that had resolved. She could not recall if she had been medicated for these attacks.

Question 1: Based on the history, what are the diagnostic possibilities for this patient?

Answer 1: This patient has nonspecific complaints that are difficult to localize entirely to the vestibular system. Moreover, her history suggests a symptom complex that has been labeled *space and motion discomfort*,[1] which refers to symptoms elicited by a specific stimulus pattern in some patients with vestibular dysfunction and in some with panic disorder. Space and motion discomfort occurs in situations characterized by inadequate or confusing visual or kinesthetic information for normal spatial orientation. Space and motion discomfort coupled with intermittent paresthesias strongly suggests an anxiety component to the patient's problem.

91

Moreover, the patient avoids heights and had suffered from panic attacks previously. Thus, this patient may have a vestibular disorder, an anxiety disorder, or both.

PHYSICAL EXAMINATION

Neurologic examination revealed square-wave jerks, that is, small, involuntary to-and-fro saccades on and off the point of visual regard. The patient was unaware of these movements. Examinations of her motor system, sensation, and coordination were normal. The patient was able to tandem walk without difficulty. Romberg's test was negative. Otologic and neuro-otologic examinations were normal, including no difficulty standing on a foam pad with the eyes closed.

LABORATORY TESTING

Videonystagmography: Ocular motor, positional, and caloric tests were normal.
Rotational testing revealed responses of normal amplitude and timing with a significant right directional preponderance.
Posturography was normal.

Question 2: In what way does the additional information from the physical examination and vestibular laboratory testing influence the diagnostic considerations?

Answer 2: The patient's square-wave jerks are a nonspecific finding often seen in the elderly, in whom they are of no clinical significance. In young adults, however, square-wave jerks are considered abnormal and may indicate a brainstem or cerebellar abnormality (see Case 41). The combination of normal caloric responses and a directional preponderance on rotational testing suggests an ongoing vestibulo-ocular asymmetry without peripheral vestibular disease. Thus, the patient may have a central nervous system abnormality. Taken together, the patient's history, physical examination, and laboratory abnormalities suggest an anxiety disorder and a central vestibular abnormality as well.

Question 3: What is *psychogenic dizziness*?

Answer 3: *Psychogenic dizziness* is a term used by many physicians synonymously with *psychic dizziness, psychiatric dizziness, psychophysiologic dizziness,* and *functional dizziness*.[2,3] The diagnosis of psychogenic dizziness is commonly based on the nature of the dizziness; lightheadedness or giddiness is said to be more likely to be psychogenic.[4] Moreover, dizziness is often diagnosed as psychogenic when it occurs in anxious or phobic individuals. This use of the term *psychogenic dizziness* can be criticized for several reasons. A large number of patients who fulfill the diagnostic criteria for a psychiatric disorder may also have vestibular dysfunction. Indeed, there is a definite association between anxiety disorders and vestibular disorders.[5] We prefer to use the term *psychiatric dizziness* for those patients in whom dizziness occurs exclusively in combination with other symptoms as part of a recognized psychiatric symptom cluster[3] (see Chapter 7). For example, dizziness that occurs as a component of the symptom cluster of panic attacks should be called psychiatric.

Question 4: What is the role of hyperventilation in the evaluation of patients with suspected anxiety disorders?

Answer 4: The hyperventilation test has been described by Drachman and Hart[6] and Nedzelski and colleagues (1986).[7] They described dizziness related to 3 minutes of hyperventilation. It is common practice to consider dizziness psychogenic if a patient's sensations can be replicated by hyperventilation. Such a practice is questionable, however. Herr and associates (1989) found that the hyperventilation test was positive in approximately 20% of patients who had diagnoses other than that of vestibular dysfunction, thereby indicating a lack of specificity of the hyperventilation test.[8] Also, recent studies have suggested that hyperventilation may induce nystagmus in patients with acoustic neuroma.[9] The sensitivity of the hyperventilation test is also unknown. Thus, although the hyperventilation test can provide the clinician with useful information, the results of this test should be interpreted with great caution.

DIAGNOSIS/DIFFERENTIAL DIAGNOSIS

The patient's symptoms of dizziness with rapid head movement coupled with abnormal vestibular laboratory studies suggest a vestibular system abnormality. Her history of space and motion discomfort, avoidance of heights, paresthesias, and a remote history of panic attacks suggests an anxiety disorder. Thus, this patient has both a vestibular disorder of uncertain etiology and anxiety.

Question 5: What is the cause-and-effect relationship, if any, between vestibular disorders and anxiety disorders?

Answer 5: Three functional mechanisms that are not necessarily exclusive might account for the association between vestibular abnormalities and anxiety disorders: the somatopsychic, psychosomatic, and neurologic linkage mechanisms.[5,10] The somatopsychic model postulates that vestibular sensations are catastrophically reinterpreted by the patient as signifying immediate danger. Agoraphobic avoidance develops as a result of this situational specificity of vestibular symptoms, for example, space and motion discomfort. The psychosomatic model postulates that vestibular dysfunction occurs as a result of anxiety or hyperventilation, perhaps by altering central vestibular processing. In favor of this mechanism are the observations that increases in vestibular responses occur with heightened arousal and hyperventilation alters vestibular responses on the rotational test and the positional test.[11–13] The neurologic linkage model[10] postulates that anxiety disorders, in combination with vestibular and audiologic dysfunction, involve abnormal activity in overlapping or interconnected areas in the brainstem, such as the locus coeruleus and the parabrachial nucleus.

TREATMENT/MANAGEMENT

Question 6: What is the appropriate treatment for this patient, who has a vestibular system abnormality and appears to have an anxiety disorder as well?

Answer 6: Treatment approaches to patients with anxiety that may be related to vestibular dysfunction are currently under development. No controlled outcome

Table Case 5–1 Medications for Anxiety Associated with Dizziness

Medication	Trade Name	Class	Dosage	Side Effects
Diazepam	Valium	Benzodiazepine	2-10 mg orally, IM, or IV every 4 to 6 hours	Lethargy
Clonazepam	Klonipin	Benzodiazepine	0.25–0.5 mg orally twice daily	Lethargy
Chlordiazepoxide	Librium	Benzodiazepine	5–10 mg orally every 6–8 hours	Drowsiness
Hydroxyzine	Vistaril, Atarax	Piperazine derivative	50–100 mg orally every 6 hours	Drowsiness, dry mouth
Imipramine	Imavate, Janimine, Presamine, SK-Pramine, Tofranil	Tricyclic antidepressant	25-100 mg orally daily	Anticholinergic effects, drowsiness
Desipramine	Norpramin, Pertofrane	Tricyclic antidepressant	25–100 mg orally daily	Anticholinergic effects, drowsiness
Amitriptyline	Amitril, Elavil, Endep	Tricyclic antidepressant	25–100 mg orally daily	Anticholinergic effects, drowsiness
Buspirone	BuSpar	Arylpiperazine	5 mg orally every 8 hours	Drowsiness, nausea

studies have been conducted. However, the vestibular disorder and the anxiety symptoms should be treated simultaneously. The vestibular disorder should be treated in the same manner as a nonspecific vestibulopathy independent of the presence of anxiety (see Case 17). The treatment of anxiety includes pharmacotherapy and behavioral therapy. Pharmacotherapy could include antianxiety agents (Table Case 5–1). Note that benzodiazepines act as both a vestibular suppressant and an anxiolytic and thus are an excellent first choice of treatment for such patients.

Question 7: Should this patient be referred to a psychiatrist for further evaluation?

Answer 7: Controlled studies are necessary to evaluate the role of psychiatric treatment for patients with both a balance disorder and a psychiatric disorder. However, psychiatric referral is definetely warranted for patients who are suffering from a clinically significant anxiety disorder, such as patients with frequent panic attacks and patients suffering from panic disorder with agoraphobia.

This patient was treated with a combination of vestibular rehabilitation therapy and clonazepam 0.25 mg by mouth, twice daily. Psychiatric consultation was deferred.

Question 8: Should this patient be referred for a course of vestibular rehabilitation therapy?

Answer 8: Vestibular rehabilitation therapy is a recognized treatment for patients with vestibular disorders (see Chapter 6). Also, a recent study has suggested that vestibular rehabilitation therapy may benefit patients with dizziness and anxiety.[14]

SUMMARY

A 43-year-old woman presented with a history consistent with both a vestibular system abnormality and an anxiety disorder. Physical examination and laboratory testing further suggested the absence of significant neurologic disease but did suggest a vestibular imbalance. The patient was treated with low-dose benzodiazepines and vestibular rehabilitation therapy.

TEACHING POINTS

1. **Anxiety often accompanies dizziness.** The cause-and-effect relationship between anxiety and dizziness is uncertain but may be related to a somatopsychic, psychosomatic, or common neurologic mechanism.
2. **Space and motion discomfort, that is, symptoms elicited by situations characterized by inadequate or confusing visual or kinesthetic information necessary for normal spatial orientation, is often seen in patients who are both anxious and dizzy.**
3. **The term *psychogenic dizziness* should be avoided in favor of the term *psychiatric dizziness*.** *Psychiatric dizziness* should be used to describe patients in whom dizziness occurs exclusively in combination with other symptoms as part of a recognized psychiatric symptom cluster. For example, dizziness that occurs as a component of the symptom cluster of panic attacks should be called psychiatric. The *term psychiatric dizziness* should not be used to describe patients who have anxiety as a component of a balance disorder.
4. **Hyperventilation is commonly used to determine whether dizziness is psychogenic.** The test is nonspecific, and the results should be interpreted with great caution.

REFERENCES

1. Jacob RG, Woody SR, Clark DB, Lilienfeld SO, Hirsch BE, Kucera GD, Furman JM, Durrant JD: Discomfort with space and motion: A possible marker of vestibular dysfunction assessed by the Situational Characteristics Questionnaire. J Psychopathol Behav Assessment 15:299–324, 1993.
2. Jacob RG, Furman JM, Balaban CD: Psychiatric aspects of vestibular disorders. In: Baloh RW, Halmagyi M (eds). Disorders of the Vestibular System. New York: Oxford University Press, 1996, pp 509–528.
3. Furman JF, Jacob RG: Psychiatric dizziness. Neurology 48(5):1161–1166, 1997.
4. Moore BE, Atkinson M: Psychogenic vertigo. Arch Otolaryngol 67:347–353, 1958.
5. Furman JF, Jacob RG: A clinical taxonomy of dizinesss and anxiety in the otoneurological setting. J Anxiety Disorders 15:9–26, 2001.
6. Drachman DA, Hart CW: An approach to the dizzy patient. Neurology 22:323–334, 1972.
7. Nedzelski JM, Barber HO, McIlmoyl L: Diagnoses in a dizziness unit. J Otolaryngol 15(2):101–104, 1986.
8. Herr RD, Zun L, Matthews JJ: A directed approach to the dizzy patient. Ann Emerg Med 18(6):664/101–672/109, 1989.
9. Minor LB, Haslwanter T, Straumann D, Zee DS: Hyperventilation-induced nystagmus in patients with vestibular schwannoma. Neurology 53(9):2158–2168, 1999.
10. Balaban CD, Jacob RG: Background and history of the interface between anxiety and vertigo. J Anxiety Disorders 15:27–51, 2001.

11. Collins WE: Arousal and vestibular habituation. In: Kornhuber HH (ed). Vestibular System Part 2: Psychophysics, Applied Aspects and General Interpretations. Berlin: Springer-Verlag, 1974, pp 361–368.
12. Theunissen EJM, Huygen PLM, Folgering HTH: Vestibular hyperreactivity and hyperventilation. Clin Otolaryngol 11:161–169, 1986.
13. Monday LA, Tetrault L: Hyperventilation and vertigo. Laryngoscope 109:1003–1010, 1980.
14. Jacob RG, Whitney SL, Detweiler-Shostak G, Furman JM: Vestibular rehabilitation for patients with agoraphobia and vestibular dysfunction: A pilot study. J Anxiety Disorders 115:131–146, 2001.

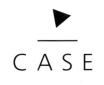
Emergency Room Management of the Dizzy Patient—Acute Cerebellar Infarction

HISTORY

A 60-year-old man presented to an emergency room with a history of several hours of vertigo. The patient related that while watching a sporting event on television he had an acute onset of vertigo, nausea, and, shortly thereafter, vomiting. The patient was unable to walk without assistance at home and was brought to the emergency department by ambulance. His vertigo had remained constant. He also complained of a mild headache. The patient had not suffered from previous episodes of vertigo. He also denied having any recent viral infections. His past medical history was significant for hypertension, which was well controlled with a beta-blocker.

Question 1: Based upon the patient's history, what are the diagnostic considerations?

Answer 1: The patient's history is consistent with an acute vestibular syndrome such as that seen with vestibular neuritis (see Cases 1, 3). However, other causes of an attack of prolonged spontaneous vertigo must also be considered, including labyrinthine ischemia, cerebellar infarction or hemorrhage, brainstem infarction or hemorrhage, multiple sclerosis, and bacterial otomastoiditis.[1] Of these, vestibular neuritis is the most common cause of an acute attack of prolonged spontaneous vertigo. However, the patient's mild headache and past medical history of hypertension increase the likelihood of central nervous system ischemia.

PHYSICAL EXAMINATION

General medical examination was normal except that the patient's blood pressure was elevated to 130/100. Neurologic examination revealed a normal mental status and normal pupillary responses with full extraocular movements. A left-beating horizontal-torsional nystagmus was noted in the primary position with fixation. The intensity of nystagmus increased with leftward gaze and decreased with rightward gaze. The remainder of the cranial nerve examination was normal including facial sensation and movement, palatal sensation and movement, and tongue movement. Motor examination revealed normal strength in all extremities. There was no pronator drift. Deep tendon reflexes were normal. Babinski's sign was absent bilaterally. Coordination testing revealed subtle difficulty with finger-to-nose testing on the right. Sensation testing was normal to all modalities. The patient was unable to walk without assistance. Romberg's test was positive; the patient fell toward the left. Otologic examination was normal. Neurotologic examination revealed an increase in the patient's left-beating nystagmus with loss of visual fixation. The head thrust testing was equivocal because of the presence of spontaneous nystagmus.

Question 2: Based upon the additional information from the physical examination, what is the most likely diagnosis?

Answer 2: The patient has an abnormal physical examination that is consistent with an acute vestibular syndrome. The patient has a vestibular nystagmus, as evidenced by the character of the nystagmus. It was horizontal-torsional, continued in the same direction with changes in gaze, and increased with loss of visual fixation. This finding strongly supports an acute loss of vestibular function on the right, and the most common cause is vestibular neuritis.

Question 3: Can an acute central nervous system abnormality present with nystagmus that appears like an acute peripheral vestibular loss?

Answer 3: Yes. Acute central vestibular disorders such as brainstem or cerebellar infarction or hemorrhage typically cause gaze-evoked nystagmus, that is, nystagmus that changes direction with a change in gaze direction. However, patients with cerebellar stroke may demonstrate nystagmus that is present in only one direction of gaze, thus appearing to have nystagmus due to an acute peripheral vestibular loss.[2]

Although a peripheral etiology seems likely in this patient, the patient's inability to walk, subtle difficulty with coordination, and falling on Romberg's test to the left rather than to the right should increase the suspicion of an acute central nervous system abnormality. Infarction or hemorrhage in the posterior fossa must seriously be considered.

Question 4: Should brain imaging be performed urgently?

Answer 4: Yes, brain imaging should be performed urgently when symptoms and signs are present that are not fully typical of acute peripheral vertigo or if the patient has known risk factors for stroke.

LABORATORY TESTING

An MRI scan of the brain revealed an infarction involving the right cerebellar hemisphere (Fig. Case 6–1).

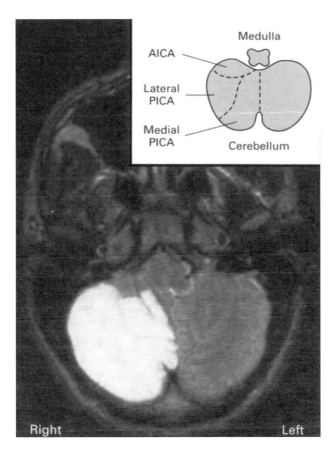

Figure Case 6–1 MRI scan of a right inferior cerebellar infarction. The inset illustrates the vascular supply to the inferior cerebellum, which is perfused by the medial and lateral branches of the posterior inferior cerebellar artery (PICA) and the anterior inferior cerebellar artery (AICA). (*Source*: With permission from Hotson JR, Baloh RW: Acute vestibular syndrome. N Engl J Med 339:680–685, 1998.[2])

DIAGNOSIS/DIFFERENTIAL DIAGNOSIS

The patient was given a diagnosis of acute cerebellar infarction.

TREATMENT

The patient received an urgent neurosurgical evaluation.

FOLLOW-UP

Following a 1-week hospitalization, the patient entered a rehabilitation center and gradually regained the ability to ambulate without assistance, although he used a cane.

Question 5: What are the common diagnoses of patients evaluated in the emergency room for dizziness?

Answer 5: A study by Alvord and Herr[3] reviewed the eventual diagnosis of 93 consecutive patients presenting to an emergency room with a primary complaint of dizziness. The distribution of diagnoses is given in Table Case 6–1. Most patients presenting to an emergency room with dizziness suffer from peripheral

Table Case 6–1 Specific Diagnoses of Patients with Dizziness in an Emergency Room

Classification	Diagnosis	n
Central	Cerebellar infarct	2
	Alcohol or drug toxicity	2
	Brain tumor	1
	Central nervous system concussion	1
	Hepatic encephalitis	1
	Hypertension	1
	Hyponatremia	1
	Multiple sclerosis	1
	Pseudotumor	1
	Total	11
Peripheral	Acute labyrinthitis	18
	Peripheral vestibular disorder	17
	Benign positional vertigo	7
	Meniere's disease	4
	Labyrinthine concussion	4
	Cervical disorder	2
	Serous otitis media	1
	Total	53
Other	Hyperventilation	3
	Psychogenesis	2
	Malingering	1
	Fumes intoxication	1
	Cystitis	1
	Migraine	1
	Total	9
Unknown	Total	20

Source: With permission from Alvord LSS, Herr RD: ENG in the emergency room: Subtest results in acutely dizzy patients. J Am Acad Audiol 5:384–389, 1994.[3]

vestibular abnormalities, but a significant number of patients present with central nervous system causes.

Question 6: What types of nonvestibular dizziness must be considered when evaluating a patient in the emergency room?

Answer 6: Table Case 6–2 provides a detailed list of the differential diagnoses for patients with nonvestibular vertigo who might be seen in an emergency room.[4]

SUMMARY

A 60-year-old man presented to an emergency room with a history of several hours of vertigo. Symptoms had begun abruptly and were associated with mild headache. The past medical history was significant for hypertension. Physical examination revealed a normal mental status, a left-beating vestibular nystagmus, a subtle difficulty with finger-to-nose testing on the right, and an inability to walk without assistance. An MRI scan of the brain revealed a cerebellar infarction. The

Table Case 6.2 Differential Diagnosis for Nonvestibular Vertigo

1. Cardiac
   a. Acute myocardial infarction
   b. Cardiac arrhythmia
   c. Cardiomyopathy
   d. Congestive heart failure
   e. Valvular heart disease
   f. Carotid sinus syndrome
2. Pulmonary/Respiratory
   a. Hypoxia
   b. Asthma
   c. COPD
   d. CHF
3. Metabolic/Endocrine
   a. Diabetes mellitus (hyper- or
      hypoglycemia)
   b. Thyroid disease (hyper- or
      hypothyroidism)
   c. Parathyroid disease (hyper- or
      hypoparathyroidism)
   d. Adrenal disease (Cushing's or
      Addison's disease)
   e. Electrolyte abnormalities
   f. Volume depletion
   g. Azotemia/uremia
	4. Gastrointestinal
	   a. Nausea and vomiting
	   b. Diarrhea
	   c. GI bleed
	5. Vascular
	   a. Coarctation of aorta
	   b. Thoracic dissection
	   c. Subclavian steal syndrome
	   d. Superior vena cava syndrome
	   e. Carotid artery stenosis
	6. Orthostatic Hypotension
	   a. Medications
	   b. Prolonged bed rest
	   c. Volume depletion
	   d. Anemia
	   e. Neurogenic disorders (autonomic
	      neuropathy)
	7. Psychogenic
	   a. Anxiety
	   b. Depression

Source: With permission from Walker JS, Barnes SB: Dizziness. Emerg Med Clin North Am 16(4):845–875, 1998.[4]

patient received an urgent neurosurgical evaluation. He gradually regained the ability to ambulate without assistance, although he used a cane.

TEACHING POINTS

1. **A diagnosis of posterior fossa infarction or hemorrhage should be considered for patients who present to an emergency room with acute onset of vertigo.**
2. **Signs of a central nervous system cause of acute vertigo may be subtle and include an inability to ambulate without assistance.**
3. **Brain imaging should be performed urgently when signs and symptoms are present that are not fully typical of acute peripheral vertigo or if the patient has known risk factors for stroke.**
4. **Nonvestibular dizziness must be considered when evaluating a patient in the emergency room.**

REFERENCES

1. Baloh RW: Dizziness: Neurological emergencies. Neurol Clin North Am 16(2):305–321, 1998.
2. Hotson JR, Baloh RW: Acute vestibular syndrome. N Engl J Med 339:680–685, 1998.
3. Alvord LSS, Herr RD: ENG in the emergency room: Subtest results in acutely dizzy patients. J Am Acad Audiol 5:384–389, 1994.
4. Walker JS, Barnes SB: Dizziness. Emerg Med Clin North Am 16(4):845–875, 1998.

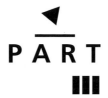

PART

III

Common Disease Case Studies

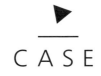

CASE

7

Benign Paroxysmal Positional Vertigo—Medical Management

HISTORY

A 45-year-old man complained of positional vertigo that had begun 6 weeks before evaluation. Symptoms occurred when he rolled over in bed to the right and when he reached above his head. There were no other neurologic or otologic symptoms. His past history was significant for a 1-day episode of severe vertigo, nausea, and vomiting that had occurred 2 months before evaluation. The family history was noncontributory. An emergency room physician at that time diagnosed labyrinthitis and prescribed promethazine, which the patient was still taking on an irregular basis. The patient had several days of nausea and severe imbalance following this acute episode; during this time, he was unable to work in his usual occupation as an attorney. Since returning to work, the patient reported a sense of mild disequilibrium and unsteadiness during quick head movements. These symptoms were gradually improving, and he was almost entirely asymptomatic at rest but still reported positional vertigo.

Question 1: Based on the patient's history, what is the most likely diagnosis?

Answer 1: This patient's history is consistent with an episode of vestibular neuritis (see Cases 1 and 3) 2 months before evaluation. He seems to have largely recovered from the vestibular neuritis but has persistent symptoms related to positional vertigo that probably are a result of benign paroxysmal positional vertigo.

105

PHYSICAL EXAMINATION

General, neurologic, and otologic examinations were normal except for impaired tandem gait. Neurotologic examination revealed no nystagmus while seated using infrared goggles, an inability to stand on a compliant foam pad with the eyes closed, and 90 degree rotation to the right on a stepping test. Dix-Hallpike maneuvers using infrared glasses were positive with the right ear down. The nystagmus was upbeating (toward the forehead) and torsional, with the upper poles of the eyes beating toward the dependent (right) ear. The nystagmus began several seconds after positioning and was accompanied by a strong sense of vertigo and nausea. It lasted for about 15 seconds, after which time the vertigo also stopped.

Question 2: How does the additional information provided by the physical examination influence this patient's diagnosis?

Answer 2: This patient manifests the characteristic symptoms and signs of benign paroxysmal positional nystagmus and vertigo, including the typical nystagmus evoked by Dix-Hallpike maneuvers. Also, the patient's abnormal neurotologic examination suggests a lingering vestibular imbalance, probably the result of the vestibular neuritis suffered 2 months earlier.

LABORATORY TESTING

Videonystagmography: Ocular motor function was normal. There was no static positional nystagmus. Dix-Hallpike maneuvers in the laboratory documented a predominantly upbeating nystagmus with the right ear down. (Note that two-dimensional videonystagmography, the technique that is currently available clinically, does not measure torsional eye movements.) Caloric irrigations revealed a significant (40%) right reduced vestibular response.

Rotational testing revealed a mild left directional preponderance.

Posturography indicated excessive sway on conditions 5 and 6, that is, a vestibular pattern.

Question 3: What is the significance of the vestibular laboratory abnormalities?

Answer 3: Taken together, these findings suggest that the patient is suffering from a partial right-sided peripheral vestibular loss, benign paroxysmal positional vertigo affecting the right ear, and ongoing vestibulo-ocular and vestibulospinal asymmetry.

The right reduced caloric response suggests that the presumed vestibular neuritis, which the patient suffered 2 months earlier, damaged afferent fibers or the sensory epithelia of the right horizontal semicircular canal. The patient's directional preponderance on rotational testing suggests an ongoing VOR asymmetry, that is, incomplete compensation for a peripheral vestibular deficit. This incomplete recovery may be based on fluctuating peripheral vestibular function on the right, chronic use of vestibular suppressants (see Case 17), or some other cause that is not obvious. The vestibular pattern on platform posturography suggests an ongoing vestibulospinal abnormality, which represents further evidence of incomplete central nervous system compensation. The nystagmus elicited during Dix-Hallpike maneuvers confirms the diagnosis of benign paroxysmal positional vertigo.

DIAGNOSIS/DIFFERENTIAL DIAGNOSIS

Question 4: Are there any conditions other than benign positional nystagmus and vertigo that should be considered?

Answer 4: Unquestionably, this patient's most likely diagnoses are resolving vestibular neuritis and benign paroxysmal positional vertigo. Other entities that can present with an acute vestibular syndrome followed by benign paroxysmal positional vertigo are labyrinthine concussion (see Cases 11 and 23) and labyrinthine infarction (see Case 30). Rarely, posterior fossa lesions can present with the typical signs and symptoms of benign paroxysmal positional vertigo,[1,2] although one or more features of the clinical presentation are often atypical, such as the direction of the nystagmus, and suggest a central nervous system abnormality.

Question 5: What features in the clinical presentation of a patient with acute vertigo followed by positional vertigo would lead to a suspicion of a posterior fossa lesion?

Answer 5: Neurologic symptoms such as numbness or weakness of the face or extremities, or visual loss associated with the onset of vertigo, should lead to the suspicion of a posterior fossa lesion. Additionally, if the neurologic examination disclosed any central nervous system signs or if the patient's Dix-Hallpike maneuvers were associated with a response atypical of benign positional nystagmus and vertigo, further evaluation, such as MRI scanning of the posterior fossa, would be warranted. Responses during the Dix-Hallpike maneuver that are atypical of benign paroxysmal positional vertigo include nystagmus that (1) is downbeating rather than upbeating in the head-hanging position, (2) occurs immediately upon positioning, (3) is not associated with vertigo, or (4) does not fatigue if the patient is repeatedly positioned.

This patient was given a diagnosis of benign paroxysmal positional vertigo.

Question 6: What is the pathophysiology of benign paroxysmal positional vertigo?

Answer 6: Benign paroxysmal positional vertigo is thought to result from malfunction of the posterior semicircular canal such that the canal becomes abnormally sensitive to gravity or linear acceleration. Malfunction of the posterior semicircular canal in benign paroxysmal positional vertigo is supported by two observations:

1. The direction of provoked nystagmus is consistent with the ocular motor connections of the dependent posterior semicircular canal. That is, excitation of the posterior semicircular canal leads to excitation of the superior oblique and contralateral inferior rectus muscles. Thus, in benign paroxysmal positional vertigo, the patient manifests a predominantly upbeating-torsional nystagmus that becomes more upbeating when gazing away from the down ear and more torsional when gazing toward the down ear.
2. Surgical sectioning of the afferent nerve to the posterior semicircular canal abolishes benign paroxysmal positional vertigo.

There are two current theories to explain why the posterior semicircular canal becomes sensitive to gravity: cupulolithiasis and canalithiasis.

Cupulolithiasis refers to the idea that detached otoconia from the utricle descend to the most inferior portion (when upright) of the labyrinth and become adherent to the cupula of the posterior semicircular canal.[3,4] These adherent particles change the specific gravity of the cupula so that it no longer is isodense with the surrounding endolymph. As a result, the posterior semicircular canal cupula becomes a gravity-sensitive organ in certain positions. Consequently, the posterior semicircular canal falsely signals continuous rotation for particular head positions, for example, tipping the head backward.

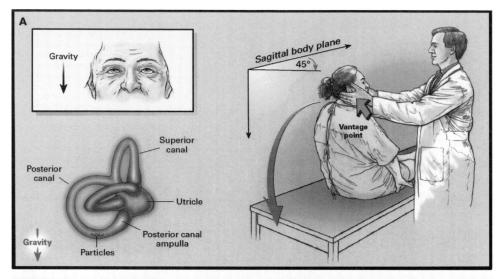

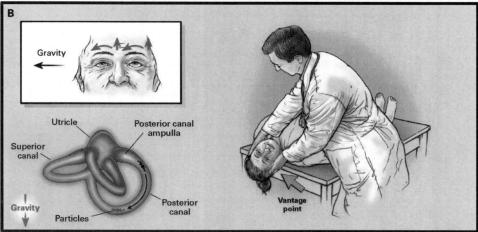

Figure Case 7–1 The Dix-Hallpike test of a patient with benign paroxysmal positional vertigo affecting the right ear. In Panel A, the examiner stands at the patient's right side and rotates the patient's head 45 degrees to the right to align the right posterior semicircular canal with the sagittal plane of the body. In Panel B, the examiner moves the patient, whose eyes are open, from the seated to the supine right-ear-down position and then extends the patient's neck slightly so that the chin is pointed slightly upward. The latency, duration, and direction of nystagmus, if present, and the latency and duration of vertigo, if present, should be noted. The arrows in the inset indicate the direction of nystagmus in patients with typical benign paroxysmal positional vertigo. The presumed location in the labyrinth of the free-floating debris thought to cause the disorder is also shown. (*Source*: With permission from Furman JM, Cass SP: Benign paroxysmal positional vertigo. N Engl J Med 341:1590–1596, 1999.[8])

Canalithiasis refers to the idea that debris, possibly degenerating otoconia or other cellular debris, becomes free-floating in the endolymph of the posterior semicircular canal (Fig. Case 7–1).[5–8] Any head movement that changes the orientation of the posterior semicircular canal with respect to gravity may cause the particles in the endolymph to move within the posterior semicircular canal. Presumably, as the particles move, the endolymph is disturbed in a manner that stimulates the posterior semicircular canal ampulla. Once the particles settle into a dependent position and stop moving, which presumably takes about 10 or 20 seconds, the abnormal stimulation ceases. When the patient returns to the upright position, the particles may again move and again cause an erroneous sensation of motion.

Both the cupulothiasis and canalithiasis theories have merit, and it is possible that both exist as pathologic conditions. However, the concept of cupulolithiasis cannot explain why the nystagmus provoked by head positioning stops after 15 to 30 seconds. If debris remained attached to the cupula, one would expect nystagmus to continue unabated for a long period of time. It is necessary to hypothesize that another mechanism, for example, central adaptation, is involved in stopping the nystagmus or that the debris is released from the cupula, in which case the debris become free-floating, as hypothesized in the concept of canalithiasis. Strong support for the canalithiasis theory includes the recent surgical observations of free-floating particles within the posterior semicircular canals of patients with benign paroxysmal positional vertigo (Fig. Case 7–2).[5] Moreover, the

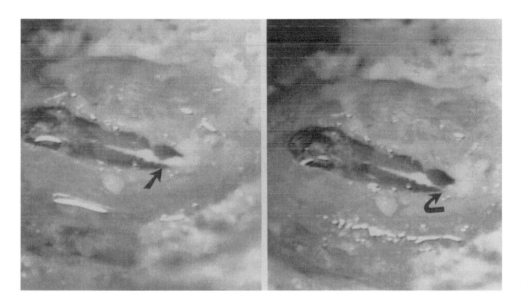

Figure Case 7–2 Free-floating endolymph particles within the posterior semicircular canal observed during surgery. The posterior semicircular canal had been opened in preparation for a canal-plugging procedure. White debris was observed within the endolymph compartment of the posterior semicircular canal. These two photographs are sequential in time and show that the particles shifted during movement of the patient's head; compare the shape and position of particles at the straight arrow with those at the curved arrow. (*Source*: With permission from Parnes LS, McClure JA: Free-floating endolymph particles: A new operative finding during posterior semicircular canal occlusion. Laryngoscope 102:988–992, 1992.[9])

latency, duration, and fatigability of the nystagmus that characterize benign paroxysmal positional vertigo can all be explained by the theory of canalithiasis without invoking other central mechanisms.

TREATMENT/MANAGEMENT

Question 7: What are the treatment options for benign positional nystagmus and vertigo? What is the role of medications such as vestibular suppressants? Should this patient continue using promethazine?

Answer 7: Benign positional nystagmus and vertigo is best treated using the particle repositioning maneuver (Fig. Case 7–3).[7,10] Previously, habituating exercises, such as those described by Brandt and Daroff[11] (Figure Case 7–4), and other physical maneuvers, such as the *liberatory* maneuver,[12] were most popular. All of these treatments are designed to relocate endolymphatic debris, which is presumed to be near or adherent to the posterior semicircular canal cupula, to the labyrinthine vestibule, where the debris no longer affects the semicircular canals and can be naturally reabsorbed. The particle-repositioning maneuver is a one-time therapy, whereas the Brandt-Daroff exercises generally require 1 to 2 weeks of twice-daily performance. During particle repositioning, mastoid vibration can be used but is probably unnecessary.[13] Posttreatment restrictions, such as staying upright for 1 to 2 days, also may not be necessary.[14,15] In the unusual patient who cannot be cured of benign paroxysmal positional vertigo with a physical maneuver or with exercises, surgical treatment is usually successful[16,17] (see Case 31).

Vestibular-suppressant medication is often helpful at the onset of benign paroxysmal positional nystagmus and vertigo, especially if it follows an acute vestibular loss, as in this patient, or if a patient is so apprehensive that he or she refuses to perform the habituating exercises if needed. However, once the acute episode of vestibular imbalance, if present, is over, vestibular-suppressant medication should be avoided, since central vestibular compensation for the peripheral vestibular loss can be delayed. If the patient expects to be exposed to excessive motion, such as prolonged car or air travel, or becomes particularly symptomatic for a brief time, meclizine, clonazepam, diazepam, or promethazine prescribed on an as-needed basis (see Case 17) may be beneficial.

A course of vestibular rehabilitation may be useful, even if the positional vertigo is cured by a repositioning maneuver, especially for a patient with evidence on physical examination or laboratory testing of an ongoing vestibular system imbalance such as a directional preponderance or abnormal posturography.

Treatment consisted of a particle-repositioning maneuver, gradual discontinuation of the patient's vestibular-suppressant medication, and a course of vestibular rehabilitation. The patient had complete relief from his positional symptoms and gradually recovered nearly normal balance. His limitations were noticed only during taxing balance tasks such as water-skiing.

Question 8: What is the natural history of benign paroxysmal positional nystagmus and vertigo? Is this patient likely to recover from this condition?

Answer 8: Benign paroxysmal positional vertigo is usually a self-limited condition. That is, without treatment, most patients recover spontaneously over several weeks or months. The typical patient with benign paroxysmal positional ver-

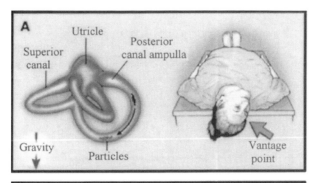

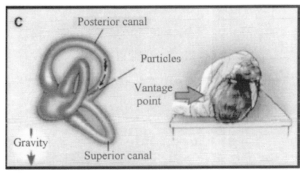

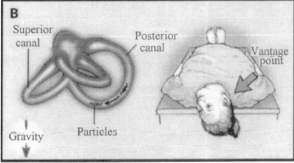

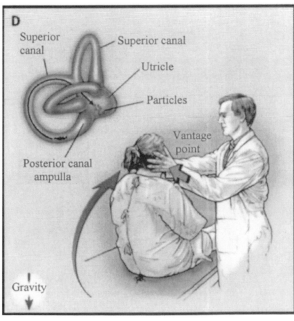

Figure Case 7–3 Bedside maneuver for the treatment of a patient with benign paroxysmal positional vertigo affecting the right ear. The presumed position of the debris within the labyrinth during the maneuver is shown in each panel. The maneuver is a three-step procedure. First, a Dix-Hallpike test is performed with the patient's head rotated 45 degrees toward the right ear and the neck slightly extended, with the chin pointed slightly upward. This position results in the patient's head hanging to the right (Panel A). Once the vertigo and nystagmus provoked by the Dix-Hallpike test cease, the patient's head is rotated about the rostral-caudal body axis until the left ear is down (Panel B). Then the head and body are further rotated until the head is face down (Panel C). The vertex of the head is kept tilted down throughout the rotation. The maneuver usually provokes brief vertigo. The patient should be kept in the final face-down position for about 10 to 15 seconds. With the head kept turned toward the left shoulder, the patient is brought into the seated position (Panel D). Once the patient is upright, the head is tilted so that the chin is pointed slightly downward. (*Source*: With permission from Furman JM, Cass SP: Benign paroxysmal positional vertigo. N Engl J Med 341:1590–1596, 1999.[8])

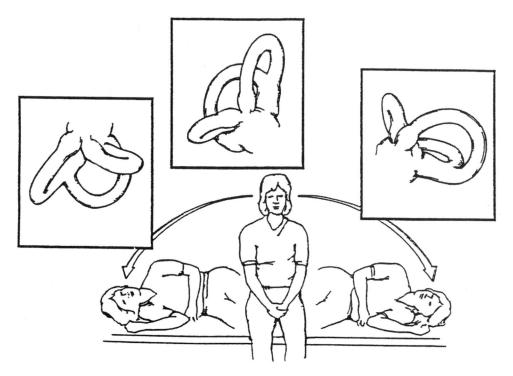

Figure Case 7–4 Brandt-Daroff exercises for benign paroxysmal positional vertigo. (*Source*: With permission from Herdman SJ: Assessment and management of benign paroxysmal positional vertigo. In: Herdman, SJ. Vestibular Rehabilitation. Philadelphia: FA Davis, 1999, p. 464.[20])

tigo seeks specialty treatment about 6 weeks after the onset of the vertigo (mean, 16 months; range, 5 days to many years).[18] It has been shown that without specific intervention, 75% of patients have spontaneous resolution of symptoms, with a mean duration of about 1 month (range, 5 to 42 days) of further symptoms.[18] Thus, for most patients, the duration of benign paroxysmal positional vertigo is about 10 weeks. However, in 25% of patients, symptoms can continue for years. The natural history of benign paroxysmal positional vertigo speaks to the value of actively treating such patients, especially since the condition can continue for years in a significant minority. Benign paroxysmal positional vertigo also may recur, often 6 months to 6 years following the initial presentation. The cumulative recurrence rate following particle repositioning is about 1% per month.[19] The patient should be advised of this possibility. Repositioning maneuvers are equally effective in treating recurrences.

SUMMARY

A 45-year-old man presented with positional vertigo following acute vestibular neuritis that had occurred 2 months before evaluation. The physical examination was consistent with benign paroxysmal positional vertigo. An ongoing vestibulo-ocular and vestibulospinal asymmetry was suggested by both the physical examination and laboratory test results. Treatment consisted of a particle-repositioning maneuver, gradual discontinuation of the patient's vestibular-suppressant medication, and a course of vestibular rehabilitation therapy. The patient had complete relief of his positional symptoms and gradually recovered nearly normal balance.

TEACHING POINTS

1. **The characteristic symptoms and signs of benign paroxysmal positional nystagmus and vertigo include a history of positionally induce vertigo and a nystagmus evoked by the Dix-Hallpike maneuver that is upbeating (fast component toward the forehead) and torsional with the upper poles of the eyes beating toward the dependent (right) ear.** The nystagmus begins several seconds after positioning and is accompanied by definite vertigo. The nystagmus lasts for about 15 seconds, after which time the vertigo also stops.

2. **Benign paroxysmal positional vertigo is thought to result from malfunction of the posterior semicircular canal such that the canal becomes abnormally sensitive to gravity or linear acceleration.** The most likely explanation for this malfunction is that debris, possibly degenerating otoconia or other cellular debris, becomes free-floating in the endolymph of the posterior semicircular canal. Any head movement that changes the orientation of the posterior semicircular canal with respect to gravity may cause these particles in the endolymph to move within the posterior semicircular canal.

3. **Benign paroxysmal positional vertigo can be seen as a sequela of other disorders, such as vestibular neuritis and labyrinthine concussion.** Benign paroxysmal positional vertigo may be only one of several manifestations of an ongoing vestibular abnormality. Patients presenting with positional vertigo should be thoroughly evaluated for other evidence of otologic disease. Patients presenting with disequilibrium for any reason should be evaluated for benign paroxysmal positional vertigo with appropriate questioning and physical examination, even if they do not present with a chief complaint of positional vertigo.

4. **Atypical positional vertigo should suggest a posterior fossa lesion.** Atypical features include any neurologic symptoms or signs that cannot be ascribed to a peripheral vestibular localization, any atypical features on the response to Dix-Hallpike maneuvers, and failure to respond to particle-repositioning maneuvers.

5. **The preferred treatment for benign paroxysmal positional vertigo is the particle-repositioning maneuver.** This is highly successful and provides complete relief in nearly all patients. Vestibular-suppressant medications can be used early in the disorder, but after several days it should be used sparingly, if at all.

6. **Benign paroxysmal positional vertigo is usually a self-limited condition.** Without specific intervention, 75% of patients have spontaneous resolution of symptoms, with a mean duration of about 1 month (range, 5 to 42 days) of further symptoms. Benign paroxysmal posi-

tional vertigo also may recur, often 6 months to 6 years following the initial presentation. The cumulative recurrence rate following particle repositioning is 1% per month.

REFERENCES

1. Watson P, Barber HO, Deck J, Terbrugge K: Positional vertigo and nystagmus of central origin. Can J Neurol Sci 8:133–137, 1981.
2. Dunniway HM, Welling DB: Intracranial tumors mimicking benign paroxysmal positional vertigo. Otolaryngol Head Neck Surg 118:429–436, 1998.
3. Schuknecht HF: Positional vertigo: Clinical and experimental observations. Trans Am Acad Ophthalmol Otolaryngol 166:319–332, 1962.
4. Schuknecht HF: Cupulolithiasis. Arch Otolaryngol 90:113–126, 1969.
5. Harbert F: Benign paroxysmal positional nystagmus. Arch Ophthalmol 84:298–302, 1970.
6. Hall SF, Ruby RRF, McClure JA: The mechanics of benign paroxysmal vertigo. J Otolaryngol 8:151–158, 1979.
7. Epley JM: The canalith repositioning procedure: For treatment of benign paroxysmal positional vertigo. Otolaryngol Head Neck Surg 107:399–404, 1992.
8. Furman JM, Cass SP: Benign paroxysmal positional vertigo. N Engl J Med 341:1590–1596, 1999.
9. Parnes LS, McClure JA: Free-floating endolymph particles: A new operative finding during posterior semicircular canal occlusion. Laryngoscope 102:988–992, 1992.
10. Parnes LS, Price-Jones R: Particle repositioning maneuver for benign paroxysmal positional vertigo. Ann Otol Rhinol Laryngol 102:325–331, 1993.
11. Brandt T, Daroff RB: Physical therapy for benign paroxysmal positional vertigo. Arch Otolaryngol 106:484–485, 1980.
12. Semont A, Greyss G, Vitte E: Curing the BPPV with a liberatory maneuver. Adv Otorhinolaryngol 42:290–293, 1988.
13. Hain TC, Helminski JO, Reis IL, Uddin MK: Vibration does not improve results of the canalith repositioning procedure. Arch Otolaryngol Head Neck Surg 126:617–622, 2000.
14. Massoud EAS, Ireland DJ: Post-treatment instructions in the nonsurgical management of benign paroxysmal positional vertigo. J Otolaryngol 25:121–125, 1996.
15. Nutti D, Nati C, Passali D: Treatment of benign paroxysmal positional vertigo: No need for post-maneuver restrictions. Otolaryngol Head Neck Surg 122:440–444, 2000.
16. Gacek RR: Transection of the posterior ampulary nerve for relief of benign paroxysmal positional vertigo. Ann Otol Rhinol Laryngol 83:596–605, 1974.
17. Parnes LS, McClure JA: Posterior semicircular canal occlusion in the normal hearing ear. Otolaryngol Head Neck Surg 104:52–57, 1991.
18. Baloh R, Honrubia V, Jacobson K: Benign positional vertigo: Clinical and oculographic features in 240 cases. Neurology 37:371–378, 1987.
19. Nunez RA, Cass SP, Furman JM: Short- and long-term outcomes of canalith repositioning for benign paroxysmal positional vertigo. Otolaryngol Head Neck Surg 122:647–652, 2000.
20. Herdman SJ: Assessment and management of benign paroxysmal positional vertigo. In: Herdman SJ: Vestibular Rehabilitation. Philadelphia: FA Davis, 1999, pp 451–475.

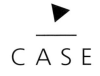

CASE
8

Migraine-Associated Dizziness

HISTORY

A 30-year-old man who worked as a bank teller presented with the chief complaint of dizziness for 6 weeks. The patient dated his symptoms to discontinuation of amitriptyline, which was being used for depression. He stated that he had discontinued it "to see if he could do without his antidepressant medication." The patient characterized his symptoms as a constant sense of lightheadedness and disequilibrium that was exacerbated by head movements and certain visual environments such as flickering lights and checkerboard patterns. He had no complaints of hearing loss, tinnitus, aural fullness, abnormal vision, weakness, loss of sensation, or incoordination. The patient stated that before he had started taking amitriptyline 2 years prior to evaluation, he had also suffered from similar dizziness complaints, although they were less severe. These previous symptoms included episodic exacerbations, occasionally associated with headache.

Question 1: What are the diagnostic considerations in this case, and what further history would be helpful?

Answer 1: This patient's dizziness and disequilibrium are nonspecific and not particularly suggestive of a peripheral vestibular disorder, given their character and time course. Many diagnostic considerations must be considered at this point in the evaluation. However, clues to the patient's diagnosis include the association with discontinuation of a tricyclic antidepressant, exacerbation by certain visual environments, and a previous history of headache. Further history should be obtained regarding precipitating factors and details of the past history of headaches and their association with dizziness. Also, any family history of a migrainous disorder would be helpful.

ADDITIONAL HISTORY

When asked about the association between his dizziness and headache, the patient said that during the previous 2 years he had suffered three or four episodes of severe unilateral throbbing headache associated with nausea, lightheadedness, and disequilibrium that were more severe than his symptoms now but similar in character. He noted that headaches were more frequent before his treatment with a tricyclic antidepressant and that most of his headaches were associated with dizziness and disequilibrium. The patient's family history was significant; his mother and his paternal aunt had suffered from migraine headaches.

Question 2: How does this additional history affect this patient's diagnosis?

Answer 2: The characteristics of the patient's headaches, coupled with the positive family history, make migraine-associated dizziness the most likely diagnosis.[1-3] A vestibulopathy unrelated to headaches is possible. Much less likely are vertebrobasilar insufficiency or a craniovertebral junction abnormality. A thorough examination and appropriate laboratory testing should be helpful in establishing a diagnosis.

Question 3: In what ways can migraine manifest itself as dizziness and disequilibrium?

Answer 3: Migraine-associated dizziness can present as a vertiginous aura preceding a migraine headache in much the same way as positive visual phenomena or auras such as scintillating scotomata and fortification spectra. Dizziness, disequilibrium, and vertigo can occur during a migraine headache or may persist following resolution of a headache.

Some patients with migraine-associated dizziness have migraine without headache, also known as *migraine equivalent*, or dizziness separate from or instead of headaches. Some patients, like this one, may experience disequilibrium between headaches, that is, more or less constantly.[4] This patient's symptoms are typical of migraine-associated dizziness, which often include dizziness and disequilibrium exacerbated by certain visual environments.

PHYSICAL EXAMINATION

The patient had normal general, neurologic, otologic, and neurotologic examinations.

Question 4: What laboratory testing, if any, would be helpful in establishing this patient's diagnosis?

Answer 4: There is no definitive laboratory test to diagnose migraine-associated dizziness, which is a diagnosis of exclusion. Nothing in the patient's history or the physical examination suggests a structural neurologic abnormality; thus, brain imaging is not indicated at this point in the evaluation. Vestibular laboratory testing might suggest an alternative diagnosis, as well as provide information regarding the status of the patient's balance system.

Audiometric testing should be performed to screen for asymmetric hearing loss that may indicate the presence of a cerebellopontine angle or brainstem neoplasm or hearing loss suggestive of endolymphatic hydrops.

Table Case 8–1 Most Common Patterns of Abnormalities on Vestibular Tests Including Electronystagmography, Rotational Testing, and Posturography in Migraine-Related Vestibulopathy (*N* = 100)

Pattern	Percent
Normal	27
Isolated directional preponderance on rotation	22
Directional preponderance on rotation + reduced vestibular response	12
Directional preponderance on rotation + abnormal posturography	9
Directional preponderance on rotation + reduced vestibular response + Abnormal posturography	6
Isolated reduced vestibular response	5
Isolated abnormal posturography	4

Source: With permission from Cass SP et al: Migraine-related vestibulopathy. Ann Otol Rhinol Laryngol 106:182–189, 1997.[8]

LABORATORY TESTING

Videonystagmography: Ocular motor, positional, and caloric tests were normal.
    Rotational testing revealed a right directional preponderance.
    Posturography was normal.
    The audiometric test was normal.

Question 5: What vestibular laboratory abnormalities have been described in patients with migraine, and how can they be explained pathophysiologically?

Answer 5: The vestibular abnormalities that have been described in patients with migraine include abnormalities on electronystagmography, rotational testing, and posturography.[5][8] Table Case 8–1 indicates the percentage of patients with migraine in our experience who have abnormal vestibular laboratory testing. By far the most common abnormality noted was a directional preponderance on rotational testing. The abnormalities in Table Case 8–1 suggest a peripheral vestibular component in some patients, such as those with a reduced vestibular response, and a central vestibular abnormality in others, such as those with a directional preponderance. A smaller but not insignificant number of patients with migraine-related dizziness show either a spontaneous or a positional nystagmus or both. Posturography abnormalities that can be ascribed to the vestibular system in patients with migraine or related dizziness are uncommon.

The pathophysiology of the vestibular abnormalities in migraine-related dizziness is uncertain. Cutrer and Baloh[1] have proposed an asymmetry in neuropeptide release at the efferent vestibular terminals. Whether such a phenomenon actually occurs is unknown. How such a mechanism accounts for vestibular abnormalities between episodes is also uncertain.

Cass et al.[8] have suggested that serotonin may play a role in the vestibular abnormalities seen with migraine, either through direct effects or through release of neuropeptides. Such activation of serotonergic or peptidergic pathways could be asymmetric, thereby producing asymmetric activation of central vestibular pathways. Alternatively, even symmetric activation of serotonergic or peptidergic pathways might produce vestibular imbalance by unmasking latent asymmetries that may be inherent in an individual's balance system.

DIAGNOSIS/DIFFERENTIAL DIAGNOSIS

This patient's diagnosis was migraine-associated dizziness. His condition was exacerbated by discontinuation of amitriptyline, which was apparently acting as an antimigrainous agent.

TREATMENT/MANAGEMENT

Question 6: What are the treatment options for a patient with migraine-associated dizziness and what factors should be considered?

Answer 6: The treatment options for patients with migraine-associated dizziness are outlined in Table Case 8–2. First, it is necessary to educate the patient regarding the association of dizziness with the underlying migrainous condition and the importance of avoiding of dietary triggers, such as tyramine-containing foods, alcohol, and caffeine, as well as avoiding stress and fatigue. Second, the underlying migrainous condition should be treated with prophylactic medications, even if headaches are not currently prominent. Our experience is that a third to half of patients respond favorably to each of the medications listed in Table Case 8–2. If the initial medication is unsuccessful, the other classes of agents should be tried in turn. Third, if the most prominent vestibular symptom is movement-associated disequilibrium, vestibular rehabilitation therapy is recommended. Fourth, if the patient reports severe space and motion discomfort (see Chapter 7), prescribe low-dose clonazepam. Finally, in patients with panic attacks or agoraphobia, we obtain a psychiatric consultation and rely on both behavioral therapy and specific medical therapy using tricyclic antidepressants or anxiolytic medications.

This patient was restarted on amitriptyline and advised regarding dietary restriction. His symptoms of dizziness resolved.

Table Case 8–2 Treatment Options for Migraine-Related Dizziness

1. Avoid dietary triggers
2. Treat underlying migraine phenomenon
   • Tricyclic antidepressants (e.g., amitriptyline 50–100 mg/day)
   • Beta blockers (e.g., propranolol 80–320 mg/day)
   • Calcium channel blockers (e.g., verapamil 80–120 mg/day)
   • Anticonvulsants (e.g., valproic acid 250–1000 mg/day)
3. Treat movement-associated disequilibrium
   • Vestibular rehabilitation therapy
4. Treat space and motion discomfort
   • Clonazepam (0.25–0.5 mg/day)
5. Treat associated anxiety or panic disorder
   • Behavioral therapy
   • Pharmacotherapy
   Tricyclic antidepressants
   Anxiolytics (e.g., benzodiazepines)

Source: Adapted with permission from Cass SP et al: Migraine-related vestibulopathy. Ann Otol Rhinol Laryngol 106:182–189, 1997.[8]

SUMMARY

A 30-year-old man presented with dizziness and disequilibrium after discontinuation of a tricyclic antidepressant. There was a past history of headache, and the patient's complaints were consistent with migraine-associated dizziness. This diagnosis was further supported by a positive family history of migraine. The patient was treated with reintroduction of amitriptyline 50 mg before sleep. This significantly reduced his daily symptoms, although he continued to have migraine headaches associated with dizziness approximately once every 6 months.

TEACHING POINTS

1. **Migraine-associated dizziness should be suspected in patients with nonspecific dizziness or vertigo associated with headache.** A past history of migraine headaches or a positive family history of migraine increases the likelihood of this disease. Patients with migraine-associated dizziness almost invariably report exacerbation of symptoms by viewing certain moving visual environments or significant motion sickness sensitivity.

2. **Migraine can manifest as dizziness and disequilibrium.** Migraine-associated dizziness can present as a vertiginous aura preceding a migraine headache in much the same way as positive visual phenomena or auras, such as scintillating scotomata and fortification spectra. Dizziness, disequilibrium, and vertigo can occur during a migraine headache. Some patients with migraine-associated dizziness have migraine without headache, also known as *migraine equivalent*, that is, dizziness separate from or instead of headaches. Some patients, like this one, may experience disequilibrium between episodes, that is, more or less constantly. This patient's symptoms are typical of migraine-associated dizziness, which often include dizziness and disequilibrium exacerbated by certain visual environments.

3. **Vestibular laboratory abnormalities may be found in migraine-associated dizziness.** A directional preponderance on rotational testing is the most common abnormality. Less often, a unilateral caloric weakness, positional nystagmus, or spontaneous nystagmus may occur.

4. **Treatment options for patients with migraine-associated dizziness are summarized in Table Case 8–2.** First, the patient should be informed about the association of dizziness with the underlying migrainous condition and the importance of avoiding dietary triggers such as tyramine-containing foods, alcohol, and caffeine. Second, the underlying migrainous condition should be treated with prophylactic antimigrainous medications even if headaches are not currently prominent. Third, if the most prominent vestibular symptom is movement-associated disequilibrium or unsteadiness, vestibular rehabilitation therapy is recommended. Fourth, if the patient reports severe space and motion discomfort, low-dose clonazepam should be prescribed. Finally, in patients with panic attacks or agoraphobia, a psychiatric

consultation should be obtained, and both behavioral therapy and specific medical therapy using tricyclic antidepressants or anxiolytic medications should be considered.

REFERENCES

1. Cutrer FW, Baloh RW: Migraine-associated dizziness. Headache 32:300–304, 1992.
2. Neuhauser H, Leopold M, von Brevern M, Arnold G, Lempert T: The interrelations of migraine, vertigo, and migrainous vertigo. Neurology 56:436–441, 2001.
3. Johnson G: Medical management of migraine-related dizziness and vertigo. Laryngoscope 108(1 pt 2):1–28, 1998.
4. Kayan A, Hood JD: Neuro-otological manifestations of migraine. Brain 107:1123–1142, 1984.
5. Toglia JU, Thomas D, Kuritzky A: Common migraine and vestibular function: Electronystagmographic study and pathogenesis. Ann Otol 90:267–271, 1981.
6. Eviatar L: Vestibular testing in basilar artery migraine. Ann Neurol 9:126–130, 1980.
7. Olsson J: Neurootologic findings in basilar migraine. Laryngoscope 101:1–41, 1991.
8. Cass SP, Ankerstjerne JDP, Yetiser S, Furman J, Balaban C, Aydogan B: Migraine-related vestibulopathy. Ann Otol Rhinol Laryngol 106:182–189, 1997.

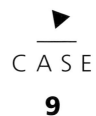

Endolymphatic Hydrops— Meniere's Disease

HISTORY

A 50-year-old female attorney was evaluated 1 week after the onset of acute vertigo. About 1 month before evaluation, the patient noticed a sense of pressure or fullness in her right ear similar to the feeling of water trapped in the ear after swimming. There was also a quiet ringing in her ear, but within a few days the fullness and ringing disappeared. A few weeks later these symptoms returned, and she also noticed difficulty hearing on the telephone with the right ear. She went to a neighborhood urgent care center, where a mild ear infection was diagnosed and treated with an oral antibiotic and a decongestant. A few days later, she woke up with an aching pressure-like pain in her ear associated with both increased ringing and decreased hearing in the ear. Suddenly, she had an episode of acute vertigo that she described as the environment whirling; it was associated with nausea and vomiting that lasted for 3 hours. She was taken to an emergency room and given an intramuscular injection of an antiemetic. The following day she felt nearly normal, with no vertigo. Her hearing loss, ringing, and fullness in the right ear had almost completely resolved. Some disequilibrium persisted. There was no significant past medical or family history.

Question 1: Based on the patient's history, what is the likely cause of these symptoms?

Answer 1: This patient's history suggests unilateral endolymphatic hydrops (see Cases 16, 21, and 25). The term *endolymphatic hydrops* is used to describe a particular pathologic condition of the inner ear characterized by swelling, or distention, of the endolymphatic compartment of the inner ear (Fig. Case 9–1). Clinically, endolymphatic hydrops is associated with recurrent vertigo and other aural

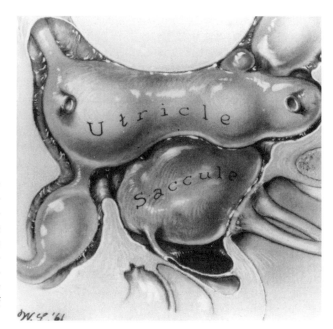

Figure Case 9–1 Dilated utricle and saccule in endolymphatic hydrops. (*Source*: Reprinted by permission of the publisher from Schuknecht HF: Pathology of the Ear. Cambridge, MA: Harvard University Press. Copyright 1974 by the President and Fellows of Harvard College.[1])

symptoms, such as tinnitus, hearing loss, and fullness or a pressure sensation in the ear. The triad of hearing loss, tinnitus, and vertigo are diagnostic of Meniere's disease.

Question 2: How does endolymphatic hydrops produce episodic symptoms of hearing loss, tinnitus, aural fullness, and vertigo?

Answer 2: The mechanism underlying episodic hearing loss and vertigo caused by endolymphatic hydrops is not entirely understood. Endolymphatic hydrops characteristically produces transient and fully reversible inner ear dysfunction early in the course of the disorder. Hearing loss, tinnitus, and aural fullness associated with endolymphatic hydrops typically lasts for hours to weeks, whereas the acute vertigo associated with endolymphatic hydrops typically lasts for at least 20 minutes, usually 2 to 4 hours, and can be followed by a day or two of mild disequilibrium. The most popular theory to explain the vertigo associated with endolymphatic hydrops is rupture of the membranous labyrinth and subsequent potassium intoxication of the vestibular hair cells.[1,2] Normally, thin, delicate membranes, such as Reissner's membrane in the cochlea or the saccular membrane in the vestibule, separate the endolymphatic space from the perilymphatic space. During endolymphatic hydrops, these membranes can rupture, allowing mixing of the high-potassium endolymph with the low-potassium perilymph. The influx of a high concentration of potassium ions into the perilymph can alter the neural discharge rate in the vestibular nerve, thereby causing nystagmus and vertigo. The direction of nystagmus observed during an acute attack of Meniere's disease is variable and complex. In the few cases where eye movements have been observed from the beginning of an attack, the slow component of the nystagmus was initially directed away from the affected labyrinth, thus suggesting abnormal excitatory neural activity in the affected ear. Seconds to minutes later, the direction of nystagmus reversed, indicating abnormally reduced neural activity in the affected labyrinth. This biphasic nystagmus response is consistent with the results of animal models of potassium perfusion into the perilymph. A third phase of nystagmus that beats toward the affected side, known as *recovery nystagmus*, also can occur days to weeks later. Recovery nystagmus is presumably related to a combination of central adaptation and recovery of vestibular function in the affected labyrinth.[3,4]

The resolution of vertigo is probably the result of a combination of restoration of normal potassium levels in the perilymph, normalization of the pressure–volume relationships within the labyrinth following membrane rupture, and central vestibular adaptation. Not uncommonly, hearing loss and aural fullness seem to improve after the vertigo spell (Lermoyez syndrome); however, for unknown reasons, aural fullness, tinnitus, and hearing loss generally follow a different, more protracted course than the vertigo.

Following repeated acute episodes, the previously reversible symptoms of Meniere's disease can become permanent and progressive. Hearing loss increases and ceases to return to normal. Tinnitus becomes invariably present, and other auditory distortions such as recruitment (sharp or loud sounds are perceived as excessively loud, even painful) and diplacusis (a given tone is heard at a different pitch in the two ears) become permanent. A permanent reduction of vestibular function also occurs. These symptoms and signs are thought to be caused primarily by progressive damage and loss of hair cells within the inner ear, not to direct involvement of the primary afferent neurons of the labyrinth.

PHYSICAL EXAMINATION

Neurologic examination was normal. Otoscopic examination was normal. On tuning-fork testing, Weber's test showed lateralization to the left, and the Rinne test was positive bilaterally. Mild diplacusis was noted. Neurotologic examination revealed no spontaneous nystagmus, a normal head thrust, and a left-beating nystagmus following head shake, Dix-Hallpike maneuvers, and normal sway while standing on foam with the eyes closed. On the stepping test, the patient marched 120 degrees to the left.

Question 3: Are the findings on this physical examination consistent with a presumptive diagnosis of Meniere's disease (endolymphatic hydrops)? Can the affected side be determined from this examination?

Answer 3: In patients with vestibular system dysfunction localized to the inner ear, the neurologic examination should be normal, as was found in this patient. The tuning-fork testing suggests a sensorineural hearing loss in the right ear. The patient's ability to stand on foam with her eyes closed indicates nearly full recovery of postural control. The nystagmus following head shake and the positive result on the stepping test, however, indicate a residual vestibular system asymmetry. Endolymphatic hydrops characteristically produces reversible changes in the inner ear. Thus, the findings on neurotologic examination depend upon when the most recent episode of vertigo occurred, because vestibular compensation (see Chapter 1) acts to reduce the symptoms and signs of any persistent peripheral vestibular injury. Immediately after an abrupt decrease in vestibular function, patients usually march on the stepping test toward the side of the affected ear. However, days to weeks following an acute spell of vertigo, patients often march toward the contralateral ear on the stepping test, suggesting that the combined influence of increasing vestibular function in the diseased ear and vestibular compensation is producing relative *overcompensation*. Thus, the physical examination of this patient supports the preliminary diagnosis of endolymphatic hydrops affecting the right ear. The diminished hearing in the right ear provides the best clue to localization, whereas the post-head-shake nystagmus and abnormal stepping test suggest a recent unilateral vestibular injury.

Question 4: What causes endolymphatic hydrops?

Answer 4: Endolymphatic hydrops represents a common pathologic response to a variety of insults to the inner ear. Etiologic factors include, but are not limited to, concurrent or preceding viral infection of the inner ear, head trauma, vascular insufficiency, syphilis, autoimmune inner ear disease, abnormal glucose metabolism, hypothyroidism, and inhalant and food allergies.[5]

The use of the terms *Meniere's disease* and *endolymphatic hydrops* can be confusing. Many prefer to define Meniere's disease as the idiopathic syndrome of endolymphatic hydrops. When the cause of endolymphatic hydrops is known, it can be clearly defined as, for example, syphilitic endolymphatic hydrops, autoimmune-related endolymphatic hydrops, and so on.

In addition to these etiologic factors, other factors thought to influence the formation of endolymphatic hydrops include excessive salt intake, stress, and excessive caffeine ingestion.

Question 5: Which laboratory studies should be ordered for this patient and why?

Answer 5: The patient's history and physical examination are both consistent with a peripheral vestibular disorder. Quantitative vestibular testing and audiometric testing should be performed to substantiate the diagnosis and to determine the affected side.

LABORATORY TESTING

Videonystagmography: Ocular motor and positional tests were normal. Caloric testing demonstrated a 35% reduced vestibular response in the right ear.

Audiometric testing (Fig. Case 9–2) revealed a unilateral low-frequency sensorineural hearing loss affecting the right ear. Hearing in the left ear was normal. Electrocochleography revealed a summating to action potential ratio of 60% in the right ear and 20% in the left ear (see Chapter 5).

Imaging: An MRI scan of the brain was normal.

Other Tests: A metabolic blood screen consisting of a complete blood count, an erythrocyte sedimentation rate, an autoimmune panel, thyroid function tests, and the fluorescent treponemal antibody absorption test (FTA-ABS) was normal.

Question 6: Why was an MRI scan performed?

Answer 6: Although the constellation of clinical symptoms is characteristic of Meniere's disease, tumors of the cerebellopontine angle, such as meningioma or acoustic neuroma, can cause similar symptoms, including fluctuating hearing loss, aural fullness, tinnitus, and dizziness. Thus, it is prudent to perform a central nervous system scan or a screening brainstem auditory-evoked potential test in cases of asymmetric hearing loss.

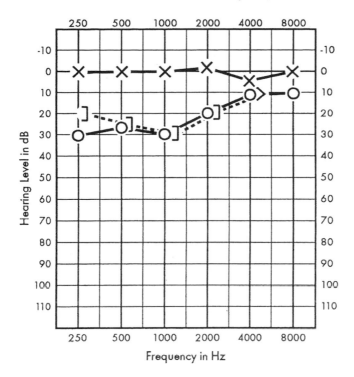

Word Recognition Score

Right : 100%
Left : 100%

		Right	Left
Air	unmasked	o—o	x—x
	masked	△—△	□—□
Bone	unmasked	‹‒‒‒‹	›‒‒‒›
	masked	E‒‒‒C	]‒‒‒]

Figure C10-2
Audiogram.

Figure Case 9–2 Audiogram.

DIAGNOSIS/DIFFERENTIAL DIAGNOSIS

This patient was given a diagnosis of Meniere's disease, or endolymphatic hydrops.

ADDITIONAL HISTORY

Further evaluation of the patient's lifestyle and habits revealed a stressful work environment that included a 10- to-12-hour workday and occasional all-nighters. In addition, the patient consumed approximately six cups of caffeinated coffee per day. Other habits that could exacerbate endolymphatic hydrops included a high-salt diet and smoking one pack of cigarettes per day.

TREATMENT/MANAGEMENT

Question 7: What medications have been shown to be efficacious in the treatment of endolymphatic hydrops?

Answer 7: Several controlled clinical trials have demonstrated the efficacy of the combination of a low-salt diet and a diuretic in the treatment of endolymphatic hydrops. The combination of hydrochlorothiazide and triamterene is widely accepted as the first choice of diuretic.[6] Oral vasodilators such as nicotinic acid and parenteral treatments such as histamine injections or papaverine have not been tested in clinical trials of endolymphatic hydrops.[7] However, based on anecdotal experiences, these medications are frequently prescribed for this condition.

Acute attacks of vertigo can be treated with antiemetic and vestibular-suppressant medications. Promethazine (25 to 50 mg) or compazine (10 mg) (oral or as a rectal suppository) are effective for mild to moderate nausea and vomiting. Meclizine (25 mg) is helpful for mild dizziness but is not generally effective for severe nausea or vomiting. Vestibular rehabilitation is not generally helpful in Meniere's disease, because the vertigo usually occurs abruptly and remits spontaneously, and most individuals report normal balance between episodes.

The initial treatment recommendations for the patient included a prescription for hydrochlorothiazide and triamterene once daily, alteration of the patient's lifestyle to include a low-salt diet, a reduction in the use of caffeine, reduced smoking, and stress reduction.

FOLLOW-UP

The patient was compliant with treatment, and she became symptom-free aside from persistent mild hearing loss and tinnitus. No major episodes of vertigo recurred.

SUMMARY

A 50-year-old female attorney presented with fluctuating aural fullness, hearing loss, and tinnitus followed by an episode of acute prostrating vertigo. The presumptive diagnosis of Meniere's disease was made on the basis of these clinical symptoms. An audiogram, electrocochleography, vestibular laboratory testing, and MRI scanning were performed to further evaluate and confirm the diagnosis. The patient was treated with a diuretic and a salt-restricted diet. This resulted in a significant reduction in her symptoms.

TEACHING POINTS

1. **The typical presentation of Meniere's disease includes fluctuating aural fullness, tinnitus, hearing loss, and recurrent bouts of vertigo.** Endolymphatic hydrops (swelling of the endolymphatic space) is the underlying pathophysiologic process of Meniere's disease.
2. **Endolymphatic hydrops can be associated with a number of metabolic, infectious, and autoimmune disorders.** Meniere's disease is defined as the idiopathic form of endolymphatic hydrops.
3. **The mechanisms of hearing loss and vertigo caused by endolymphatic hydrops are uncertain.** Possibly, endolymphatic hydrops causes

rupture of intralabyrinthine membranes and mixing of endolymph and perilymph with concomitant potassium intoxication.

4. **The medical treatment of endolymphatic hydrops includes the combination of a diuretic and dietary salt restriction.**

REFERENCES

1. Schuknecht HF: Pathology of the Ear. Cambridge, MA: Harvard University Press, 1974.
2. Brown DH, McClure JA, Downar-Zapolski Z: The membrane rupture theory of Meniere's disease—is it valid? Laryngoscope 98:599–601, 1988.
3. McClure JA, Copp JC, Lycett P: Recovery nystagmus in Meniere's disease. Laryngoscope 91:1727–1737, 1981.
4. Bance M, Mai M, Tomlinson D, Rutka J: The changing direction of nystagmus in acute Meniere's disease: Pathophysiological implications. Laryngoscope 101:197–201, 1991.
5. Paparella MM: The cause (multifactorial inheritance) and pathogenesis (endolymphatic malabsorption) of Meniere's disease and its symptoms (mechanical and chemical). Acta Otolaryngol (Stockh) 99:445–451, 1985.
6. Jackson CG, Glasscock ME, Davis WE: Medical management of Meniere's disease. Ann Otol 90:142–147, 1981.
7. Cass SP: Role of medications in otological vertigo and balance disorders. Semin Hearing 12:257–269, 1991.

CASE

10

Disequilibrium of Aging

HISTORY

An 80-year-old woman presented with a complaint of disequilibrium when walking. The patient noted occasional lightheadedness but had no complaint of vertigo, hearing loss, or tinnitus. She did not complain of positional sensitivity when lying supine. Her symptoms had been present for several years but had been especially noticeable in the last 6 months. The patient dated the onset of her problem to cataract surgery in the right eye that resulted in a marked improvement in her vision. The patient's family confirmed that her balance had been gradually worsening for several years, and she had become more sedentary. Her primary care physician ordered a computed tomography (CT) scan of the head, which revealed a small (0.5 cm) meningioma in the falx cerebri without evidence of a mass effect. A magnetic resonance imaging (MRI) scan confirmed this finding and revealed diffuse increased signal intensity in the deep white matter. The patient was using meclizine, 25 mg twice daily, without obvious benefit.

Question 1: Based on this patient's history, what are the diagnostic considerations, and what further information would be helpful in the evaluation of this patient?

Answer 1: This patient's history suggests a nonspecific abnormality of the balance system. With the information available, it is difficult to localize the problem to the vestibular system. Further information regarding the patient's past medical history, medication use, any remote history of a vestibular disorder, family history, and habits such as smoking and alcohol consumption would all be helpful. Additionally, a physical examination is likely to provide helpful information.

ADDITIONAL HISTORY

The patient had a history of essential hypertension for the past 20 years and was being treated with a diuretic. There was no remote history of dizziness or disequilibrium. The patient had smoked one pack of cigarettes per day for 40 years but had quit 15 years ago and consumed about one ounce of ethanol daily.

The patient has no family history of balance disorder.

PHYSICAL EXAMINATION

The patient's general examination was normal. Neurologic examination revealed no specific abnormalities of cranial nerves aside from difficulty pursuing a slowly moving target. Examination of the motor and sensory systems was normal. Coordination was normal. However, the patient had a slightly widened base to her gait and was unable to tandem walk without assistance. Otologic examination was normal. Neurotologic examination was normal, except that she was quite unsteady on a compliant foam surface with the eyes open or eyes closed, but she did not fall.

Question 2: Based on the history and physical examination, what is this patient's likely diagnosis? What laboratory tests might assist in making the diagnosis?

Answer 2: This patient has no obvious cause for disequilibrium, although several factors might be contributing, including age, probable atherosclerotic disease considering the risk factors of hypertension and tobacco use, recent cataract surgery that changed her vision, and a diminished level of activity.

Further information from laboratory tests may be helpful. Vestibular laboratory testing would provide information regarding the presence of a vestibular system abnormality. An MRI scan has already been performed. The patient was found to have evidence of small-vessel disease. Her small falcine meningioma is probably asymptomatic. If not already assessed by the patient's primary care physician, her metabolic, hematologic, and thyroid status should be determined.

LABORATORY TESTING

Videonystagmography: Ocular motor testing revealed difficulty performing smooth pursuit. There was a direction-changing positional nystagmus of 4 degrees per second, which was considered borderline abnormal for an 80-year-old patient. Caloric irrigations revealed symmetric responses somewhat larger than average amounting to about 30 degrees per second peak slow component velocity for each irrigation.

Rotational testing revealed responses of normal magnitude and symmetry with an increased phase lead. Trapezoidal rotations revealed a time constant of about 9 seconds, which is somewhat short. Posturography testing indicated excessive sway in all conditions in a nonspecific pattern. Also, the patient had an inability to adapt to repeated platform rotations.

Audiometric testing revealed a mild sensorineural hearing loss, worse at higher frequencies, which was seen bilaterally.

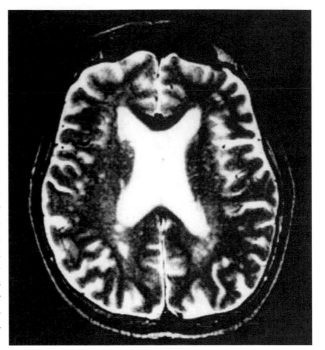

Figure Case 10–1 Magnetic resonance image of white matter lesions in a patient with disequilibrium of aging. (*Source*: With permission from Baloh RW, Yue Q, Socotch TM, Jacobson KM: White matter lesions and disequilibrium in older people. I. Case-control comparisons. Arch Neurol 52(10):970–974, 1995.[3])

MRI scanning of the brain revealed diffuse nonspecific deep white matter changes on T2 imaging (Fig. Case 10–1).

Vestibular laboratory test results suggest a nonspecific central vestibular, possibly cerebellar, abnormality because of the abnormally large caloric responses and abnormal timing of rotational responses. The MRI findings also are nonspecific. These findings may be simply an effect of age.

DIAGNOSIS/DIFFERENTIAL DIAGNOSIS

Question 3: Based on the information available, what is this patient's likely diagnosis?

Answer 3: The patient's disequilibrium cannot be ascribed to a single causative factor. Such older patients with deep white matter changes have been given a diagnosis of "disequilibrium of aging," "presbyastasis" and "disequilibrium of the elderly."[1–4]

Presumably, such patients have disequilibrium caused primarily by abnormal sensory processing by the central nervous system and abnormal control mechanisms for balance. Their problem is worsened by abnormal sensory signals, an aged musculoskeletal system with a concomitant decreased range of motion, and diminished strength.

Question 4: What is the influence of age on vestibular function?

Answer 4: Although balance function is known to be adversely affected by aging, manifested by an increase in the incidence of falls in the elderly,[5] the cause of this decline is not known. Many structures in the peripheral vestibular system are known to be affected by increased age. Specifically, vestibular hair cell degeneration,[6] saccular otoconia degeneration,[7] changes in vestibular hair cell synaptic membranes,[8] a decline in the number of vestibular ganglion cells,[9] and a decline in the number of vestibular fibers[10] are all associated with increased age. Aging also influences central vestibular function. There are modest changes in vestibulo-ocular function[11-14]; a reduction in the ability to combine visual and vestibular signals, that is, impaired visual–vestibular interaction; and a preserved ability to modify (adapt) vestibular reflexes in response to altered visual input.[12] Postural sway also increases with advanced age, particularly under circumstances that require vestibular sensation such as standing on a compliant surface with a distorted visual surround.[15]

This patient was given a diagnosis of disequilibrium of aging.

TREATMENT/MANAGEMENT

This patient was enrolled in a vestibular rehabilitation therapy program that emphasized gait training. Vestibular-suppressant medications were discontinued. The patient's disequilibrium improved slightly.

SUMMARY

An 80-year-old woman presented with gradually worsening balance during walking without specific complaints of vertigo. The patient had a past medical history of hypertension. Physical examination did not suggest a specific localization for her disequilibrium. Laboratory studies suggested cerebrovascular disease and nonspecific vestibular system impairment. A diagnosis of disequilibrium of aging was given. Treatment consisted of discontinuation of vestibular-suppressant medications and vestibular rehabilitation therapy.

TEACHING POINTS

1. **Aging affects the vestibular system.** In the vestibular periphery, otoconia, hair cells, and ganglion cells and nerve fibers degenerate with increasing age. Centrally, there is a decline in vestibular processing that includes a reduction in the ability to combine visual and vestibular signals and a decline in the ability to modify (adapt) vestibular reflexes.
2. *Disequilibrium of aging*, **also known as** *presbyastasis*, **is a term used to describe the condition of elderly patients who present with imbalance and disequilibrium that cannot be ascribed to a particular disease state or to a single causative factor.** White matter lesions on MRI scans have been associated with this condition. Presumably, such patients have disequilibrium based on abnormal sensory input, abnormal sensory processing by the central nervous system, abnormal control mechanisms for balance, and an aged musculoskeletal system with a concomitant decreased range of motion and diminished strength.

3. **Vestibular rehabilitation therapy may benefit patients with disequilibrium of aging.** Despite physical limitations and the decline of sensory function and sensorimotor processing, such individuals should be counseled regarding prevention of falls, including use of a cane if necessary, and the use of appropriate home safety devices such as rails in the bathroom.

REFERENCES

1. Jenkins HA, Furman JM, Gulya AJ, Honrubia V, Linthicum FH, Mirka A: Disequilibrium of aging. Otolaryngol Head Neck Surg 100:272–282, 1989.
2. Belal A, Glorig A: Disequilibrium of ageing (presbyastasis). J Laryngol Otol 100:1037–1041, 1986.
3. Baloh RW, Yue Q, Socotch TM, Jacobson KM: White matter lesions and disequilibrium in older people. I. Case-control comparisons. Arch Neurol 52(10):970–974, 1995.
4. Whitman GT, Tang T, Lin A, Baloh RW: A prospective study of cerebral white matter abnormalities in older people with gait dysfunction. Neurology 57(6):990–994, 2001.
5. Tinetti ME, Speechley M, Ginter SG: Risk factors for falls among elderly persons living in the community. N Engl J Med 319:1701–1707, 1988.
6. Rosenhall U, Rubin W: Degenerative changes in the human vestibular sensory epithelia. Acta Otolaryngol 79:67–80, 1975.
7. Ross MD, Peacor D, Johnsson LG, Allard LF: Observations on normal and degenerating human otoconia. Ann Otol 85:310–326, 1976.
8. Engstrom H, Ades HW, Engstrom B, Gilchrest D, Bourne G: Structural changes in the vestibular epithelia in elderly monkeys and humans. Adv Otorhinolaryngol 22:93–110, 1977.
9. Richter, E: Quantitative study of human Scarpa's ganglion and vestibular sensory epithelia. Acta Otolaryngol 90:199–208, 1980.
10. Bergstrom B: Morphology of the vestibular nerve. II. The number of myelinated vestibular nerve fibers in man at various ages. Acta Otolaryngol 76:173–179, 1973.
11. Baloh RW, Jacobson KM, Socotch TM: The effect of aging on visual-vestibuloocular responses. Exp Brain Res 95:509–516, 1993.
12. Paige GD: Senescence of human visual–vestibular interactions. J Vestib Res 2:133–151, 1992.
13. Peterka R, Black F, Schoenhoff M: Age-related changes in human vestibulo-ocular reflexes: Sinusoidal rotation and caloric tests. J Vestib Res 1:49–59, 1990.
14. Furman JF, Redfern MS: Effect of aging on the otolith-ocular reflex. J Vestib Res 11:91–103, 2001.
15. Peterka R, Black F: Age-related changes in human posture control: Sensory organization tests. J Vestib Res 1:73–85, 1990.

Labyrinthine Concussion

HISTORY

A 44-year-old woman who worked as a travel agent complained of dizziness and disequilibrium that were present constantly but fluctuated from day to day. The patient dated the onset of her symptoms to head trauma sustained during a motor vehicle accident 10 months before evaluation. The car that she was driving was struck on the passenger side, causing the left side of her head to strike the inside of the passenger compartment. The patient had no loss of consciousness at the time of the accident. She was particularly symptomatic during rapid head movement and had difficulty ambulating in dimly lit environments. Headaches occurred irregularly. The patient noted that hearing in the right ear was not as good as in the left. Symptoms were not exacerbated by Valsalva maneuvers such as coughing, sneezing, or straining during bowel movements. There was no positional dizziness. There was no anxiety, insomnia, undue fatigue, or personality change. There was no significant past medical history. The family history was noncontributory.

A CT scan of the head obtained by the patient's primary care physician was within the normal limits. The patient had used meclizine, obtaining some relief, but she continued to experience dizziness and disequilibrium.

Question 1: Based on the patient's history, what is the likely diagnosis?

Answer 1: This patient is likely to have suffered from a labyrinthine concussion caused by head trauma during the motor vehicle accident.[1] Other considerations include perilymphatic fistula (see Case 52), brainstem concussion, and cervicogenic vertigo (see Case 53). Other possibilities include conditions that may be unrelated to the motor vehicle accident or exacerbated by it, such as a prior compensated peripheral vestibulopathy or a central nervous system disorder such as demyelinating disease or a mass lesion. The latter two conditions are unlikely, but for uncertain reasons they can sometimes come to light following head trauma and so must be considered.

PHYSICAL EXAMINATION

The general and neurologic examinations were normal. Otologic examination revealed normal-appearing tympanic membranes with normal mobility on pneumatic otoscopy. During tuning forks examination using 512 and 1024 Hz forks, Weber's test lateralized to the left and the Rinne tests were positive bilaterally, indicating a possible sensorineural type of hearing loss on the right. Neuro-otologic examination revealed spontaneous left-beating nystagmus with infrared glasses, normal head thrust testing, negative Dix-Hallpike maneuvers, no cervical nystagmus, difficulty standing on a compliant foam surface with the eyes closed, a normal stepping test, and no nystagmus observed with infrared glasses during hyperventilation, tragal stimulation, Valsalva maneuvers, or pneumatic otoscopy.

LABORATORY TESTING

Videonystagmography: Ocular motor function was normal. A spontaneous left-beating vestibular nystagmus of 6 degrees per second was present. There was no positional nystagmus. Caloric irrigations revealed a right-reduced vestibular response of 35%.

Rotational testing revealed a mild left-directional preponderance.

Posturography indicated excessive sway only on Condition 6.

Audiometric testing revealed a mild to moderate right-sided sensorineural hearing loss that was greatest in the higher frequencies (Fig. Case 11–1). Hearing in the left ear was normal. Results of electrocochleography, which was performed to evaluate the possibility of posttraumatic endolymphatic hydrops (see Cases 9, 16, 21, 25) or perilymphatic fistula (see Case 52), was normal.

A CT scan of the brain was normal.

Question 2: Based on the patient's history, physical examination, and laboratory studies, what is the most likely diagnosis?

Answer 2: The most likely diagnosis is labyrinthine concussion on the right as a result of head trauma suffered during a motor vehicle accident. This diagnosis is supported by the combination of the asymmetric sensorineural hearing loss in the right ear and a right unilateral reduced vestibular response on caloric testing. The fact that the patient described hitting the side of her head against the passenger compartment seems inconsistent with the right-sided audiovestibular loss. However, because the exact mechanism of injury in labyrinthine concussion is not well known, the fact that head trauma occurred is more important than the side of the head impact. Further, the concept of *coup-contracoup injuries* provides a possible explanation for the laterality of the patient's findings. There is also a possibility that a combination of central and peripheral dysfunction is causing the present symptoms (see Case 2).

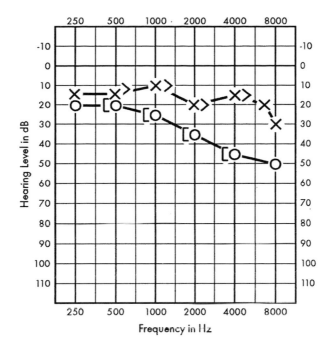

Figure Case 11–1 Audiogram.

Word Recognition Score				Right	Left
	Air	unmasked		O——O	✕——✕
		masked		△——△	□——□
Right : 90%	Bone	unmasked		◄---◄	►---►
Left : 96%		masked		⊏---⊏	⊐---⊐

Question 3: What is the pathophysiologic basis for labyrinthine concussion?

Answer 3: The mechanism of injury in labyrinthine concussion is poorly understood.[2,3] Possible mechanisms of concussive injury to the labyrinth include pressure *shock waves* transmitted directly to the labyrinth by the skull, implosive barotrauma in the form of acoustic energy, and barometric pressure waves transmitted via the tympanic membrane and the ossicular chain to the labyrinth. Explosive pressure changes can also occur from sudden shifts of the brain or intracranial fluids. Sudden intracranial pressure changes can be transmitted to the labyrinth via the cochlear aqueduct, endolymphatic sac, or cribriform regions of the internal auditory canal that transmit eighth cranial nerve fibers into the labyrinth. Sudden pressure shifts of the labyrinthine fluids can cause hemorrhage or tears of fine labyrinthine membranes, allowing intermixing of perilymph and endolymph and local metabolic disturbances that could result in the formation of endolymphatic hydrops. Sudden pressure shifts can also damage hair cell stereocilia, the organ of Corti, or the various specialized cupular structures, cause collapse or fibrosis of the endolymphatic membranes, or cause the loss of hair cells themselves.

Question 4: Why is this patient still symptomatic 10 months following the trauma?

Answer 4: The patient has not compensated for her peripheral vestibular loss. As discussed in Case 3, impaired compensation for a peripheral vestibular lesion may be a result of one or more of several causes. This patient may be experiencing erroneous or fluctuating peripheral vestibular input as a result of labyrinthine trauma. It is possible that the central vestibular system has more difficulty compensating for erroneous or fluctuating vestibular signals from the peripheral end organ than for a complete or fixed peripheral vestibular deficit. Following any significant head injury, subtle central nervous system dysfunction that could impair central compensatory processes is also possible. No abnormalities of vision or proprioception are noted, and thus these causes are unlikely to be contributing to the current balance dysfunction. Inadequate sensory input as a result of sedentary behavior also is possible and could have impaired compensation.

Question 5: What conditions other than impaired compensation for a peripheral vestibular lesion may underlie persistent dizziness following head trauma?

Answer 5: Conditions other than impaired compensation for a peripheral vestibular lesion that may underlie persistent dizziness following head trauma include benign paroxysmal positional vertigo (see Cases 7, 22, 25, 31, 39), perilymphatic fistula (discussed in Case 52), and brainstem or cerebral concussion. This patient is unlikely to be suffering from benign paroxysmal positional vertigo, considering the absence of a history of positional vertigo and negative Dix-Hallpike maneuvers. Perilymphatic fistula is more difficult to rule out, but the patient does not report fluctuation of hearing loss, nor are her symptoms exacerbated by coughing, sneezing, or straining during bowel movements, and no symptoms or signs were induced by tragal stimulation, Valsalva maneuvers, or pneumatic otoscopy. Electrocochleography may be positive in either endolymphatic hydrops or perilymphatic fistula but was negative in this patient. Nevertheless, perilymphatic fistula should remain a possibility because of the inherent difficulty in diagnosing perilymphatic fistula (see Case 52). The patient is unlikely to have suffered from a brainstem contusion because neurologic signs are absent. However, it is possible that some degree of the patient's impaired compensation may relate to a mild brainstem concussion. The patient is unlikely to have suffered from a significant cerebral concussion since there are no complaints of abnormal memory or personality change. Her headaches, however, suggest the possibility of a mild cerebral concussion, although the headaches could be the result of head trauma without cerebral concussion.

DIAGNOSIS/DIFFERENTIAL DIAGNOSIS

The patient was given a diagnosis of labyrinthine concussion.

TREATMENT/MANAGEMENT

Because the patient was symptomatic primarily during rapid head movement and while ambulating in dimly lit environments, she was treated with vestibular rehabilitation therapy. She was also given a vestibular suppressant, meclizine 25 mg, to be used on an as-needed basis up to three times per day, only when she was particularly symptomatic. The patient was also advised that recovery might be prolonged because of the possibility of a brainstem concussion and that improvement could continue for up to 2 years. The plan was to discontinue meclizine as soon as possible following the hoped-for successful treatment with vestibular rehabilitation therapy.

FOLLOW-UP

The patient's symptoms gradually decreased and her balance improved noticeably following vestibular rehabilitation therapy. At the 6-month follow-up visit, she was using meclizine only a few days each month when her symptoms seemed worse.

SUMMARY

A 44-year-old woman complained of 10 months of dizziness that began following a motor vehicle accident in which she struck the side of her head against the inside of the passenger compartment. The patient's laboratory test results suggested a mild unilateral reduced vestibular response and a sensorineural hearing loss on the same side. These findings suggested a labyrinthine concussion. The patient's persistent symptoms suggested impaired compensation, may have been based on abnormal or fluctuating peripheral vestibular function or sedentary behavior, and may have been compounded by a mild brainstem concussion. Treatment consisted of vestibular rehabilitation therapy and a vestibular-suppressant agent to be used for a short time only on an as-needed basis.

TEACHING POINTS

1. **The differential diagnosis for posttraumatic dizziness includes posttraumatic benign paroxysmal positional vertigo, posttraumatic endolymphatic hydrops, labyrinthine concussion, perilymphatic fistula, brainstem concussion, and cervical-related vertigo.** Other possibilities include conditions that may be unmasked by the trauma, such as a prior compensated peripheral vestibulopathy or a central nervous system disorder such as demyelinating disease or a mass lesion.
2. **A diagnosis of labyrinthine concussion is suggested by the presence of symptoms or signs of inner ear dysfunction such as asymmetric sensorineural hearing loss, tinnitus, and a unilateral reduced vestibular response on caloric testing following head trauma.**
3. **Prolonged dizziness following head trauma may relate to impaired compensation for a trauma-related peripheral vestibular lesion.** Impaired compensation may be based on aberrant or fluctuating peripheral vestibular input as a result of labyrinthine trauma, subtle central nervous system dysfunction, inadequate sensory input as a result of sedentary behavior, or subclinical damage to the contralateral ear. Following head trauma, other conditions such as benign paroxysmal positional vertigo, perilymphatic fistula, and brainstem or cerebral concussion also may underlie persistent dizziness.

4. **The pathophysiology of labyrinthine concussion is poorly understood.** Possible mechanisms of injury include (1) implosive barotrauma in the form of acoustic energy or barometric pressure waves transmitted via the skull, the tympanic membrane, or the ossicular chain to the labyrinth; (2) explosive pressure changes from sudden shifts of the brain or intracranial fluids; or (3) sudden pressure shifts of labyrinthine fluids that can cause hemorrhage or tears of fine labyrinthine membranes, allowing intermixing of perilymph and endolymph and local metabolic disturbances.

REFERENCES

1. Fitzgerald DC: Head trauma: hearing loss and dizziness. J Trauma 40(3):488–496, 1996.
2. Schuknecht HF, Neff WD, Perlman HD: An experimental study of auditory damage following blows to the head. Ann Otol Rhinol Laryngol 60:273–289, 1951.
3. Schuknecht HF: A clinical study of auditory damage following blows to the head. Ann Otol Rhinol Laryngol 59:331–359, 1950.

CASE
12

Vertebrobasilar Insufficiency

HISTORY

A 70-year-old man presented with episodic dizziness. The patient's symptoms had been particularly troublesome during the last 6 weeks. He described spontaneous episodes occurring about twice a week, characterized by the acute onset of vertigo and a tendency to fall to the right, lasting for seconds to a few minutes. There were no clear precipitating factors such as changes in head position. The patient had no complaints of hearing loss or tinnitus. His past history was significant for hypertension and peptic ulcer disease. Current medications included an angiotensin converting enzyme inhibitor and an H_2 blocking agent.

Question 1: What are the diagnostic considerations in this case, and what further historic information would be helpful in establishing a diagnosis?

Answer 1: This patient's symptoms are suggestive of an episodic dysfunction of peripheral vestibular function such as Meniere's disease (see Cases 9, 16, 21, 25) or benign paroxysmal positional vertigo (see Cases 7, 22, 25, 31, 39). The absence of symptoms related to changes in head position makes benign paroxysmal positional vertigo less likely. The absence of associated otologic symptoms such as hearing loss or tinnitus makes Meniere's disease less likely. The patient's age and history of hypertension suggest the possibility of vertebrobasilar insufficiency, although a structural abnormality of the posterior fossa is another diagnostic possibility. A thorough history regarding associated neurologic complaints would be helpful in establishing a diagnosis. A family history would also be helpful.

139

Table Case 12–1 Initial Symptoms of Vertebrobasilar Insufficiency

Symptoms	Percentage
Vertigo	48
Visual hallucinations	10
Drop attacks or weakness	10
Visceral sensations	8
Visual field defects	6
Diplopia	5
Headaches	3
Other	8

Source: Adapted with permission from Baloh RW, Honrubia V: Clinical Neurophysiology of the Vestibular System, ed 2. Philadelphia: FA Davis, 1990, p. 221.[9]

ADDITIONAL HISTORY

Upon careful questioning, the patient noted that with several of his vertiginous episodes he had experienced circumoral paresthesias and, on one occasion, double vision. His family related that during some of the patient's episodes his speech was often difficult to understand, and he walked "like he was drunk." The patient had no family history of neurologic or otologic disease.

Question 2: What are the characteristic features of vertebrobasilar insufficiency, and what information would be helpful in establishing this as the patient's diagnosis?

Answer 2: Although vertigo alone is rarely a symptom of vertebrobasilar insufficiency,[1–3] especially if the vertigo is chronic,[4] Grad and Baloh[5] have indicated that vertigo alone can be the presenting sign of vertebrobasilar insufficiency. Table Case 12–1 presents the initial symptoms of vertebrobasilar insufficiency. Note that vertigo appears in this list. Patients with vertebrobasilar insufficiency can experience vertigo in isolation for up to 1.5 years.[5] Table Case 12-2 lists associated symptoms in patients with vertebrobasilar insufficiency.

A complete physical examination and brain imaging are likely to add additional diagnostic information to this case.

PHYSICAL EXAMINATION

The patient had entirely normal general, neurologic, and otologic examinations, with the exception of several "soft" neurologic signs, including a very mild left pronator drift and an equivocal Babinski sign on the left. The patient had a slightly widened base to his gait and had difficulty tandem walking. Neurotologic examination, including Dix-Hallpike maneuvers, was normal, with the exception of difficulty standing on a compliant foam surface with the eyes closed.

LABORATORY TESTING

Videonystagmography: Ocular motor, positional, and caloric tests were normal. The rotational test was normal.

Table Case 12–2 Symptoms Associated with Vertebrobasilar Insufficiency

Symptoms	Percentage
Visual dysfunction	69
Drop attacks	33
Unsteadiness, incoordination	21
Extremity weakness	21
Confusion	17
Headache	14
Hearing loss	14
Loss of consciousness	10
Extremity numbness	10
Dysarthria	10
Tinnitus	10
Perioral numbness	5

Source: Adapted with permission from Grad A, Baloh RW: Vertigo of vascular origin. Arch Neurol 46:218–284, 1989.[5]

Audiometric testing revealed bilateral high-frequency sensorineural hearing loss.

An MRI scan of the head revealed an old infarction of the right frontal lobe, a right internal carotid artery occlusion, and bilateral white matter hyperintensities in the periventricular white matter. There were no obvious abnormalities in the brainstem or cerebellum.

DIAGNOSIS/DIFFERENTIAL DIAGNOSIS

Question 3: Based on the history, physical examination, and laboratory studies, what is this patient's most likely diagnosis and why?

Answer 3: The patient's episodes are not typical of benign paroxysmal positional vertigo, and Dix-Hallpike maneuvers were negative. There was no acute syndrome to suggest vestibular neuritis. A vestibular-only form of Meniere's disease (see Case 9) is possible, but the patient's episodes are brief compared to typical episodes of endolymphatic hydrops, there is no associated hearing loss or tinnitus, and some of the patient's episodes are associated with neurologic deficits. Migraine-associated dizziness (see Cases 8, 21, 24) is also a diagnostic possibility, but there is no prior history of headache or family history of migraine. Thus, the patient is probably suffering from vertebrobasilar insufficiency, considering the combination of symptoms that characterize his attacks, his history of hypertension, and evidence of cerebrovascular disease on brain imaging. However, this diagnosis is not certain.

The patient was given a diagnosis of vertebrobasilar insufficiency.

TREATMENT/MANAGEMENT

The patient was treated with an antiplatelet agent. The frequency of his vertiginous episodes decreased markedly, but episodes of dizziness still occurred occasionally.

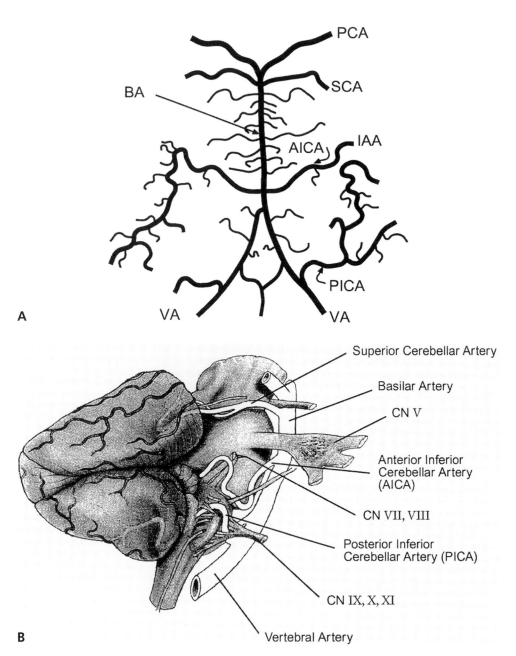

Figure Case 12–1 Blood supply to the brainstem and cerebellum. (A) Schematic drawing of the vertebrobasilar arterial tree. PCA = posterior cerebral artery; SCA = superior cerebellar artery; AICA = anterior inferior cerebellar artery; IAA = internal auditory canal artery; PICA = posterior inferior cerebellar artery; VA = vertebral artery; BA = basilar artery. (B) Drawing highlighting each of the three neurovascular complexes of the posterior fossa. The upper complex is related to the superior cerebellar artery; the middle complex is related to the anterior inferior cerebellar artery; the lower complex is related to the posterior inferior cerebellar artery. [(A) *Source*: Modified with permission from Oas JG, Baloh RW: Vertigo and the anterior inferior cerebellar artery syndrome. Neurology 42:2274–2279, 1992. (B) *Source*: With permission from Rhoton AL: Microsurgical anatomy of posterior fossa cranial nerves. In: Barrow DL (ed). Surgery of the Cranial Nerves of the Posterior Fossa. Park Ridge: American Associations of Neurological Surgeons, 1993, p. 2.[8])]

142

Question 4: What is the vascular supply of the vestibular system? What is the pathophysiologic basis for this patient's vertiginous episodes?

Answer 4: Figure Case 12–1A is a schematic diagram of the vertebrobasilar system. Note that the posterior-inferior cerebellar artery, which arises from the vertebral artery, supplies the vestibular nuclei, while the anterior-inferior cerebellar artery, which arises from the basilar artery, supplies the vestibulocerebellum and gives rise to the internal auditory artery (labyrinthine artery), which, in turn, gives rise to the anterior vestibular artery.

Ischemia in the vertebrobasilar arterial system can cause vestibular symptoms due to peripheral vestibular dysfunction, central vestibular dysfunction, or both (Fig. Case 12–1B). Because the vestibular nuclei are supplied by the posterior-inferior cerebellar artery, a brief interruption of the vertebral artery or of the posterior-inferior cerebellar artery itself can cause transient symptoms similar to those experienced in Wallenberg's syndrome (see Case 29). Because the anterior-inferior cerebellar artery supplies the labyrinth and the vestibulocerebellum, a brief interruption of this artery can also lead to episodic vestibular symptoms (see also Case 30). Baloh[6] has hypothesized that the vertigo seen with vertebrobasilar insufficiency is probably related to labyrinthine ischemia. For much of the blood supply to the vestibular system, the arteries are end-arterial (see Chapter 1), and therefore the opportunity for collateral circulation is limited. This is especially true for the blood supply to the peripheral vestibular system, as well as for the small perforating arteries that supply the brainstem. It should be noted that there is much variability in the vertebrobasilar system, which may lead to variability in presentation.

SUMMARY

A 70-year-old man presented with episodic vertigo lasting for minutes and occasionally associated with double vision, slurred speech, and ataxic gait. The patient had a past history of hypertension. Examination revealed "soft" neurologic signs, and brain imaging revealed evidence of cerebrovascular disease. The patient was given the diagnosis of vertebrobasilar insufficiency and treated with an antiplatelet agent.

TEACHING POINTS

1. **The blood supply of the vestibular system is derived from the basilar artery.** It includes (1) the posterior-inferior cerebellar artery, which arises from the vertebral artery and supplies the vestibular nuclei; (2) the anterior-inferior cerebellar artery, which arises from the basilar artery and supplies the vestibulocerebellum; and (3) the internal auditory artery, which arises from the anterior-inferior cerebellar artery and gives rise to the anterior vestibular artery, which supplies the vestibular apparatus.
2. **Ischemia in the vertebrobasilar artery system can cause vestibular symptoms due to peripheral vestibular dysfunction, central vestibular dysfunction, or both.** For much of the blood supply to the vestibu-

lar system, the arteries are end-arterial and therefore the opportunity for collateral circulation is limited, especially for the blood supply to the peripheral vestibular system.

3. **A diagnosis of vertebrobasilar insufficiency should be reserved for patients who have clearly defined episodes of transient neurologic symptoms and signs that can be localized to the posterior circulation.** Vertebrobasilar insufficiency can present with many different neurologic symptoms. Even if vertigo is not the presenting complaint of vertebrobasilar insufficiency, eventually most patients with vertebrobasilar insufficiency experience vertigo on one or more occasions.

4. **Isolated vertigo, especially if chronic, is rarely a symptom of vertebrobasilar insufficiency.** However, vertigo associated with definitive neurologic symptoms, especially in a patient with risk factors for cerebrovascular disease, should lead to a consideration of vertebrobasilar insufficiency.

REFERENCES

1. Ferbert A, Bruckmann H, Drummen R: Clinical features of proven basilar artery occlusion. Stroke 21(8):1135–1142, 1990.
2. Estol C, Caplan LR, Pressin MS: Isolated vertigo: An uncommon manifestation of vertebrobasilar ischaemia. Cerebrovasc Dis 6(Suppl 2):161, 1996.
3. Gomez CR, Cruz-Flores S, Malkoff MD, Sauer CM, Burch CM: Isolated vertigo as a manifestation of vertebrobasilar ischemia. Neurology 47(1):94–97, 1996.
4. Fisher CM: Vertigo in cerebrovascular disease. Arch Otolaryngol 85:529–534, 1967.
5. Grad A, Baloh RW: Vertigo of vascular origin. Arch Neurol 46:281–284, 1989.
6. Baloh RW: Otological aspects of cerebrovascular disease. In: Toole JF (ed). Handbook of Clinical Neurology, Vol 11: Vascular Diseases, Part III. New York: Elsevier Science, 1989, pp. 129–135.
7. Oas JG, Baloh RW: Vertigo and the anterior inferior cerebellar artery syndrome. Neurology 42: 2274–2279, 1992.
8. Rhoton AL: Microsurgical anatomy of posterior fossa cranial nerves. In: Barrow DL (ed). Surgery of the Cranial Nerves of the Posterior Fossa. Park Ridge: American Association of Neurological Surgeons, 1993, pp 1–103.
9. Baloh RW, Honrubia V: Clinical Neurophysiology of the Vestibular System, ed 2. Philadelphia: FA Davis, 1990.

Benign Recurrent Vertigo of Childhood

HISTORY

A 13-year-old boy presented with a chief complaint of 4 months of dizziness occurring once or twice each week. The patient described a spinning sensation associated with a feeling of imbalance and a tendency to fall. He also noted that if he disregarded these symptoms and continued his normal activities, he became nauseated and on two occasions had vomited. The patient had no complaint of hearing loss or tinnitus and did not describe fullness in the ears. His school performance was excellent, but he had experienced some recent difficulty in gym class and in performing extracurricular sports.

Question 1: Based on the patient's history, what are the diagnostic considerations?

Answer 1: By far the most common causes of episodic vertigo in childhood is benign recurrent vertigo of childhood,[1–3] also known as *benign paroxysmal vertigo of childhood*, which is believed to have a migrainous basis.[2] Infrequently, endolymphatic hydrops (see Cases 9, 16, 21, 25) can be present in childhood. Less likely disorders include perilymphatic fistula (see Case 52), a seizure disorder (see Case 47), and an anxiety disorder (see Case 5). Benign paroxysmal positional vertigo (see Cases 7, 22, 25, 31, 39) should not be confused with benign recurrent vertigo of childhood; the former is rare in children. Unusual metabolic abnormalities such as ornithine transcarbamylase deficiency[4] can present with episodic dizziness, as can familial periodic ataxia. Structural lesions in the posterior fossa, including mass lesions, and malformations such as a Chiari malformation would not be expected to produce episodic symptoms but should be concluded.

145

Question 2: What further historical information will be helpful in establishing a diagnosis of benign recurrent vertigo of childhood?

Answer 2: Associated historical features often include motion sickness; an apparent relationship between vertiginous episodes and certain foods such as aged cheese and chocolate, possibly because of their tyramine or phenylethylamine (vasoactive amines) content[4]; and a positive family history of migraine. Patients may also be bothered by certain visual environments such as flickering candles or open spaces.[5]

ADDITIONAL HISTORY

The patient had a history of car sickness, especially when riding in the back seat. He did not notice a particular association between dizziness episodes and diet. There was a strong family history of migraine on the maternal side; the patient's mother and maternal aunt suffered from throbbing headaches associated with photophobia, phonophobia, and nausea. Also, the patient's mother remembered having car sickness and avoiding amusement parks during her childhood.

PHYSICAL EXAMINATION

The patient's general, neurologic, otologic, and neurotologic examinations were normal.

LABORATORY TESTING

Videonystagmography test results were normal.

Rotational testing revealed a left directional preponderance.

Audiometry testing was scheduled because of the possibility of endolymphatic hydrops or some other associated cochlear abnormality. The results were normal.

MRI scanning of the brain, which had been ordered by the patient's pediatrician, was normal.

Question 3: Are the vestibular laboratory findings in this patient consistent with a diagnosis of benign recurrent vertigo of childhood?

Answer 3: This patient's laboratory studies suggest an ongoing vestibulo-ocular imbalance without evidence of peripheral vestibular involvement. Moreover, there was no evidence of auditory system involvement or of a structural abnormality of the central nervous system. Taken together, these findings make the diagnosis of benign recurrent vertigo of childhood most likely. Although Basser's original description of benign recurrent vertigo of childhood[3] suggested that unilateral caloric reduction was important in making this diagnosis, subsequent studies have not suggested this as a diagnostic criterion.[6] A review of vestibular laboratory findings in patients with migraine suggests that a directional preponderance on rotation is a common finding (see Case 8).[7–9]

Table Case 13–1 Foods That
May Provoke Migraine

Foods containing tyramine
   Aged cheeses
   Chianti wine
   Pickled herring
   Dried smoked fish
   Sour cream
   Yogurt
   Yeast extracts
   Chicken liver
Chocolate
Citrus fruits
Dairy products
Onions
Nuts
Beans
Caffeine (excess, withdrawal)
Avocado
Banana
Food additives
Nitrates (e.g., in hot dogs, luncheon meats)
Monosodium glutamate
Aspartame artificial sweetener

Source: Adapted with permission from American
Council for Headache, Constantine LM, Scott S:
Migraine: The Complete Guide. New York: Dell,
1994, p 66.[10]

DIAGNOSIS/DIFFERENTIAL DIAGNOSIS

This patient was diagnosed as having benign recurrent vertigo of childhood, presumably a manisfestation of a migrainous disorder.

TREATMENT/MANAGEMENT

Based on the frequency of attacks, propranolol, 20 mg three times daily, was prescribed. The patient was also advised to reduce his intake of foods known to provoke migraine[10] (see Table Case 13–1). He responded well to this intervention, and the frequency and severity of his attacks were markedly reduced. Other medications effective in treating childhood migraine, such as periactin, calcium channel blockers, and anticonvulsants, could also have been tried.[2]

SUMMARY

A 13-year-old boy presented with episodic vertigo associated with nausea and two episodes of vomiting. The patient had a history of car sickness and a family history of migraine. The MRI scan and the audiometry test were normal. Vestibular laboratory testing showed a normal caloric test and vestibulo-ocular asymmetry on rotational testing. The patient was given a diagnosis of benign recurrent vertigo of childhood. Treatment consisted of dietary restriction of migraine-provoking foods and a prescription for a beta blocker. The patient responded well to this intervention, the frequency and severity of his attacks were markedly reduced.

TEACHING POINTS

1. **Causes of episodic vertigo in childhood include benign recurrent (paroxysmal) vertigo of childhood, endolymphatic hydrops, perilymphatic fistula, seizure disorder, and anxiety disorder.** Several metabolic, anatomic, and degenerative disorders may also present with episodic dizziness. These include ornithine transcarbamylase deficiency, cranial-cervical junction malformations such as Chiari malformation and familial periodic ataxia.

2. **Benign recurrent vertigo of childhood is the most common cause of vertigo in childhood and is probably a childhood manifestation of migraine.** The diagnosis of benign recurrent vertigo of childhood is established by the presence of episodic vertigo in a child without auditory symptoms in conjunction with associated historical features such as motion sickness sensitivity, an apparent relationship between vertiginous episodes and certain foods such as aged cheese and chocolate, and a positive family history of migraine.

3. **Vestibular test results in benign recurrent vertigo of childhood usually include evidence of an ongoing vestibulo-ocular imbalance without evidence of peripheral vestibular involvement.** Unilateral caloric reduction is sometimes found but is not important for this diagnosis. Directional preponderance on rotational testing is a common finding.

4. **Treatment of benign recurrent vertigo of childhood includes the identification and avoidance of dietary triggers.** Potentially beneficial medications that may be tried in more severe cases include propranolol, periactin, amitriptyline, and depakote.

REFERENCES

1. Russell G, Abu-Arafeh I: Paroxysmal vertigo in children—an epidemiological study. Int J Pediatr Otorhinolaryngol 49(Suppl 1):S105–S107, 1999.
2. Abu-Arafeh I, Russell G: Paroxysmal vertigo as a migraine equivalent in children: A population-based study. Cephalalgia 15(1):22–25, 1995.
3. Basser L: Benign paroxysmal vertigo of childhood. Brain 87:141–152, 1964.
4. Hockaday JM (ed): Migraine in Childhood. London: Butterworths, 1988.
5. Davidoff RA: Migraine: Manifestations, Pathogenesis, and Management. Philadelphia: FA Davis, 1995.
6. Lanzi G, Balottin U, Fazzi E, Tagliasacchi M, Manfrin M, Mira E: Benign paroxysmal vertigo of childhood: A long follow-up. Cephalalgia 14:458–460, 1994.
7. Toglia J, Thomas K, Kuritzky A: Common migraine and vestibular function electronystagmographic study and pathogenesis. Ann Otol 90:267–271, 1981.
8. Kayan A, Hood J: Neuro-otological manifestations of migraine. Brain 107:1123–1142, 1984.
9. Cass SP, Furman JM, Ankerstjerne K, Balaban C, Yetiser S, Aydogan B: Migraine-related vestibulopathy. Ann Otol Rhinol Laryngol 106(3):182–189, 1997.
10. American Council for Headache, Constantine LM, Scott S: Migraine: The Complete Guide. New York: Dell, 1994.

Multisensory Disequilibrium

HISTORY

A 55-year-old man who owned a clothing store presented with the chief complaint of disequilibrium. The patient dated the onset of his problem to a vertiginous episode experienced 6 months before evaluation. Since that time, he had noted difficulty with ambulation, especially in dimly lit environments, and great difficulty while trying to shower. He had no complaint of vertigo since recovery from the single vertiginous episode 6 months before evaluation and no complaints of hearing loss or tinnitus. The patient did not report positional sensitivity.

The patient's past history was significant for insulin-dependent diabetes mellitus for 10 years. There was no family history of a balance problem.

Question 1: Based on the history provided, what are the diagnostic considerations, and what further historical information would be helpful in reaching a diagnosis?

Answer 1: This patient's history is consistent with a balance system abnormality. A diagnostic consideration is residual dysfunction from his vertiginous episode 6 months previously. The patient's lack of vertigo and difficulty with ambulation suggest that he may not have compensated for a peripheral vestibular loss (see Case 1). Also, his diabetes mellitus may have caused visual loss, proprioceptive loss, or both. Thus, along with vestibular dysfunction, the patient may be suffering from a combination of sensory deficits. He should be asked about diabetic retinopathy, any symptoms suggestive of a peripheral neuropathy, and more details of the vertiginous episode 6 months before presentation.

ADDITIONAL HISTORY

The patient's vertiginous episode 6 months previously was associated with the acute onset of vertigo, nausea, and vomiting. He had severe gait ataxia and was bedridden for nearly a day. The patient did not require hospitalization or intravenous hydration despite his insulin-dependent diabetes mellitus, but he was nauseated and had a poor appetite for 3 days, after which he noticed disequilibrium when walking. His gait instability improved somewhat, but by 2 weeks after the acute vertiginous episode, his symptoms had become constant. He was evaluated by his primary care physician, was told that he had "labyrinthitis," and was given meclizine. The meclizine provided symptomatic relief of dizziness for the first month after the vertiginous episode. Because the medication caused him to feel lethargic, he discontinued its use, with no worsening of his dizziness or imbalance.

The patient had required laser treatments in both eyes in the past for diabetic retinopathy but had not required such treatment in the last year. He also reported numbness and tingling in both feet that was more or less constant but was especially noticeable when he was cold. The patient also occasionally had a sense of burning in the feet that was annoying when he was trying to fall asleep. He was using gabapentin, 100 mg three times daily, for this complaint.

PHYSICAL EXAMINATION

The patient had a normal general examination without postural hypotension. Funduscopic examination revealed evidence of diabetic nonproliferative retinopathy. On neurologic examination, extraocular movements were full, without nystagmus. On neurotologic examination, no nystagmus was seen with infrared glasses. Motor system examination and coordination were normal. Decreased vibratory sensation below the knee bilaterally was noted. The patient made several errors during assessment of joint position in both feet. Ankle jerks were absent. His gait was wide-based, and he was very cautious when walking. He did not veer to the right or to the left, nor was there a reeling quality to his walk. Romberg's test was negative. Otologic examination was normal.

However, the patient could not stand on a compliant foam surface with his eyes open or closed. On the stepping test his gait was wide-based and ataxic but without significant deviation.

LABORATORY TESTING

Videonystagmography revealed no spontaneous or positional nystagmus. Caloric testing revealed absent responses during alternate bithermal testing on the left, with reduced responses of 6 degrees per second peak velocity for both warm and cold irrigation on the right. Ice-water irrigation of the left ear revealed that responses were present but markedly reduced. Ice-water irrigation of the right ear was not performed.

Rotational testing revealed symmetric responses of reduced magnitude with an increased phase lead at low frequency (0.02 and 0.05 Hz) and a short time constant of 9 seconds.

Posturography indicated excessive sway on conditions 4, 5, and 6, that is, a surface dependence pattern (see Chapter 4).

Audiometric testing showed a bilateral sensorineural hearing loss of mild to moderate degree that was worse at the high frequencies. Word recognition was well preserved bilaterally.

MRI scanning of the brain showed nonspecific periventricular white matter changes.

Question 2: How does the information from the physical examination alter the diagnostic considerations in this case?

Answer 2: The physical examination suggests that the patient has diabetic retinopathy and a peripheral neuropathy, probably the result of diabetes. On examination, the patient had no evidence of an ongoing vestibular asymmetry, with no spontaneous nystagmus and no veering of gait. Thus, although impaired sensation other than vestibular function predisposes to impaired compensation, the patient's physical examination does not suggest poor compensation. Rather, he may be suffering from the combined effects of loss of several sensory modalities that are important for balance.

DIAGNOSIS/DIFFERENTIAL DIAGNOSIS

Question 3: Based on the history, physical examination, and laboratory tests, what is this patient's likely diagnosis?

Answer 3: This patient is likely to be suffering from multisensory disequilibrium[1] caused by diabetes mellitus. He has a history consistent with an acute vestibular syndrome, possibly from diabetic vascular disease, with involvement of either the vestibular labyrinth or the vestibular nerve. Laboratory testing confirms a bilateral reduction that is worse on the left. The history of tingling and burning paresthesias, decreased sensation in the feet, and absent ankle jerks supports the conclusion that a peripheral neuropathy exists.

Question 4: What is multisensory disequilibrium? In what clinical settings is it often seen?

Answer 4: Multisensory disequilibrium is a condition wherein a patient is suffering from dysfunction in all three of the sensory systems most important for balance, that is, vestibular, visual, and somatic and proprioceptive sensation. Such patients typically complain of unstable gait worsened by environments that further impair or distort their sensory input, such as dimly lit environments, slanted surfaces, soft or compliant surfaces, or moving surfaces such as walkways or escalators.[2]

Like patients with vestibular system abnormalities, those with multisensory disequilibrium may find it helpful to lightly touch a wall or furniture while standing or walking indoors or lightly touch a companion while walking outdoors. Such patients also may benefit from carrying a walking stick, which can provide supplemental proprioceptive information regarding spatial orientation through the upper extremities.

Multisensory disequilibrium is most commonly seen in patients with diabetes mellitus because the disease can cause vestibulopathy, retinopathy, and peripheral neuropathy. In addition to diabetes, multisensory disequilibrium can be seen with any combination of disorders that impair all three sensory modalities that are important for balance.

This patient was given a diagnosis of multisensory disequilibrium due to diabetes mellitus.

TREATMENT/MANAGEMENT

Question 5: What is the treatment of patients with multisensory disequilibrium?

Answer 5: The treatment of patients with multisensory disequilibrium is aimed at increasing the amount of sensory input available and training such patients how to best use their remaining sensory inputs to control balance. Vestibular-suppressant medications should be discontinued. Refractive errors should be corrected. If patients have cataracts, they should be evaluated by an ophthalmologist for possible surgery. A cane should be prescribed for patients with multisensory disequilibrium to add to their somatosensory input. Medication use should be scrutinized for the presence of any agents known to impair central nervous system function, and these medications also should be discontinued if possible.

Ergonomic factors should be optimized, including proper footwear, night lights in the home, removal of throw rugs, and installation of handrails. Also, these patients should be referred for vestibular rehabilitation therapy, including gait training (see Chapter 6).

This patient was advised not to use meclizine or any other vestibular-suppressant medication. A cane was prescribed for him, and he was referred for a course of vestibular rehabilitation therapy. With these measures, his disequilibrium improved somewhat.

SUMMARY

A 55-year-old man with a history of diabetes mellitus presented with a complaint of disequilibrium that had persisted for 6 months after a vertiginous episode. Physical examination suggested evidence of diabetic retinopathy and peripheral neuropathy. Laboratory testing confirmed the presence of a bilateral peripheral vestibular loss coupled with a vestibular asymmetry. The patient was given the diagnosis of multisensory disequilibrium. Treatment consisted of discontinuation of vestibular-suppressant medication, the use of a cane, enrollment in a course of vestibular rehabilitation therapy, and counseling regarding the benefit of using proper footwear, night lights in the home, removal of throw rugs, and the installation of handrails.

TEACHING POINTS

1. **The three sensory systems most important for balance are vestibular, visual, and somatic-proprioceptive sensation.**
2. **Multisensory disequilibrium is a combined dysfunction of vestibular, visual, and somatic-proprioceptive sensation.** Patients with mul-

tisensory disequilibrium typically complain of unstable gait worsened by environments that further impair or distort their sensory input, such as dimly lit environments, slanted surfaces, soft or compliant surfaces, or moving surfaces such as walkways or escalators.

3. **Diabetes mellitus is a common cause of multisensory disequilibrium because the disease can cause vestibulopathy, retinopathy, and peripheral neuropathy.** In addition to diabetes, multisensory disequilibrium can be seen with any combination of disorders that impair all three sensory modalities important for balance, such as a combination of peripheral vestibulopathy, impaired vision from cataracts, and peripheral neuropathy.

4. **Supplemental proprioceptive information regarding spatial orientation via the upper extremities may benefit patients with multisensory disequilibrium.** Patients often find it helpful to lightly touch a wall or furniture while standing or walking indoors or to touch a companion while walking outdoors. Such patients also may benefit from carrying a walking stick.

5. **The treatment of multisensory disequilibrium is aimed at increasing the amount of sensory input available and training patients how to best use their remaining sensory inputs to control balance.**

REFERENCE

1. Drachman DA, Hart CW: An approach to the dizzy patient. Neurology 22:323–334, 1972.
2. Brandt T, Daroff R: The multisensory physiological and pathological vertigo syndromes. Ann Neurol 7:195–203, 1980.

CASE

15

Recurrent Vestibulopathy

HISTORY

A 51-year-old man complained of episodic dizziness. The patient stated that he had had three discrete episodes of dizziness during the past 3 years. The most recent one had occurred 6 weeks before evaluation. He related that during his episodes he experienced severe vertigo associated with nausea and vomiting. He was bedridden during each of these episodes for several hours and had great difficulty with ambulation for several additional hours. For the first 1 to 2 days following each episode, he had a mild sense of disequilibrium but was able to return to his work as a field service representative. He had no associated hearing loss, tinnitus, or fullness in the ears. There was no loss of vision, double vision, numbness, weakness, or alteration in the level of consciousness. The patient required an emergency room visit for two of the three episodes for control of nausea and vomiting. He was asymptomatic between episodes. There was no history of migraine headaches and no significant past medical history. The patient had no family history of otologic or neurologic disease, including no history of migraine. An MRI scan requested by the patient's primary care physician was within normal limits.

Question 1: Based on the patient's history, what are the diagnostic considerations?

Answer 1: The clinical syndrome demonstrated by this patient consists of multiple episodes of vertigo lasting for minutes to hours without auditory or neurologic symptoms. This syndrome has been termed *recurrent vestibulopathy*. Other diagnostic considerations include a vestibular-only form of Meniere's disease (see Cases 9, 16, 21, 25), recurrent vestibular neuritis (see Cases 1 and 3), migraine-related vestibulopathy (see Cases 8, 21, and 24,), and benign paroxysmal posi-

154

tional vertigo (see Cases 7, 22, 25, 31, 39). There was little to suggest a central nervous system abnormality because of the isolated nature of the patient's vertigo. However, vertebrobasilar insufficiency (see Case 12), although unlikely, should be considered in the differential diagnosis. Other considerations include perilymphatic fistula (see Case 52), panic disorder (see Case 5), and a seizure disorder (see Case 47).

PHYSICAL EXAMINATION

Physical examinations, including general, neurologic, otologic, and neurotologic evaluations, were normal.

LABORATORY TESTING

Videonystagmography: Ocular motor, caloric, and positional tests were normal. The audiometric test was normal.

DIAGNOSIS/DIFFERENTIAL DIAGNOSIS

Question 2: This patient's symptoms are characteristic of the syndrome termed *recurrent vestibulopathy*.[1,2] How can this diagnosis be confirmed?

Answer 2: The diagnosis of recurrent vestibulopathy cannot be confirmed and is both a provisional diagnosis and a diagnosis of exclusion.[1,2] As noted previously, recurrent vertigo can be seen in Meniere's disease (endolymphatic hydrops), recurrent vestibular neuritis, benign paroxysmal positional vertigo, perilymphatic fistula, migraine-related vestibulopathy, vertebrobasilar insufficiency, panic disorder, and seizure disorder. These entities can usually be ruled out by a careful history and a physical examination. However, some of these entities, such as recurrent vestibular neuritis, migraine-related vestibulopathy, and endolymphatic hydrops, are difficult, if not impossible, to rule out definitively. This uncertainty is reflected in the fact that in approximately 30% of patients with a provisional diagnosis of recurrent vestibulopathy, another specific diagnosis will become clear over time, most commonly endolymphatic hydrops, benign paroxysmal positional vertigo, or migraine-related vestibulopathy.[2]

Question 3: What is the cause of recurrent vestibulopathy?

Answer 3: The cause of recurrent vestibulopathy is not known, and the nonspecific name was originally chosen to reflect the unknown underlying pathophysiology. The signs and symptoms that typify recurrent vestibulopathy are most similar to those of vestibular neuritis, except that patients with vestibular neuritis have more prolonged vertigo (days rather than minutes to hours) and chronic vestibular symptoms (weeks to months rather than days) than patients with recurrent vestibulopathy. Thus, it has been hypothesized that recurrent vestibulopathy represents a milder form of vestibular neuritis or migraine-related vestibulopathy. Although the precise mechanism of vestibular neuritis is unknown, there is evidence to support viral-induced injury to the vestibular nerve[3] (see Cases

1 and 3). Given the similarities of vestibular neuritis and recurrent vestibulopathy, similar viral-related mechanisms may be involved in both clinical syndromes.[4-6] As discussed in Case 8, the mechanism of migraine-related dizziness also is unknown.

This patient was given a diagnosis of recurrent vestibulopathy.

TREATMENT/MANAGEMENT

There is no specific treatment for recurrent vestibulopathy. Antinausea and antiemetic agents should be prescribed to prevent a needless emergency room visit. Agents such as oral promethazine and prochlorperazine suppositories should be in the patient's possession and used when appropriate.

SUMMARY

A 51-year-old man presented with recurrent vertigo without hearing loss, tinnitus, ear fullness, or any neurologic complaints. There was no past medical history or family history to suggest a particular disorder such as migraine or panic attacks. Laboratory studies, including caloric testing and brain imaging, were normal. The patient was given the provisional diagnosis of recurrent vestibulopathy and was given prescriptions for antinausea agents to be used only on an as-needed basis.

TEACHING POINTS

1. **Recurrent vestibulopathy is a clinical syndrome that consists of multiple episodes of vertigo lasting for minutes to hours without auditory or neurologic signs or symptoms.**
2. **Recurrent vestibulopathy is a diagnosis of exclusion.** Several other disorders that can cause recurrent vertigo, such as Meniere's disease (endolymphatic hydrops), recurrent vestibular neuritis, benign paroxysmal positional vertigo, perilymphatic fistula, migraine-related vestibulopathy, vertebrobasilar insufficiency, panic disorder, and seizure disorder, should be excluded before diagnosing recurrent vestibulopathy.
3. **Recurrent vestibulopathy may be a provisional diagnosis.** Approximately 30% of patients given this diagnosis develop a condition that warrants a more specific diagnosis, most commonly endolymphatic hydrops, benign paroxysmal positional vertigo, or migraine-related vestibulopathy.
4. **The cause of recurrent vestibulopathy is not known.** A reversible viral or immune-related injury to the vestibular nerve has been hypothesized.
5. **Treatment for recurrent vestibulopathy is nonspecific.** Antinausea and antiemetic agents should be prescribed for the patient to have on hand in the event of an episode of acute vertigo.

REFERENCES

1. LeLiever WC, Barber HO: Recurrent vestibulopathy. Laryngoscope 91:1–6, 1981.
2. Rutka JA, Barber HO: Recurrent vestibulopathy: Third review. J Otolaryngol 15:105–107, 1986.
3. Ishiyama A, Ishiyama GP, Lopez I, Eversole LR, Honrubia V, Baloh RW: Histopathology of idiopathic chronic recurrent vertigo. Laryngoscope 106:1340–1346, 1996.
4. Dix MR, Hallpike CS: The pathology, symptomatology and diagnosis of certain common disorders of the vestibular system. Proc R Soc Med 45:15–28, 1952.
5. Coats AC: Vestibular neuronitis. Acta Otolaryngol 251(Suppl):1–32, 1969.
6. Schuknecht HF, Kitamura K: Vestibular neuritis. Ann Otol Rhinol Laryngol 78(Suppl):1–19, 1981.

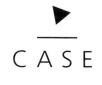

CASE

16

Meniere's Disease—
Surgical Management

HISTORY

A 36-year-old woman who worked as a cashier in a large grocery store presented with a complaint of recurrent bouts of vertigo that had occurred every 7 to 14 days for 6 months before evaluation. The spells consisted of severe rotatory vertigo, nausea, and often retching or vomiting that usually lasted for a few hours. For 1 or 2 days after the acute vertigo, she felt somewhat unsteady and dizzy when moving her head. Subsequently, her symptoms resolved within several days. The episodes of vertigo occurred irregularly and without an obvious precipitant. She reported being quite embarrassed on a number of occasions when incapacitating vertigo occurred suddenly at work. One year before evaluation, the patient had suffered a few spells of vertigo and was evaluated by her primary care physician, who thought that the vertigo might possibly be caused by Meniere's disease. The physician prescribed meclizine and a diuretic, with a low-salt diet. The patient had faithfully used the diuretic and restricted her salt intake and was symptom free for about 6 months. She felt quite frustrated by the return of the episodic vertigo.

In addition to the episodes of vertigo, the patient reported the recent onset of some hearing disturbances in her right ear. She described her hearing as sometimes muffled or clogged, with intermittent tinnitus, and fullness in her right ear before the vertigo. On the day of the evaluation, the patient noticed that loud noises sounded abnormally sharp and almost painful.

PHYSICAL EXAMINATION

The neurologic examination was normal, except that the patient had increased sway on Romberg's test. Gait was normal. Otologic examination was normal. Pressure changes induced in the external auditory canal by pneumatic otoscopy produced no dizziness or nystagmus. Neurotologic examination revealed no spontaneous nystagmus. The patient had a normal head thrust test, normal Dix-Hallpike tests, normal stability on foam with the eyes open and closed, and an abnormal stepping test with 100 degrees of rotation to the right.

DIAGNOSIS/DIFFERENTIAL DIAGNOSIS

Question 1: What is this patient's most likely diagnosis?

Answer 1: This patient is likely to have Meniere's disease (see Cases 9, 21, 25). The symptoms of recurrent vertigo, hearing loss, tinnitus, and aural fullness are characteristic of this disease. However, Meniere's disease is a clinical diagnosis. No test is absolutely diagnostic of this disease, and the presence of endolymphatic hydrops can be proved with certainty only by postmortem histologic examination of the temporal bones. It is important that the term *Meniere's disease* not be used to describe all forms of dizziness, but be restricted to patients who manifest the full symptom complex described above. Patients manifesting only part of the syndrome, such as Meniere-like vertigo without hearing loss, tinnitus, and aural fullness without vertigo, can be described as possibly having Meniere's disease. In these individuals, the true diagnosis often becomes evident over time.

This patient was given the diagnosis of Meniere's disease.

Question 2: What are the options for treating this patient?

Answer 2: It is essential that treatable causes of endolymphatic hydrops, such as immunologic, allergic, metabolic, and endocrine disorders, infectious diseases, and central nervous system abnormalities, be considered and ruled out. A number of factors such as stress, smoking, excessive salt intake, and the use of alcohol and caffeine are known to be capable of exacerbating Meniere's disease, and the patient should be encouraged to adjust her lifestyle accordingly. The use of a diuretic and dietary salt restriction is an effective treatment of Meniere's disease.[1] Other medications that have been used include vasodilators, vestibular suppressants, and calcium channel blockers. It is estimated that about 20% of individuals with Meniere's disease will eventually fail medical therapy.[1] Individuals such as this patient, who have failed medical therapy, are faced with providing symptomatic relief of each episode or considering surgical intervention, which will now be discussed.

Question 3: What surgical procedures are available to treat vertigo caused by Meniere's disease?

Answer 3: The surgical alternatives for treating vertigo caused by Meniere's disease include endolymphatic sac surgery, labyrinthectomy, and vestibular nerve section. It is essential that the patient understand that none of these procedures reduce the hearing loss, tinnitus, or aural fullness associated with Meniere's disease. In fact, any otologic surgical procedure, including endolymphatic sac sur-

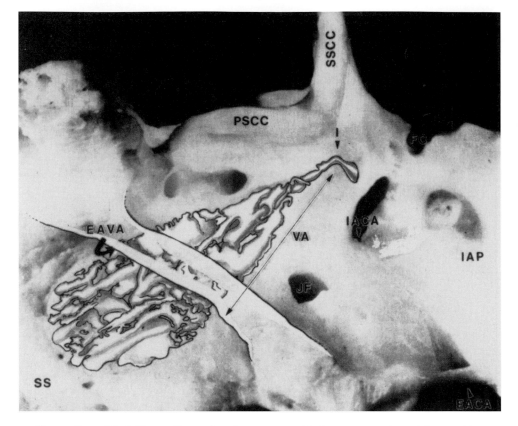

Figure Case 16–1 Three-dimensional computer-aided reconstruction of the vestibular aqueduct and endolymphatic sac anatomically positioned within a microdissected left human temporal bone. VA = vestibular aqueduct; EAVA = external aperture of the vestibular aqueduct; FC = facial canal; EACA = external aperture of the cochlear aqueduct; IACA = internal aperture of the cochlear aqueduct; IAP = internal auditory canal; JF = jugular foramen; PSCC = posterior semicircular canal; SS = sigmoid sinus; SSCC = superior semicircular canal. (*Source*: With permission from Wackym PA et al: Re-evaluation of the role of the human endolymphatic sac in Meniere's disease. Otolaryngol Head Neck Surg 102:732–744, 1990.[11])

gery and vestibular nerve section, may cause further hearing loss. Labyrinthectomy always produces complete deafness.

Endolymphatic sac surgery presumably reduces vertigo by affecting the underlying pathologic process of endolymphatic hydrops, that is, by reducing endolymphatic pressure.[2] The endolymphatic sac is illustrated in Figure Case 16–1. Endolymphatic sac surgery is a safe and uncomplicated procedure. It is usually performed as outpatient surgery and requires only 3 to 5 days of postsurgical convalescence. Unfortunately, its success rate for control of vertigo ranges between 50% and 70%. Many surgeons recognize that this low success rate approximates what would be expected from a placebo procedure and thus do not routinely recommend sac surgery.[3] Interestingly, despite its relatively low success rate, patients often choose to undergo sac surgery because of the prospect of improving their vertigo without undergoing a more involved surgical procedure.

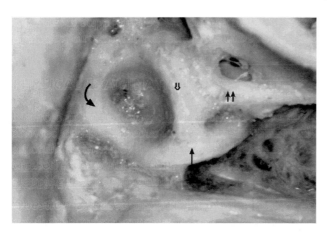

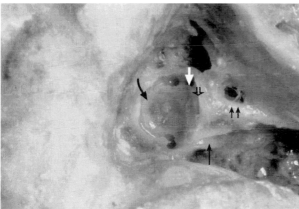

Figure Case 16–2 (A) Gross anatomic view of the semicircular canals from a microdissected right human temporal bone. (B) Surgical labyrinthectomy performed by opening each of the canals and the vestibule, with direct visualization and removal of the neuroepithelium. Curved arrow = superior semicircular canal; open arrow = horizontal semicircular canal; straight arrow = posterior semicircular canal; double arrows = facial nerve; white arrow = vestibule.

The goal of both labyrinthectomy and vestibular nerve section is to ablate permanently all vestibular function in the ear affected by Meniere's disease. The dysfunctional ear then can no longer produce vertigo because the vestibular apparatus has been destroyed (labyrinthectomy) or disconnected from the brain (vestibular nerve section). Labyrinthectomy is a highly successful procedure (90% to 95% vertigo control) and has a relatively low risk, but it always results in permanent loss of hearing in the treated ear.[4] Surgical labyrinthectomy is illustrated in Figure Case 16–2. The advantages of labyrinthectomy include brief operating time, technical ease, and the ability to visualize clearly and remove all vestibular neuroepithelium, which ensures the reliable control of vertigo.

Vestibular nerve section is also highly successful (85% to 90% vertigo control) and has the advantage that hearing is usually preserved in the treated.[5,6] Vestibular nerve section is illustrated in Figure Case 16–3. The disadvantage is that vestibular nerve section is a more complicated procedure, and although the incidence of complications is low, the potential complications can be severe.

Another form of treatment, chemical labyrinthectomy, is also available.[7] In chemical labyrinthectomy, an ototoxic medication that is preferentially toxic to vestibular but not auditory hair cells, such as gentamicin, is injected into the middle ear space (Fig. Case 16–4). Once in the middle ear, the medication reaches the inner ear through the round window membrane and exerts a toxic effect on the

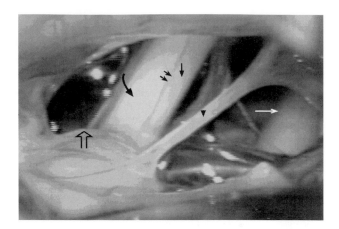

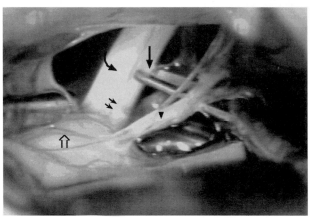

Figure Case 16–3 (A) Surgical view of the vestibular and cochlear nerves through a small craniotomy posterior to the left mastoid. (B) Selective vestibular nerve section is performed using micro-scissors. Note the small blood vessel running on the posterior surface of the vestibular-cochlear nerve complex, which helps to define the plane between the vestibular and cochlear nerve bundles. (C) Completed vestibular nerve section. Open arrow = cerebellar flocculus; curved arrow = cochlear division of the eight cranial nerve; double black arrows = blood vessel demarcating the border between the cochlear and vestibular divisions of the eighth cranial nerve; white arrow = fifth cranial nerve; arrowhead = strand of arachnoid tissue.

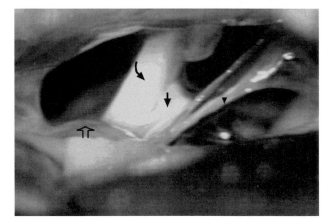

vestibular hair cells, resulting in ablation of vestibular function in the ear. Chemical labyrinthectomy is performed in the physician's office using topical anesthesia.

Control of vertigo with chemical labyrinthectomy appears to be similar to that achieved with vestibular nerve section. Hearing loss induced by chemical labyrinthectomy occurs in about 25% of patients compared to about 5% of patients following vestibular nerve section. It is unclear, however, if the long-term

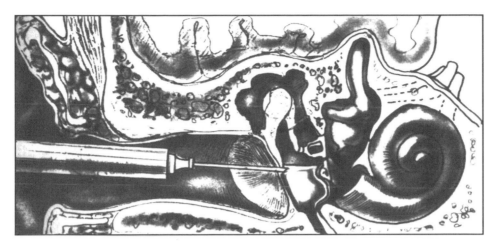

Figure Case 16–4 Schematic view of the injection of gentamicin into the middle ear space for chemical labyrinthectomy. (*Source*: With permission from Monsell EM et al: Chemical labyrinthectomy: Methods and results. In: Brackmann DE (ed): Otologic Surgery. Philadelphia: WB Saunders, 1994, p 517.[7])

hearing results differ among patients undergoing vestibular neurectomy, chemical labyrinthectomy, and the natural progression of hearing loss that characterizes Meniere's disease.

Patients with profound loss of hearing are ideal candidates for surgical or chemical labyrinthectomy. Patients with normal or nearly normal hearing are ideal candidates for vestibular nerve section. The patient and surgeon need to discuss the pros and cons of labyrinthectomy and vestibular nerve section. Our general belief is that younger patients (under age 65) with good hearing should first consider vestibular nerve section. This conclusion recognizes that (1) hearing in Meniere's disease typically fluctuates over time and could improve spontaneously after surgery; (2) individuals with a long life expectancy have a chance of unexpectedly losing hearing in their contralateral ear. If this happens, any hearing that is preserved may be of critical importance; and (3) speech reception threshold and word recognition levels do not fully describe all the beneficial aspects of hearing. *Useful* hearing is difficult to define and must be individualized.

Older patients (over age 65) who have moderate to severe hearing loss that has stopped fluctuating and who do not receive any benefit from using a hearing aid are generally better candidates for labyrinthectomy.

In the setting of bilateral Meniere's disease or unilateral Meniere's disease complicated by a contralateral hearing loss of any cause, treatment decisions regarding surgical treatment can be complex.

Question 4: What are the characteristics of patients with Meniere's disease for whom surgery is an appropriate treatment option?

Answer 4: As a general rule, the following three criteria should be met before considering surgery for vertigo. First, the vertigo should be caused by unilateral peripheral vestibular dysfunction, and the offending ear must be localized with certainty. Meniere's disease is one of the most common forms of unilateral peripheral vestibular dysfunction, and the affected side is usually unambiguously identified by the presence of unilateral hearing loss, tinnitus, and aural fullness. Second, the vertigo should be disabling to the patient. There are no hard-and-fast rules to determine disability, and each patient's situation and desires must be considered individually. Third, there should be no signs or symptoms of central vestibular system dysfunction that could impair vestibular compensation (see Chapter 1 and Cases 1 and 3).[8,9] Central nervous system dysfunction can be detected by the neurologic portion of the physical examination and confirmed by vestibular function testing. Aging also adversely affects vestibular compensation, and therefore the patient's age, both chronologic and physiologic, must be considered before recommending surgery.

Question 5: At what stage in a patient's clinical course should surgery be considered for Meniere's disease?

Answer 5: Surgical candidates should have failed at least a 6-month trial of medical therapy (diuretic and dietary salt restriction), and the vertigo should be disabling to the patient. Vertigo caused by Meniere's disease is usually incapacitating, producing violent spinning vertigo, loss of postural control, nausea, and often vomiting. These episodes usually last for a few hours, and most patients need to rest or sleep afterward. When these episodes are frequent, employment, family life, and personal well-being are threatened and surgical intervention is appropriate. As noted above, Meniere's disease should not be bilateral and there should be no evidence of central nervous system dysfunction. Younger individuals with financial and family responsibilities are more likely to feel disabled by the recurrent vertigo and often seek a surgical remedy earlier in their disease than nonworking or retired individuals, who can usually tolerate this condition without much disruption of their lifestyle. Thus, because Meniere's disease is not a life-threatening disorder, surgical intervention should be emphasized only when vertigo is causing a significant and unacceptable change in a patient's lifestyle.

Question 6: What laboratory testing is indicated before surgery for Meniere's disease?

Answer 6: Vestibular function testing is indicated to search for evidence of coexisting central nervous system dysfunction and to assess function in both the affected and unaffected ears. Central nervous system dysfunction is a contraindication to surgery because of its potential adverse effect on postsurgical vestibular compensation, which is required for a successful clinical outcome. Also, it is helpful to know whether the contralateral ear has normal caloric function. Moreover, the degree of caloric weakness in the affected ear can be used to estimate the severity of the postsurgical acute vestibular syndrome. If the ear to be operated on has absent responses preoperatively, the patient's immediate postoperative vestibular imbalance may be mild because the patient probably already has compensated for a unilateral vestibular deficit.

An audiogram is indicated to (1) confirm the involved ear and to be sure it fits into a Meniere-type pattern; (2) to document the amount and usefulness of the remaining hearing to the patient because, as noted above, this information is an important factor in deciding which surgical procedure to consider; and (3) to assess whether the contralateral ear is also affected by endolymphatic hydrops.

Brainstem auditory-evoked potentials or brain imaging is also indicated in all patients before surgical intervention to assess the central nervous system.

LABORATORY TESTING

Videonystagmography: Ocular motor function including saccades, pursuit, and optokinetic nystagmus was normal. A low-amplitude left-beating spontaneous vestibular nystagmus was noted. There was no positional nystagmus. Caloric irrigation revealed a very significant (>50%) right reduced vestibular response.

Rotational testing revealed normal gain and phase, with a mild left directional preponderance. Posturography was normal.

Audiometric testing showed normal hearing in the left ear and a mild low-frequency sensorineural hearing loss in the right ear. Word recognition scores were 100% in each ear.

An MRI scan of the brain with and without gadolinium enhancement was normal.

TREATMENT/MANAGEMENT

The patient elected to undergo right selective vestibular nerve section. The surgical procedure was performed without complications and required approximately 3 hours. After surgery, the patient remained in the hospital for 4 days. On the first postoperative day, the patient was very nauseated and vomited when she rolled over in bed. She stayed in bed the entire day and required intravenous hydration and intramuscular antiemetics. Interestingly, she stated that an acute attack of Meniere's disease was worse than the way she felt after surgery. Third-degree left-beating vestibular nystagmus, that is, a horizontal-torsional left-beating vestibular nystagmus that was present in all fields of gaze but worst on leftward gaze, was noted. On the second postoperative day, she was able to get out of bed, ambulate with assistance, and drink fluids without vomiting. Her gait was wide-based and slow. She consistently veered to the right and restricted her head movement. Examination of her extraocular movements revealed the presence of second-degree vestibular nystagmus, that is, a nystagmus that was like the third-degree nystagmus seen the previous day except that now it was present only with gaze straight ahead and to the left. There was no nystagmus on rightward gaze. On consultation with a physical therapist, the patient was instructed regarding the use of head, eye, and body exercises to promote vestibular compensation (see Chapter 6). The patient was discharged home on the fourth postoperative day. On the day of discharge, a first-degree vestibular nystagmus was noted, that is, a nystagmus that was present only on gaze to the left but absent on rightward or straight-ahead gaze. The patient was able to return to work about 1 month later.

Question 7: Can Meniere's disease occur in both ears?

Answer 7: Yes. Estimates in the literature of the incidence of bilateral Meniere's disease in patients with initially unilateral symptoms range between 5% and 50%. This wide range of estimates largely reflects the criteria used to determine if Meniere'disease was present in the opposite ear. A reasonable estimate is that 5% of patients with unilateral disease will develop the complete symptom triad of Meniere's disease in the opposite ear. Up to 50% of patients may describe symptoms in the opposite ear such as tinnitus, aural fullness, or hearing loss that may possibly be related to Meniere's disease.

Question 8: Can bilateral Meniere's disease occur many years following the onset of unilateral Meniere's disease?

Answer 8: Yes; however, in most patients with bilateral Meniere's disease, the two ears become symptomatic within 2 years of one another.

Question 9: Are patients with bilateral Meniere's disease treated differently?

Answer 9: Yes. In patients with bilateral Meniere's disease, a thorough search for autoimmune disease of the ear, Cogan's syndrome, and allergic, leutic, and metabolic causes of ear disease should be undertaken. Oral immunosuppressive therapy for at least 6 weeks should be tried. Ablative procedures should be avoided if possible. Endolymphatic sac decompression and shunting can be used when one of the ears can be clearly identified as the active offending ear. In patients with persistent and disabling symptoms, intramuscular streptomycin therapy can be used.

Question 10: What is intramuscular streptomycin therapy?

Answer 10: Intramuscular streptomycin[10] can produce a bilateral reduction of vestibular function and can be used to treat vertigo caused by simultaneously active Meniere's disease in both ears, vertigo in a patient with bilateral Meniere's disease when the active ear cannot be determined, Meniere's disease in an only hearing ear, and Meniere's disease in the second ear when the first ear has been previously treated with an ablative procedure. Intramuscular streptomycin must be given in a controlled manner to produce subtotal vestibular ablation, with the dose titrated to control episodes of acute vertigo while stopping short of complete bilateral loss of vestibular function.

SUMMARY

A 36-year-old woman presented with a 1-year history of recurrent vertigo. She was diagnosed as having unilateral Meniere's disease. Medical therapy was unsuccessful. She was treated with surgery consisting of a selective vestibular nerve section. Her hearing was unchanged. Vertiginous episodes ceased. The patient underwent vestibular rehabilitation with a physical therapist and returned to work 1 month following surgery.

TEACHING POINTS

1. **Meniere's disease is characterized by recurrent vertigo, hearing loss, tinnitus, and aural fullness.** Meniere's disease is a clinical diagnosis, and no test is absolutely diagnostic for it. Meniere's disease may be considered the idiopathic form of endolymphatic hydrops. It is essential that known treatable causes of endolymphatic hydrops such as metabolic, endocrine, and infectious diseases be considered and ruled out. Several factors such as stress, excessive salt intake, and use of tobacco, alcohol, and caffeine can exacerbate Meniere's disease.
2. **Medical treatment of Meniere's disease includes the use of a diuretic and dietary salt restriction.** However, about 20% of individuals with Meniere's disease will eventually fail medical therapy.

3. **Surgical treatment for Meniere's disease includes endolymphatic sac surgery, labyrinthectomy, and vestibular nerve section.** It is essential that the patient understand that none of these procedures reduce the hearing loss, tinnitus, or aural fullness associated with Meniere's disease. Surgical candidates should have failed at least a 6-month trial of medical therapy (diuretic and dietary salt restriction), and the vertigo should be disabling to the patient.

4. **Chemical labyrinthectomy, an alternative to surgery, is a new non-surgical procedure.** It produces ablation of vestibular function without surgery or general anesthesia. This procedure consists of instillation of an ototoxic agent, typically an aminoglycoside antibiotic, into the middle ear. Chemical labyrinthectomy is especially applicable to elderly or infirm patients with disabling vertigo.

5. **Vestibular function testing in Meniere's disease may uncover coexisting central nervous system dysfunction.** Central nervous system dysfunction is a contraindication to surgery because of its potential adverse effect on postsurgical vestibular compensation, which is required for a successful clinical outcome.

6. **The incidence of bilateral Meniere's disease is between 5% and 50%.** A reasonable estimate is that 5% of patients with unilateral disease will develop the complete symptom triad of Meniere's disease in the opposite ear. Up to 50% of patients may describe symptoms in the opposite ear such as tinnitus, aural fullness, or hearing loss that may possibly be related to Meniere's disease. Bilateral Meniere's disease occur many years following the onset of unilateral Meniere's disease. However, in most patients with bilateral Meniere's disease, the two ears become symptomatic within 2 years of one another.

7. **In patients with bilateral Meniere's disease, a thorough search for autoimmune disease of the ear, Cogan's syndrome, and allergic, leutic, and metabolic causes of ear disease should be undertaken.** Oral immunosuppressive therapy for at least 6 weeks should be tried. Ablative procedures should be avoided if possible. In patients with persistent and disabling symptoms, intramuscular streptomycin therapy can be used.

REFERENCES

1. Jackson CG, Glasscock ME, Davis WE: Medical management of Meniere's disease. Ann Otol 90:142–147, 1981.
2. Monsell EM, Wiet RJ: Endolymphatic sac surgery: Methods of study and results. Am J Otol 9:396–402, 1988.
3. Silverstein H, Smouha E, Jones R: Natural history vs. surgery for Meniere's disease. Otolaryngol Head Neck Surg 100:6–16, 1989.
4. Kemink JL, Telian SA, Graham MD, Joynt L: Transmatoid labyrinthectomy: Reliable surgical management of vertigo. Otolaryngol Head Neck Surg 101:5–10, 1989.
5. Silverstein H, Norell H: Retrolabyrinthine vestibular neurectomy. Otolaryngol Head Neck Surg 90:778–782, 1982.
6. Monsell EM, Wiet RJ, Young NM, Kazan RP: Surgical treatment of vertigo with retrolabyrinthine vestibular neurectomy. Laryngoscope 98:835–839, 1988.
7. Monsell EM, Cass SP, Rybak LP: Chemical labyrinthectomy: Methods and results. In: Brackmann DE (ed). Otologic Surgery. Philadelphia: WB Saunders, 1994, pp 509–518.

8. Monsell EM, Brackmann DE, Linthicum FH: Why do vestibular destructive procedures sometimes fail? Otolaryngol Head Neck Surg 99:472–479, 1988.

9. Konrad HR: Intractable vertigo—When not to operate. Otolaryngol Head Neck Surg 95:482–484, 1986.

10. Langman AW, Kemink JL, Graham MD: Titration streptomycin therapy for bilateral Meniere's disease. Ann Otol Rhinol Laryngol 99:923–926, 1990.

11. Wackym PA, Linthicum FH Jr, Ward PH, House WF, Micevych PE, Bagger-Sjoback D: Re-evaluation of the role of the human endolymphatic sac in Meniere's disease. Otolaryngol Head Neck Surg 102:732–744, 1990.

CASE

17

Nonspecific Vestibulopathy

HISTORY

A 30-year-old female data processor presented with a chief complaint of dizziness and disequilibrium. The patient's complaints were of approximately 1 year's duration, worse in the last several months, especially premenstrually. There was a constant sense of dizziness and disequilibrium, with periodic exacerbations lasting for several days. There was no positional dizziness. When the patient was symptomatic, she noticed that rapid head movements were bothersome and that looking at her computer screen at work caused discomfort, including mild nausea and "eye strain." She had no neurologic complaints. The patient walked regularly for exercise and noticed that, when symptomatic, she veered slightly both to the right and to the left. There was no history of headache and no family history of migraine headache. The patient had no complaint of hearing loss or tinnitus and no complaint of fullness, pain, or stuffiness in the ears. She was evaluated extensively by her primary care physician, with no diagnosis reached. An MRI scan revealed that the cerebellar tonsils were 2 mm below the foramen magnum, without evidence of compression of brainstem or caudal midline cerebellar structures. The patient noted some increase in symptoms in shopping malls and grocery stores but was able to carry on her homemaking activities. She had not experienced panic attacks. The patient used meclizine on an as-needed basis. This provided some relief, but she was still symptomatic.

Question 1: Based on the patient's history, what is the differential diagnosis?

Answer 1: This patient has a symptom complex that is nonspecific but does suggest some impairment of the balance system. Although she has a Chiari malformation by imaging criteria, it is unlikely to be symptomatic, considering her his-

169

tory and the lack of compression of posterior fossa structures.[1] However, a physical examination will be helpful in establishing whether a Chiari malformation could be causing some or all of the patient's symptoms (see Case 40). Because the patient benefited from meclizine, she may have a vestibular system abnormality, a mild anxiety condition, or both. From the information available, there are many conditions that are unlikely, including endolymphatic hydrops, benign paroxysmal positional vertigo, migraine-related dizziness, and multiple sclerosis. It is unlikely that a definitive diagnosis will be reached.

PHYSICAL EXAMINATION

The patient's general, neurologic, otologic, and neurotologic examinations were normal, with the exception of some difficulty standing on a compliant foam surface with the eyes closed. The patient's gait had a slightly widened base.

LABORATORY TESTING

Videonystagmography: Ocular motor, positional, and caloric tests were normal.
   A mild right directional preponderance was seen on rotational testing.
   Posturography indicated minimally excessive sway on conditions 5 and 6.
   The blood tests including metabolic, hematologic, rheumatologic, and thyroid tests were normal.

DIAGNOSIS/DIFFERENTIAL DIAGNOSIS

Question 2: Based on all of the information available, what diagnosis can be given to this patient?

Answer 2: This patient does not have a well-defined disease process. This patient's evaluation does not suggest a symptomatic Chiari malformation (see Case 40). Based upon the history and laboratory abnormalities, the patient could be given the diagnosis of *vestibulopathy* of unknown origin. This is a diagnosis of exclusion, so it must be remembered that other conditions that are difficult to rule out, such as migraine, are possibilities. Follow-up care may allow a specific diagnosis.
   This patient was given the diagnosis of nonspecific vestibulopathy.

TREATMENT/MANAGEMENT

Question 3: What are the treatment options for a patient with nonspecific vestibulopathy?

Answer 3: In patients in whom a specific diagnosis cannot be made but in whom vestibular system involvement is highly suspected, treatment may consist of one or more of the modalities listed in Table Case 17–1. The choice of medication will depend on the physician's judgment about the importance and predominance of

Table Case 17–1
Treatment Modalities
for Nonspecific
Vestibulopathy

Antinausea agents
Vestibular-suppressant agents
Antianxiety agents
Antidepressants
Vestibular rehabilitation therapy

symptoms of nausea, dizziness, anxiety, depression, or a functional impairment of balance.[2]

Medications commonly used to decrease dizziness and nausea are listed in Table Case 17–2. Note that these medications have multiple effects. Specifically, medications used to decrease nausea may also reduce dizzines, and drugs used to decrease dizziness often have antinausea properties. The primary action of these medications and their major side effects are also listed in Table Case 17–2.

Some patients respond favorably to antianxiety or antidepressant medications even when their complaints of dizziness are quite prominent. We have also found that adding a sympathomimetic agent such as pseudoephedrine to agents that cause lethargy, such as promethazine hydrochloride, can be useful. In our experience, prochlorperazine should be reserved for patients with acute vestibular symptoms, such as those experienced during the very early stages of vestibular neuritis or during a severe episode of endolymphatic hydrops. We have found little use for transdermal scopolamine in patients with vestibulopathy. In addition to the minimal relief provided, there is frequently a complaint of anticholinergic side effects including blurred vision, which may actually worsen the symptoms of dizziness. Also, discontinuation of scopolamine can be problematic.

The patient was given oral clonazepam, 0.25 mg twice daily. She was also encouraged to increase her physical activity. She had some relief of symptoms but continued to experience mild dizziness and disequilibrium.

SUMMARY

A 30-year-old woman presented with nonspecific dizziness and disequilibrium of a constant nature with periodic exacerbations. The patient's evaluation did not reveal a specific diagnosis but suggested a vestibular system abnormality that could not definitely be localized to the central or peripheral vestibular system. Treatment was therefore symptomatic. The patient was given oral clonazepam, 0.25 mg twice daily. She was also encouraged to increase her physical activity. She had some relief of symptoms but continued to experience mild dizziness and disequilibrium.

TEACHING POINTS

1. *Vestibulopathy of unknown origin* and *nonspecific vestibulopathy* are terms used to describe a complex of nonspecific symptoms that sug-

Table Case 17–2 Medications Commonly Used to Reduce Dizziness, Vertigo, and Associated Nausea

Generic Name	Trade Name	Class	Dosage	Primary Symptom Treatment	Side Effects
Prochlorperazine	Compazine	Phenothiazine	10 mg orally or IM every 6 hours or 25 mg rectally every 12 hours	Nausea	Extrapyramidal reactions, drowsiness, anticholinergic effects
Promethazine with pseudoephedrine	Phenergan	Phenothiazine	25 mg orally or rectally every 6 hours (promethazine) 60 mg orally every 6 hours (pseudophedrine)	Nausea	Extrapyramidal reactions, drowsiness Restlessness
Meclizine	Antivert, Bonine	Piperazine (H_1-blocking agent)	25 mg orally every 4 to 6 hours	Dizziness	Drowsiness
Dimenhydrinate	Dramamine	Ethanolamine (H_1-blocking agent)	50 mg orally every 4 to 6 hours	Dizziness	Drowsiness
Scopolamine	Transerm Scop	Amine antimuscarinic	0.5 mg adhesive skin patches every 3 days	Dizziness	Dry mouth, blurred vision, drowsiness, disorientation
Cyclizine	Marezine	Piperzine (H_1-blocking agent)	50 mg orally or IM every 4 to 6 hours	Dizziness	Drowsiness
Clonazepam	Klonopin	Benzodiazepine	0.25–0.5 mg orally twice daily	Dizziness	Lethargy
Diazepam	Valium	Benzodiazepine	2–10 mg orally, IM, or IV every 4 to 6 hours	Dizziness	Lethargy
Trimethobenzamine	Tigan	Substituted ethanolamine	250 mg orally every 6 to 8 hours or 200 mg rectally or IM	Nausea	Extrapyramidal reaction (unusual)
Diphenhydramine	Benadryl	Ethanolamine (H_1-blocking agent)	25–50 mg orally, IM, or IV every 6 hours	Nausea	Drowsiness
Hydroxyzine	Vistaril, Atarax	Piperazine derivative	25–100 mg orally every 8 hours	Nausea	Drowsiness

gest some impairment of the balance system but do not fit any recognized vestibular syndromes.

2. **Nonspecific vestibulopathy is a diagnosis of exclusion.** Conditions that should be considered and ruled out include Meniere's disease (endolymphatic hydrops), benign paroxysmal positional vertigo, migraine-related dizziness, anxiety and panic disorders, and potential central nervous system abnormalities such as multiple sclerosis, Chiari malformation, or neoplasm. Follow-up care is important because a specific diagnosis may become evident over time.

3. **Treatment options for nonspecific vestibulopathy include medications and a course of vestibular rehabilitation therapy.** The choice of treatment depends on the physician's judgment about the importance and predominance of symptoms of nausea, dizziness, anxiety, depression, or a functional impairment of balance. Medications commonly used to decrease dizziness, vertigo, and nausea are listed in Table Case 17–2.

REFERENCES

1. Weber PC, Cass SP: Neurotologic manifestation of Chiari 1 malformation. Otolaryngol Head Neck Surg 109:853–860, 1993.
2. Cass SP: Role of medications in otological vertigo and balance disorders. Semin Hearing 12:257–269, 1991.

Chronic Otitis Media

HISTORY

A 45-year-old male insurance agent presented with 1 week of disequilibrium that had started after 1 day of vertigo, nausea, and vomiting 3 days following the onset of a malodorous discharge and pain in his left ear. Since resolution of the acute spell of vertigo, the patient had had disequilibrium that varied in intensity. He noted occasional staggering but otherwise was only mildly unsteady. The patient did not complain of any positional symptoms but felt mildly lightheaded and dizzy even at rest. In addition, he reported that recently he could provoke brief vertigo by putting his finger in his left ear to relieve itching. He also occasionally noticed momentary vertigo when he heard a loud sound. The patient reported a lifelong history of recurrent ear infections and had undergone mastoid surgery on the left ear at age 10 years. Medicated ear drops were prescribed for him by his primary care physician before evaluation.

Question 1: Based on the patient's history, what are the diagnostic considerations?

Answer 1: The history of chronic ear infections and the occurrence of a malodorous discharge immediately preceding the onset of vertigo suggest that the patient's vertigo may be related to infection involving the middle ear and mastoid. Considering his long history of middle ear problems, the patient may simply be experiencing an acute exacerbation of chronic otitis media, or there may be an ongoing chronic middle ear infection related to recurrent cholesteatoma (see later). Alternatively, the patient's complaints may have no relationship whatever to past and present middle or outer ear problems. If so, the differential diagnosis is broad.

174

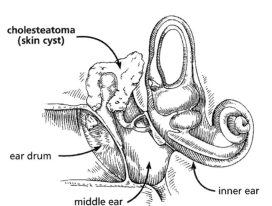

cholesteatoma (skin cyst)

ear drum

middle ear

inner ear

Figure Case 18–1 Schematic drawing of the ear drum, cholesteatoma within the middle ear space, and the inner ear. The cholesteatoma is shown causing erosion of the lateral semicircular canal, resulting in a bony fistula. (*Source*: Modified with permission from Glasscock ME et al: Handbook of Vertigo. New York: Raven Press, 1990.[6])

Question 2: What is a cholesteatoma of the ear?

Answer 2: A cholesteatoma of the ear is a skin cyst that behaves like a localized tumor (Fig. Case 18–1). It causes destruction of bone and predisposes to repeated acute middle ear and mastoid infections. Cholesteatoma of the ear is usually found in the presence of chronic middle ear infection (chronic otitis media).

Question 3: How do chronic otitis media and cholesteatoma cause vertigo?

Answer 3: An acute exacerbation of chronic otitis media can cause vertigo and dizziness as a result of bacterial toxins contained in the inflammatory exudate of the middle ear reaching the vestibular labyrinth, usually by transmission through the round window membrane. This process is referred to as *serous labyrinthitis* and also may be associated with sensorineural hearing loss primarily affecting the high frequencies. Cholesteatoma of the ear may cause dizziness by creating a perilymphatic fistula as a result of erosion of the bony vestibular labyrinth (Fig. Case 18–1). The combination of an erosive perilymphatic fistula and otitis media can cause both serous labyrinthitis and bacterial labyrinthitis.[1–4]

Question 4: How can an acute exacerbation of chronic otitis media be distinguished from a cholesteatoma of the ear?

Answer 4: Chronic otitis media and cholesteatoma of the ear cannot be distinguished on the basis of the history. Diagnosis of a cholesteatoma of the ear can be made by debridement of the external ear followed by an otologic examination using an operative microscope by a physician skilled in the management of otologic disease. If a cholesteatoma is found, CT imaging is indicated to aid in evaluating the bony labyrinth for erosion and fistula formation. Imaging studies are not indicated before cleaning and examining the ear.

PHYSICAL EXAMINATION

The patient's general and neurologic examinations were normal, including a negative Romberg's test and normal gait. He was able to stand on compliant foam with his eyes open but not with his eyes closed, indicating an ongoing vestibular system abnormality. On the stepping test, the patient rotated 120 degrees to the

left. Compression of the tragus produced both nystagmus and a sensation of vertigo. Otologic examination revealed a malodorous yellow discharge draining from
the left ear, a tympanic membrane perforation, and thickened polypoid mucosa
in the middle ear space. With the operative microscope, the ear was cleaned using suction and debrided to reveal minimal bony erosion of the external auditory
canal wall and a large cholesteatoma pocket with a moist cholesteatoma matrix
overlying the area of the lateral semicircular canal. On tuning fork examination,
the Weber's test showed lateralization to the right. The Rinne test was positive
on the right, but no abnormality was detected on the left.

Question 5: What do the results of the physical examination suggest about the
cause of this patient's vertigo?

Answer 5: The presence of a large cholesteatoma with active inflammation overlying the lateral semicircular canal suggests that the patient's vertigo may be
caused by the presence of fistulization of the lateral semicircular canal. The vertigo and nystagmus induced by pressure changes in the external auditory canal
using pneumatic otoscopy or tragal pressure are known as *Hennebert's symptoms
and signs* and are highly suggestive of bony labyrinthine fistula. The tuning fork
tests suggest a profound sensorineural hearing loss in the left ear.

Question 6: What is the value of vestibular laboratory testing at this point in the
evaluation of this patient?

Answer 6: The presence of a cholesteatoma and a positive Hennebert's sign
strongly suggest that a bony fistula in the left ear is the source of the patient's
vestibular symptoms. The profound sensorineural hearing loss in the left ear further suggests that the fistula has produced both auditory and vestibular damage.
Although caloric testing can provide information regarding responsiveness of the
vestibular labyrinth, vestibular laboratory testing is not indicated because of the
presence of the severe acute infection. Also, vestibular testing in the setting of an
acute middle ear infection is very uncomfortable and does not provide further
significant information needed for diagnosis at this time.

Question 7: What is the value of obtaining a CT scan at this point in the patient's
evaluation? What is the value of MRI?

Answer 7: A high-resolution CT scan of the temporal bone can define the bony
architecture of the vestibular labyrinth and mastoid and can confirm the presence
of a bony labyrinthine fistula. In addition, other potentially life-threatening conditions such as a sigmoid sinus thrombosis or a dural abscess may be detected.
A CT scan is indicated rather than MRI because of the ability of CT to image the
bony anatomy of the labyrinth; MRI of the temporal bone could reveal widespread
inflammation but could not provide the anatomic detail necessary to confirm the
diagnosis of a bony labyrinthine fistula.

LABORATORY TESTING

Vestibular laboratory function testing was deferred because of the presence of
acute infection and discharge.

Audiometric testing showed normal hearing in the right ear but profound
sensorineural hearing loss in the left ear.

A CT scan of the temporal bones confirmed the presence of a bony fistula of the horizontal semicircular canal.

DIAGNOSIS/DIFFERENTIAL DIAGNOSIS

The patient was given the diagnosis of chronic otitis media with cholesteatoma formation and a fistula of the horizontal semicircular canal.

TREATMENT/MANAGEMENT

Following debridement of the ear, the patient was placed on an oral antibiotic and medicated otic drops. He was asked to return in 1 week for further debridement and examination.

The patient returned in 1 week with significant improvement in his symptoms. The drainage had greatly diminished, and the dizziness had been reduced but had not disappeared completely. Otologic examination revealed significant improvement in the amount of discharge and inflammation present in the middle ear and mastoid space, which was visible because of the previous surgery at age 10. The patient's medications were changed from medicated otic drops to daily boric acid irrigation of the ear. He was counseled about the need for future revision mastoid surgery, which was performed.

Question 8: What constitutes surgery for cholesteatoma? When is surgery indicated for a patient who presents with vertigo and is found to have otitis media and a cholesteatoma? Should this patient be advised to undergo repeat mastoid surgery?

Answer 8: Surgery for cholesteatoma consists of opening the mastoid cavity and excising the cholesteatoma or widely exteriorizing the cholesteatoma skin cyst.[5] If a bony fistula of a semicircular canal is found, the skin covering the fistula is usually not dissected off the fistula because this can cause further deterioration of hearing and vestibular symptoms. However, by preventing the further progression and inflammation associated with the cholesteatoma, further acute vertiginous symptoms are usually eliminated. Unfortunately, in this case there is no treatment for the hearing loss, which is permanent.

Surgery is indicated for a patient with a cholesteatoma that is not *self-cleaning,* that is, that produces repeated acute infections, or that is associated with complications such as vertigo, hearing loss, facial nerve paralysis, or central nervous system complications such as meningitis, dural venous sinus thrombosis, or a dural abscess. In this patient's case, there is a large cholesteatoma that has produced a bony labyrinthine fistula with concomitant hearing loss and vertigo. If this cholesteatoma is treated only medically, it is likely that the patient will undergo additional repeated acute attacks of vertigo, suffer persistent imbalance, and be at risk for central nervous system complications of bacterial infection.

Question 9: What is the proper treatment of patients with chronic otitis media that is not associated with cholesteatoma?

Answer 9: Acute exacerbations of chronic otitis media are treated primarily with frequent debridement, local antibiotics, and oral antibiotics. Occasionally, tympanoplasty and mastoid surgery are required, but only after the failure of local care.

SUMMARY

A 45-year-old man with a previous history of chronic ear disease and mastoid surgery at age 10 years presented with disequilibrium following the onset of acute vertigo after 3 days of a malodorous discharge from his left ear. The patient's ear was debrided, revealing the presence of a cholesteatoma. He had a positive Hennebert's sign and a profound loss of hearing in the left ear, suggesting the presence of a bony labyrinthine fistula. A fistula of the horizontal semicircular canal was confirmed by CT imaging. Treatment consisted of repeated debridement and ototopic agents followed by a revision mastoidectomy.

TEACHING POINTS

1. **Acute otitis media or an acute exacerbation of chronic otitis media can cause vertigo and dizziness as a result of bacterial toxins contained in the middle ear inflammatory exudate reaching the vestibular labyrinth, usually by transmission through the round window membrane.** This process is referred to as *serous labyrinthitis* and may also be associated with sensorineural hearing loss primarily affecting the high frequencies.

2. **A cholesteatoma of the ear is a skin cyst that behaves like a localized tumor. It causes destruction of bone and predisposes to repeated acute middle ear infections.** Cholesteatoma of the ear is often found in the presence of chronic middle ear infection and can cause dizziness by creating a perilymphatic fistula as a result of erosion of the bony vestibular labyrinth. The combination of an erosive perilymphatic fistula and otitis media can cause both serous labyrinthitis and bacterial labyrinthitis.

3. **A bony labyrinthine fistula should be considered in a patient with a history of chronic otitis media who presents with Hennebert's symptoms and signs, vertigo, and nystagmus induced by pressure changes in the external auditory canal.** A high-resolution CT scan of the temporal bone can define the bony architecture of the vestibular labyrinth and mastoid and should be used to confirm the presence of a bony labyrinthine fistula. An MRI scan of the temporal bone can reveal widespread inflammation but cannot provide the anatomic detail necessary to confirm the diagnosis of a bony labyrinthine fistula.

4. **Treatment of vertigo caused by acute otitis media in an otherwise normal ear includes drainage and both topical and oral antibiotics.**

5. **Treatment of vertigo associated with an acute exacerbation of chronic otitis media or cholesteatoma requires repeated debridement of the ear, a combination of oral and topical antibiotics, and CT imaging of the ear.** Surgery is indicated for a patient with a cholesteatoma that is not self-cleaning, that is, that produces repeated acute infections, or that is associated with complications such as vertigo, hearing loss, facial nerve paralysis, or central nervous system complications such as meningitis, dural venous sinus thrombosis, or a dural abscess.

REFERENCES

1. Paparella M, Sugiura S: The pathology of suppurative labyrinthitis. Ann Otol Rhinol Laryngol 76:554–586, 1967.
2. Walby PA, Barrerra A, Schuknecht HF: Cochlear pathology in chronic suppurative otitis media. Ann Otol Rhinol Laryngol 103(Suppl):3–19, 1983.
3. Meyerhoff WL, Kim CS, Paparella MM: Pathology of chronic otitis media. Ann Otol 87:749–760, 1978.
4. Paparella MM, Morizono T, Le CT, Mancini F, Sipila P, Choo YB, Liden G, Kim CS: Sensorineural hearing loss in otitis media. Ann Otol Rhinol Laryngol 93:623–629, 1984.
5. Sheehy JL, Brackmann DE, Graham MD: Cholesteatoma surgery: Residual and recurrent disease. Ann Otol Rhinol Laryngol 86:1–12, 1977.
6. Glasscock ME, Cueva RA, Thedinger BA: Handbook of Vertigo. New York: Raven Press, 1990.

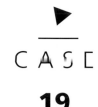

CASE

19

Cerebellar Degeneration

HISTORY

A 65-year-old man presented with a gradually worsening course of disequilibrium and gait instability. The patient did not complain of vertigo, hearing loss, or tinnitus. His problem had been present for at least 5 years and possibly for as long as 10 years, with gradually increasing difficulty with balance while walking, especially on uneven surfaces while hunting. He did not notice any particular worsening of his balance in dimly lit environments. There was some exacerbation of symptoms with rapid head movements. There were no symptoms with position change. The patient had no past medical history of importance and used no medication. His family history was significant; his mother, who died in her early 80s, had suffered from a gradually worsening balance problem and became wheelchair-bound in her middle to late 70s.

Question 1: Based on the patient's history, what are the diagnostic considerations and what further historical information would be helpful?

Answer 1: This patient has a nonspecific balance complaint. There is little in the history to suggest a peripheral vestibular process. Rather, the patient's complaint of abnormal gait suggests a central nervous system, possibly a cerebellar, disorder. Further, the gradual worsening of the patient's problem suggests a degenerative disorder, especially because of the positive family history, but a mass lesion must also be considered. A multisensory disequilibrium should also be considered, although there is nothing in the history that suggests sensory system involvement.

It would be helpful to learn more about the patient's ethanol use and any information regarding toxic exposures. A more detailed family history would also be helpful.

180

FURTHER HISTORY

The patient denied significant ethanol consumption. There was no past medical history of pancreatitis, seizures, or cirrhosis of the liver. The family history was significant; for his mother and maternal uncle had had a late-onset balance disorder. The patient's older brother was killed in World War II, and his 60-year-old sister had no balance complaints.

PHYSICAL EXAMINATION

The patient had no postural hypotension. Neurologic examination revealed full extraocular movements. However, pursuit tracking was not smooth, and a bilateral horizontal gaze-evoked nystagmus was seen. Motor examination was normal. Coordination testing showed very mild abnormalities of rapid alternating movements, finger-to-nose movements, and heel-knee-shin movements. Sensation was normal. The patient's gait was extremely wide-based, and the patient was ataxic and unable to tandem walk. He had great difficulty standing with his feet together even with his eyes open, so Romberg's test could not be performed. Otologic examination was normal. Neurotologic examination revealed no spontaneous nystagmus, a normal head thrust, and no positional or positioning nystagmus. Stance on foam could not be assessed, and the stepping test could not be performed.

Question 2: Based on the history and physical examination, what laboratory tests would provide further information regarding this patient's problems?

Answer 2: The patient's history and physical examination suggest a central nervous system abnormality, probably affecting the cerebellum. Diagnostic considerations include cerebellar degeneration (unlikely to be due to alcoholism) and a posterior fossa mass lesion. Other conditions to be considered, although unlikely, include vasculitis, a paraneoplastic process, or a structural abnormality such as a Chiari malformation. Thus, MRI of the brain with special attention to the posterior fossa is appropriate. Additionally, vestibular laboratory testing specifically to assess cerebellar function should be considered.

LABORATORY TESTING

Videonystagmography: Ocular motor testing revealed normal velocity saccades with overshoot dysmetria, impaired pursuit, dysrhythmic optokinetic nystagmus, that is, irregular quick component generation, and no spontaneous nystagmus.

Rotational testing indicated symmetric responses of high-normal response amplitude with an abnormally large phase lead. Nystagmus dysrhythmia, that is, an irregular pattern of quick and slow components of nystagmus, was also noted on rotational testing. Visual–vestibular interaction testing (see Chapter 4) was abnormal in that there was difficulty suppressing vestibular responses while viewing a head-fixed target during sinusoidal rotation, and the magnitude of the nystagmus during rotation while viewing earth-fixed stripes was not significantly greater than the magnitude of nystagmus elicited by rotation in darkness.

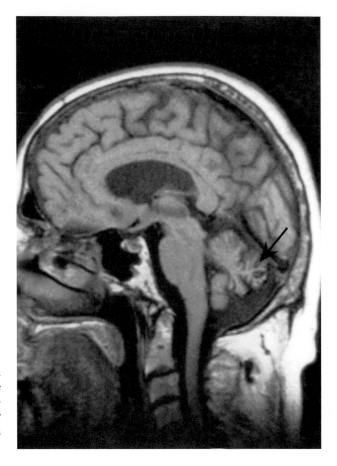

Figure Case 19–1 Note on this sagittal MRI scan that the midline cerebellum is atrophied (arrow). The cerebellar vermian sulci are larger than normal.

Posturography indicated moderately excessive sway in all conditions in a nonspecific pattern.

An MRI scan of the brain showed midline cerebellar degeneration (Fig. Case 19–1). There was obvious involvement of the anterior cerebellar vermis and a suggestion of loss of tissue in the caudal midline cerebellum. No other abnormalities were seen on the MRI scan.

The screening blood studies including hematologic, metabolic, rheumatologic, and thyroid studies were normal.

Question 3: Under what circumstances is visual–vestibular interaction testing useful?

Answer 3: Visual–vestibular interaction testing is useful as an adjunct to quantitative vestibular laboratory testing when information is needed regarding the patient's ability to modify vestibular reflexes with vision. Visual–vestibular interaction is a particularly sensitive measure when searching for evidence of an abnormality of the vestibulocerebellum.[1] Although most patients with abnormalities of visual–vestibular interaction also have abnormalities of ocular pursuit, several studies have indicated that visual–vestibular interaction provides information beyond that which can be obtained from measuring pursuit.[2] In this patient's case, abnormal visual–vestibular interaction confirms the suspicion of abnormal central vestibular processing and suggests involvement of the cerebellar flocculus in the degeneration syndrome.

DIAGNOSIS/DIFFERENTIAL DIAGNOSIS

Question 4: Based on the history, physical examination, and laboratory studies, what is the localization of this patient's abnormality and what is its likely etiology?

Answer 4: The patient's history, physical examination, and laboratory studies all point toward an abnormality of cerebellar function. The MRI scan documents loss of midline cerebellar tissue, and quantitative laboratory testing documents ocular motor and vestibulo-ocular abnormalities. The most likely diagnosis is adult-onset cerebellar degeneration. Because saccades were of normal velocity and there were no corticospinal tract findings on neurologic examination, this patient does not have olivopontocerebellar atrophy. Given the family history, the patient appears to have a dominantly inherited form of parenchymal cerebellar atrophy.

The patient was given the diagnosis of adult-onset cerebellar degeneration, probably dominantly inherited.

Question 5: What are the clinical and genetic features of the dominantly inherited ataxias, and what role might genetic testing have in this patient?

Answer 5: There are numerous dominatly inherited spinocerebellar ataxias (SCA) that have been identified clinically and genetically. Table Case 19–1 lists the SCAs currently identified, with some of their clinical and genetic features. Another cere-

Table Case 19–1 Clinical Features of the Autosomal Dominant Spinocerebellar Ataxias

Disorder	Distinguishing Features	Gene Locus and Protein
SCA1	Pyramidal signs, peripheral neuropathy	6p22 CAG repeats, ataxin-1
SCA2	Slow sacccades; less often myoclonus, areflexia	12q24 CAG repeats, ataxin-2
SCA3	Slow saccades, persistent stare, extrapyramidal signs, peripheral neuropathy	14q32 CAG repeats, ataxin-3
SCA4	Sensory neuropathy	16q22
SCA5	Early onset but slow progression	11
SCA6	May have very late onset; mild; may lack family history, nystagmus	19p13 CAG repeats, alpha 1A P/Q calcium channel Subunit
SCA7	Macular degeneration	3p12 ataxin-7
SCA8	Mild disease	13q21 CTG repeats
SCA9	Not categorized	
SCA10	Generalized or complex partial seizures	22q13 ATTCT repeats
SCA11	Mild disease	15q14
SCA12	Tremor, dementia	15q14 CAG repeats in 5' region, protein phosphatase 2A
SCA13	Mental retardation	19q13
SCA14	Intermittent myoclonus with early-onset disease	19q13
DRPLA	Chorea, seizures, myoclonus, dementia	12p CAG repeats, atrophin-1

Source: Modified with permission from Opal P, Zoghbi HY: The spinocerebellar ataxias. UptoDate OnLine 9.3, November 15, 2001.[3]

bellar disorder whose genetic basis has been elucidated is episodic ataxia type II (EA 2), which presents with primarily episodic cerebellar dysfunction.[4] This patient does not clearly fit the picture of any of the known disorders on a purely clinical basis. While genetic testing may uncover a specific genetic abnormality, there are no known treatments that would be based on such information.

TREATMENT/MANAGEMENT

The patient was treated by discontinuation of vestibular-suppressant medications, a home safety consultation, and referral to a physical therapist for gait training. These measures were associated with a slight improvement in the patient's balance.

SUMMARY

A 65-year-old man presented with a gradually worsening course of disequilibrium and gait instability. The patient's complaints did not suggest a peripheral vestibular disorder. The family history was positive for a late-onset balance disorder. Examination suggested cerebellar system abnormalities. Brain imaging showed midline cerebellar degeneration. Vestibular laboratory testing indicated abnormal visual–vestibular interaction. The patient was given the diagnosis of adult-onset cerebellar degeneration, probably dominantly inherited. Symptomatic treatment consisted of vestibular rehabilitation therapy and discontinuation of vestibular-suppressant medication.

TEACHING POINTS

1. **A neurodegenerative disorder should be considered in patients with a gradual onset and worsening of imbalance in the absence of vertigo.** Other diagnostic considerations for patients with progressively severe symptoms include a posterior fossa mass lesion, vasculitis, a paraneoplastic process, or a structural abnormality such as a Chiari malformation. If a degeneration syndrome is suspected, a family history should be obtained to determine whether or not other family members have had similar difficulties.
2. **Cerebellar degeneration may be associated with pontine abnormalities.** Thus, patients should be examined carefully for signs of pontine involvement such as slowing of saccadic eye movements and for signs of corticospinal tract involvement. In this way, it can be determined whether they have an isolated olivocerebellar degeneration or olivopontocerebellar atrophy because pontine involvement causes saccadic slowing and corticospinal tract signs. This categorization may be important because olivopontocerebellar atrophy has a worse prognosis than olivocerebellar degeneration.
3. **Vestibular laboratory manifestations of cerebellar dysfunction may include saccadic dysmetria, impaired pursuit and optokinetic nys-**

tagmus, and nystagmus dysrhythmia, that is, an irregular pattern of quick components of nystagmus.

4. **Visual–vestibular interaction testing in the vestibular laboratory provides a quantitative assessment of the patient's ability to modify vestibular reflexes with vision.** Visual–vestibular interaction is a particularly sensitive measure when searching for evidence of an abnormality of the vestibulocerebellum, particularly the flocculus. Although most patients with abnormalities of visual–vestibular interaction also have abnormalities of ocular pursuit, several studies have indicated that visual–vestibular interaction provides information beyond that which can be obtained from measuring pursuit.

5. **Several different genetic abnormalities have been discovered that cause dominantly inherited SCA.** Unfortunately, such testing has no treatment implications.

REFERENCES

1. Baloh RW, Honrubia V: Clinical Neurophysiology of the Vestibular System, ed. 3. New York: Oxford University Press, 2001.
2. Chambers BR, Gresty MA: The relationship between disordered pursuit and vestibulo-ocular reflex suppression. J Neurol Neurosurg Psychiatry 46:61–66, 1983.
3. Opal P, Zoghbi HY: The spinocerebellar ataxias. UptoDate Online 9.3, November 15, 2001.
4. Baloh RW, Yue Q, Furman JF, Nelson SF: Familial episodic ataxia: Clinical heterogeneity in four families linked to chromosome 19p. Ann Neurol 41:8, 1997.

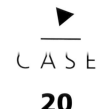

CASE

20

Multiple Sclerosis

HISTORY

A 40-year-old woman presented with a chief complaint of blurred vision, light-headedness, and imbalance. There was no complaint of hearing loss or tinnitus. The patient had a past medical history of multiple sclerosis with intermittent exacerbations. She had suffered from optic neuritis on several occasions. Additionally, she had suffered intermittent exacerbations characterized by weakness, incoordination, and urinary dysfunction. The patient recovered to a large extent from each of these episodes and was able to continue her work as a licensed practical nurse. One week before evaluation, the patient awoke with vertigo. She noticed a sense of disorientation worsened by head movement and had severe imbalance while attempting to walk. There was no change in any of her other neurologic functions. The patient's symptoms had decreased slightly during the week before evaluation. The family history was noncontributory.

Question 1: Based on the history, what is the likely cause of the patient's symptoms?

Answer 1: This patient's symptoms of vertigo and imbalance suggest a vestibular system abnormality. Multiple sclerosis could be an underlying cause of the patient's condition if there is a lesion in central vestibular structures. Additionally, she could be suffering from a peripheral vestibular abnormality independent of her multiple sclerosis. In this case, the patient's central nervous system abnormalities might be interfering with compensation for a peripheral vestibular deficit (see Case 3).

186

PHYSICAL EXAMINATION

The patient's general examination was normal. Eye movement examination revealed a left-beating nystagmus on left gaze. There was no evidence of internuclear ophthalmoplegia or gaze paresis and no vertical nystagmus. The patient had normal strength and sensation. Coordination testing revealed an abnormal finger-to-nose test response in the left upper extremity. Otherwise, there was no abnormality of coordination. Deep tendon reflexes were brisk and symmetric. Plantar responses were flexor bilaterally. Gait was mildly ataxic, with a negative Romberg's test. Otologic examination was normal. Neurotologic examination revealed a left-beating nystagmus in the primary position using infrared glasses. The patient was unable to stand on a compliant foam surface without assistance and fell toward the right. The stepping test was wide-based and ataxic, without significant rotation.

Question 2: Based on the history and physical examination, what is this patient's likely diagnosis?

Answer 2: The physical examination suggests the presence of a vestibular abnormality. The patient also has signs of central nervous system involvement, with an abnormal finger-to-nose test response on the left and gaze-evoked nystagmus on leftward gaze, which might have been the result of an accentuated vestibular nystagmus. The ataxic gait could be a result of either a vestibular system or a cerebellar system abnormality or both. Thus, the patient has evidence of combined peripheral and central vestibular abnormalities.

LABORATORY TESTING

Videonystagmography: A spontaneous left-beating nystagmus was recorded. There was a direction-fixed left-beating positional nystagmus. Caloric responses revealed a right reduced vestibular response of 50%.

Rotational testing revealed increased phase lead with a normal amplitude of responses. A left directional preponderance was noted.

Posturography indicated excessive sway on conditions 3, 5, and 6, that is, a combined vestibular deficit and visual dependence pattern (see Chapter 2).

Audiometric testing showed normal hearing in the left ear. The right ear showed a mild to moderate high-frequency sensorineural hearing loss. Word recognition scores were normal bilaterally (Fig. Case 20–1).

An MRI scan of the brain revealed a vestibular root entry-zone lesion on the right (Fig. Case 20–2). The scan also indicated numerous periventricular white matter hyperintensities on weighted images.

DIAGNOSIS/DIFFERENTIAL DIAGNOSIS

Question 3: Based on the information from the laboratory tests in addition to the information from the history and physical examination, what is this patient's likely diagnosis?

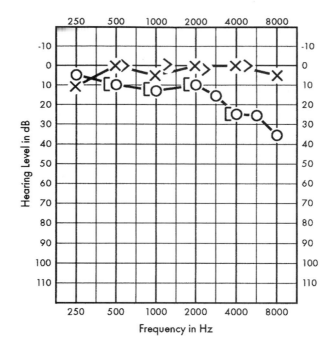

Figure Case 20–1 Audiogram.

Answer 3: This patient has evidence of vestibular system involvement based on the history, physical examination, and vestibular laboratory testing. The MRI scan indicates a vestibular root entry-zone lesion. Thus, the patient is likely to have symptoms of dizziness and disequilibrium due to multiple sclerosis, which can account for both the peripheral and central vestibular symptoms and signs.

Question 4: Should this patient's eighth nerve root entry-zone lesion be considered a peripheral or central vestibular abnormality?

Answer 4: A root entry-zone lesion should be considered a peripheral vestibular abnormality on the basis of function because damage is limited to afferent vestibular activity. Structurally, of course, a root entry-zone lesion, because it is intra-parenchymal, is a central nervous system abnormality and thus could be labeled a central vestibular lesion. Moreover, patients with root entry-zone lesions due to multiple sclerosis often have a much more prolonged recovery period than patients with peripheral vestibular ailments. This prolongation of recovery probably results from lesions other than that at the root entry zone that impair compensation, although there may be some inherent characteristic of a root entry-zone lesion that causes compensation to differ from that following lesions of the vestibular end organ or vestibular nerve.

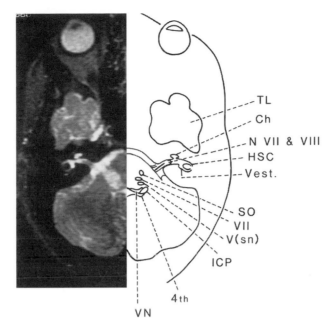

Figure Case 20–2 Axial magnetic resonance image showing the high signal intensity typical of multiple sclerosis in the region of the eighth nerve root entry zone. A line drawing of the major anatomic structures of the brain stem is shown for comparison. TL = temporal lobe; Ch = cochlea; N VII & VIII = cranial nerves 7 and 8; HSC = horizontal semicircular canal; Vest = labyrinthine vestibule; SO = superior olive; VII = facial nucleus; V(sn) = trigeminal nucleus and spinal-trigeminal tract; ICP = inferior cerebellar peduncle; 4th = fourth ventricle; VN = vestibular nuclei. (*Source*: With permission from Furman JM et al: Eighth nerve signs in a case of multiple sclerosis. Am J Otolaryngol 10:376–381, 1989.[3])

This patient was given the diagnosis of demyelination of the vestibular nerve root entry zone caused by multiple sclerosis.

Question 5: What are the common vestibular and ocular motor symptoms and signs associated with demyelinating disease?

Answer 5: Demyelinating disease, most notably multiple sclerosis, can present with the acute onset of vertigo, as in this case. Statistically, about 5% of patients with multiple sclerosis suffer from vertigo as their first neurologic symptom,[1] but most suffer from vertigo or disequilibrium at some time during the disease.[2] Patients with root entry-zone lesions may exhibit asymmetric vestibular function, including spontaneous nystagmus, a unilateral reduced vestibular response on caloric testing, a directional preponderance on caloric and/or rotational testing, and abnormal platform posturography.[3,4] These patients often suffer from blurred vision. Patients with multiple sclerosis whose lesions do not affect the root entry zone may also have evidence of vestibulo-ocular, vestibulospinal, or balance abnormalities as a result of brainstem and cerebellar lesions that affect central vestibular structures, notably the vestibular nuclei.[5] Symptoms may be exacerbated by optic neuritis and posterior column disease, which may affect visual and somatosensory inputs important for balance.

Typical eye movement abnormalities associated with multiple sclerosis include internuclear ophthalmoplegia with dissociated nystagmus, gaze evoked nystagmus, vertical nystagmus (see Case 40), positional nystagmus, abnormal accuracy of saccades, and, occasionally, pendular nystagmus (see Case 42) (see Grenman[2] for a review).

TREATMENT/MANAGEMENT

The patient was referred to a vestibular rehabilitation therapy program[6] and given a short (2-week) trial of meclizine. Her dizziness and lightheadedness gradually resolved and her balance slowly improved, but she still had a wide-based gait.

SUMMARY

A 40-year-old woman with a history of multiple sclerosis complained of a vertiginous episode 1 week before evaluation, followed by persistent disequilibrium. Physical examination and vestibular laboratory testing suggested a combined peripheral and central vestibular abnormality. MRI disclosed a vestibular root entry-zone lesion, as well as numerous small areas of increased signal intensity. The patient was thought to have a vestibular system problem due to multiple sclerosis with both peripheral and central features. Vestibular-suppressant medication, prescribed for a period of 2 weeks, reduced her dizziness. A course of vestibular rehabilitation therapy produced a small but definite improvement in balance.

TEACHING POINTS

1. **Vertigo and imbalance in patients with multiple sclerosis may indicate a lesion in central vestibular structures.** A peripheral vestibular abnormality independent of multiple sclerosis should also be considered.
2. **A root entry-zone lesion, because it is intraparenchymal, is a central nervous system abnormality and, strictly speaking, is a central vestibular lesion.** However, a root entry-zone lesion often behaves as a peripheral vestibular abnormality because damage is limited to afferent vestibular activity.
3. **Both peripheral and central vestibular symptoms and signs can be seen in patients with multiple sclerosis.** A lesion that includes the vestibular root entry zone in addition to other brainstem structures interrupts vestibular afferents in the lateral brainstem, causing abnormalities indistinguishable from those due to an end-organ lesion.
4. **Prolonged recovery is seen in patients with root entry-zone lesions caused by multiple sclerosis.** This protracted recovery probably results from lesions other than those at the root entry zone that impair compensation.
5. **Multiple sclerosis can present with vestibular and ocular motor symptoms and signs.** About 5% of patients with multiple sclerosis suffer from vertigo as their first neurologic symptom.

6. **Eye movement abnormalities associated with multiple sclerosis include internuclear ophthalmoplegia, gaze-evoked nystagmus, vertical nystagmus, saccadic dysmetria, and pendular nystagmus.**

REFERENCES

1. McAlpine D: Symptoms and signs, brain-stem multiple sclerosis. In: Multiple Sclerosis: A Reappraisal McAlpine D, Lumsden CE, Acheson ED (Eds.) London: Churchill Livingstone, 1972, pp 164–196.
2. Grenman R: Involvement of the audiovestibular system in multiple sclerosis. An otoneurologic and audiologic study. Acta Otolaryngol 420(Suppl):1–95, 1985.
3. Furman JM, Durrant JD, Hirsch WL: Eighth nerve signs in a case of multiple sclerosis. Am J Otolaryngol 10:376–381, 1989.
4. Williams NP, Roland PS, Yellin W: Vestibular evaluation in patients with early multiple sclerosis. Am J Otol 18:93–100, 1997.
5. Bronstein AM, Rudge P: Vestibular involvement in spasmodic torticollis. J Neurol Neurosurg Psychiatry 49:290–295, 1986.
6. Kasser SL, Rose DJ, Clark S: Balance training for adults with multiple sclerosis: Multiple case studies. Neurol Rep 23(1):5–12, 1999.

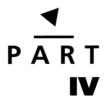

PART IV

Multiple Diagnosis Case Studies

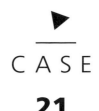
Meniere's Disease and Migraine

HISTORY

A 57-year-old woman presented with the complaints of vertigo, right-sided hearing loss, right-sided tinnitus, and right-sided ear fullness that had been occurring intermittently during the previous 2 years. The patient had been evaluated by an otolaryngologist, who diagnosed Meniere's disease. She was treated with a combination of hydrochlorothiazide and triamterene and was advised to reduce her sodium intake. However, her headaches worsened, so she discontinued the medication. Her episodes of vertigo, hearing loss, and tinnitus typically lasted for about 30 minutes and were associated with nausea and occasional vomiting. Until recently, the patient was essentially asymptomatic between episodes. However, during the previous 6 months, she noted intermittent disequilibrium usually associated with headache. The patient indicated that this disequilibrium was not at all like her prior episodes of vertigo, which continued to occur approximately once every 2 months. During the episodes of disequilibrium, she also noted a rocking sensation that was exacerbated by lying down. Bending her head forward or engaging in physical activity also worsened symptoms, which included nausea and veering of her gait to the right. Preceding one of the patient's episodes was an aura of flashing lights. Prior to the onset of her episodic disequilibrium 6 months prior to evaluation, the patient suffered from severe headaches every few months. Recently, however, the headaches had lessened in severity, increased in frequency, and were often associated with disequilibrium. Aside from the visual aura noted above, there was no complaint of changes in vision and no complaint of numbness, weakness, or alteration in level of consciousness. The patient's past medical history was significant for hypertension not currently requiring treatment. The family history was significant; her mother had had migraine headaches, and a paternal uncle had experienced dizziness of unknown cause.

Question 1: Based upon the patient's history, what are the diagnostic considerations?

Answer 1: The patient's history is consistent with both Meniere's disease and migraine-related dizziness. Her history of episodic vertigo accompanied by unilateral hearing loss, tinnitus, and ear fullness virtually assures a diagnosis of Meniere's disease (see Cases 9, 16, 25). The patient's more recent complaint of episodic disequilibrium in association with headache strongly suggests migraine-related dizziness (see Case 8). Other diagnostic considerations such as benign paroxysmal positional vertigo (see Cases 7, 22, 25, 31, 39) or a structural lesion of the central nervous system seem unlikely.

PHYSICAL EXAMINATION

Neurologic and otologic examinations were normal. Neurotologic examination revealed no spontaneous nystagmus and a normal head thrust. Dix-Hallpike testing disclosed no signs or symptoms with the left ear down. However, with the right ear down, the patient experienced a sense of dizziness without vertigo or nystagmus. While standing on a foam pad with her eyes closed, the patient complained of feeling dizzy and displayed unsteadiness, but she did not lose her balance.

Question 2: What are the diagnostic problems associated with the combination of Meniere's disease and migraine-related dizziness?

Answer 2: Both Meniere's disease and migraine-related dizziness are associated with episodic vestibular symptoms. In fact, Neuhauser et al.[1] suggested that the diagnostic criteria for migrainous vertigo include episodic vestibular symptoms of moderate severity such as rotational vertigo or other illusory self or object motion. Thus, because the defining characteristics of Meniere's disease and migraine-related dizziness overlap, it may be difficult or impossible in some patients to reach a definitive diagnosis based on the history alone.[2] Another problem in diagnosis is overlap in the situations that can exacerbate symptoms. Patients with migraine-related dizziness may experience head motion intolerance and sensitivity to visual motion. The same complaints can be seen in some patients with Meniere's disease between attacks. Another issue is that of disease onset. In patients with combined Meniere's disease and migraine-related dizziness, the onset of these disorders may not occur simultaneously. In fact, most patients manifest one condition prior to the other, as in this patient, who suffered from typical Meniere's disease–related symptoms for 18 months before manifesting migraine-related dizziness. Still another issue is synergy. Attacks of Meniere's disease may serve as a trigger for migraine and migraine-related dizziness. This phenomenon would obviously preclude defining whether a particular episode was related solely to Meniere's disease or migraine-related dizziness.

Studies have indicated an increased incidence of migraine in patients with Meniere's disease[3] and an increased incidence of hearing loss and tinnitus in patients with migraine[4] and basilar artery migraine,[5] suggesting that there is more than a chance co-occurrence of these disorders.

Question 3: Based upon the additional information from the physical examination, what are the diagnostic considerations for this patient?

Answer 3: The patient's physical examination is nonspecific but suggests ongoing balance problems due to the symptoms experienced during Dix-Hallpike testing and during assessment of postural sway on a compliant surface. Benign paroxysmal positional vertigo was absent. Also, the patient's normal neurologic examination argues against a structural central nervous system lesion. Thus, the patient is likely to be suffering from both Meniere's disease and migraine-related dizziness.

LABORATORY TESTING

Videonystagmography revealed normal ocular motor function, no positional nystagmus, and a right reduced vestibular response of 35%.

Rotational testing revealed a mild right directional preponderance.

Audiometric testing revealed a low-frequency sensorineural hearing loss on the right.

Hearing on the left was normal.

The MRI scan was normal.

Question 4: Based upon the information available from the history, physical examination, and laboratory testing, what are the most likely diagnostic considerations?

Answer 4: The laboratory tests support a diagnosis of right-sided Meniere's disease because of both the reduced caloric response and the low-frequency sensorineural hearing loss on the right. However, several studies have indicated that a unilateral caloric reduction can be seen in patients with migraine related dizziness.[4-6] The asymmetric rotational responses could be based on the patient's Meniere's disease. Alternatively, this laboratory abnormality could support the diagnosis of migraine-related dizziness. Note that the asymmetry is in the opposite direction from that seen with acute peripheral vestibular lesions. Thus, laboratory testing supports the diagnosis of Meniere's disease, migraine-related dizziness, or both.

DIAGNOSIS/DIFFERENTIAL DIAGNOSIS

The patient was given the diagnosis of a combination of Meniere's disease and migraine-related dizziness.

TREATMENT

Question 5: What are the treatment issues in a patient with the diagnosis of Meniere's disease and migraine-related dizziness?

Answer 5: The issues that pertain to the treatment of any patient with two diagnoses are (1) whether to treat one disorder prior to treating the other or whether to treat both simultaneously and (2) the conflicts, if any, between the treatments for the two disorders. In patients with both Meniere's disease and migraine-related dizziness, it is prudent to treat both disorders simultaneously. The treatment for Meniere's disease includes a salt-restricted diet and a diuretic. Typically, these remedies have no effect on a patient's migraine-related dizziness. In fact, as noted above, successful treatment of Meniere's disease in a patient who also has migraine-related dizziness may reduce the migraine-related dizziness due to a reduction of Meniere's disease–related vertiginous episodes, which may act as potential migraine triggers. The medications used for the treatment of migraine, and in particular migraine-related dizziness, would not be expected to exacerbate or interfere with the treatment of Meniere's disease.

This patient was treated for Meniere's disease with a low-sodium diet and another trial of a diuretic. She was also treated for migraine-related dizziness by being told to reduce her dietary intake of foods that might be provoking migraine[6] and by prescribing clonazepam, 0.25 mg orally twice a day, and imipramine, 25 mg orally at hour of sleep.

Question 6: How is this patient's prognosis affected by having two balance disorders, Meniere's disease and migraine-related dizziness?

Answer 6: It is not known whether the combination of Meniere's disease and migraine-related dizziness influences the natural history or efficacy of the treatment for these disorders. In our experience, as patients improve, both disorders are often reduced.

FOLLOW-UP

The patient was reevaluated 3 months following the initial assessment. She had experienced only a single brief episode of true vertigo. Her disequilibrium also was improved but persisted. The patient was referred for vestibular rehabilitation, which led to further improvement but not complete alleviation of her imbalance.

SUMMARY

A 57 year-old woman presented with the complaints of vertigo, right-sided hearing loss, right-sided tinnitus, and right-sided ear fullness that had been occurring intermittently during the previous 2 years. During the previous 6 months, the patient noted intermittent disequilibrium usually associated with headache. She indicated that this disequilibrium was not at all like her prior episodes of vertigo, which continued to occur approximately once every 2 months. The family history was significant for migraine headaches. Physical examination was nonspecific but suggested an ongoing balance problem. Videonystagmography revealed a right reduced vestibular response. The MRI scan was normal. The patient was given the diagnosis of a combination of Meniere's disease and migraine-related dizziness. She was treated for both conditions.

TEACHING POINTS

1. **Both Meniere's disease and migraine-related dizziness are associated with episodic vestibular symptoms.** Because the defining characteris-

tics of these conditions overlap, it may be difficult or impossible in some patients to reach a definitive diagnosis based on the history alone.

2. **A unilateral caloric reduction can be seen in patients with Meniere's disease and in patients with migraine-related dizziness.** Also, asymmetric rotational responses can be due to migraine-related dizziness or a recent episode of Meniere's disease.

3. **For patients with both Meniere's disease and migraine-related dizziness, it is prudent to treat both disorders simultaneously.**

4. **It is not known whether the combination of Meniere's disease and migraine-related dizziness influences the natural history or efficacy of treatment for these disorders.**

REFERENCES

1. Neuhauser H, Leopold M, von Brevern M, Arnold G, Lempert T: The interrelations of migraine, vertigo, and migrainous vertigo. Neurology 56:436–441, 2001.
2. Dimitri PS, Wall C, Oas JG, Rauch SD: Application of multivariate statistics to vestibular testing: Discriminating between Meniere's disease and migraine associated dizziness. J Vestib Res 11(1):53–65, 2001.
3. Rassekh CH, Harker LA: The prevalence of migraine in Meniere's disease. Laryngoscope 102:135–138, 1992.
4. Kayan A, Hood JD: Neuro-otological manifestations of migraine. Brain 107:1123–1142, 1984.
5. Olsson JE: Neurotologic findings in basilar migraine. Laryngoscope 101(Suppl 52):1–41, 1991.
6. Cass SP, Furman JM, Ankerstjerne JKP, Balaban C, Yetiser S, Aydogan B: Migraine-related vestibulopathy. Ann Otol Rhinol Laryngol 106:182–189, 1997.

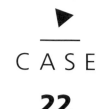

Benign Paroxysmal Positional Vertigo and Anxiety Disorder

HISTORY

A 39-year-old male salesman presented with the chief complaint of disequilibrium and positional dizziness for the preceding 6 months. Symptoms had started abruptly following a viral upper respiratory tract infection. The patient felt as if he were walking on a cloud. Subsequently, he noted dizziness when looking up or turning in bed. He also related having panic attacks several times each week. The patient had no prior psychiatric history and had no recent changes in his family or work situation. His panic attacks were characterized by dizziness, pounding in the chest, numbness and tingling in the fingers, difficulty breathing, air hunger, sweating, nausea, and a fear that he might die. Besides having symptoms of positional vertigo and intermittent panic attacks, the patient worried excessively about having future attacks. He had mild disequilibrium that provoked fear, and had discomfort in certain environments such as shopping malls, grocery stores, and congested traffic. The patient's only medication was diazepam, 2 mg twice daily. The family history was not contributory.

Question 1: Based upon the patient's history, what diagnoses should be considered?

Answer 1: The patient's history suggests the diagnosis of benign paroxysmal positional vertigo. It also suggests an anxiety disorder, specifically panic disorder. The diagnosis of benign paroxysmal positional vertigo is suggested by the definite positional nature of the patient's complaints. Panic disorder is suggested by the patient's attacks of fearfulness associated with typical autonomic symptoms of panic attacks. The patient's complaints of discomfort in shopping malls and grocery stores suggest space and motion discomfort (Chapter 7), which can be seen in anxiety-prone individuals with vestibular disorders.

PHYSICAL EXAMINATION

Neurologic and otologic examinations were normal. Neurotologic examination revealed no spontaneous nystagmus, a normal head thrust, and excessive sway without falling while standing on a compliant foam pad with the eyes closed. Dix-Hallpike testing with the left ear down revealed no signs or symptoms. However, with the right ear down, the patient complained of vertigo, and typical upbeating-torsional nystagmus of benign paroxysmal positional vertigo was observed. However, within 10 seconds of reaching the head-hanging-right position, the patient began to hyperventilate, and he demanded that the infrared goggles he was wearing be removed and that he be returned to the seated position. Upon returning to the seated position, the patient continued to hyperventilate for about 1 minute, during which time he complained of symptoms comparable to those that he experienced during his typical panic attacks.

Question 2: Based upon the patient's physical examination, what are the diagnostic considerations?

Answer 2: The patient's physical examination confirms a diagnosis of right-sided benign paroxysmal positional vertigo. Additionally, the patient's emotional reaction to Dix-Hallpike testing suggests that he has an anxiety disorder and that some, if not all, of his panic attacks are induced by positional vertigo. Thus, the patient appears to have a combination of benign paroxysmal positional vertigo and panic disorder.

LABORATORY TESTING

Videonystagmography revealed normal ocular motor testing, no persistent positional nystagmus, and a 30% right reduced vestibular response on caloric testing. Rotational testing revealed a mild left directional preponderance. Square-wave jerks were noted throughout the eye movement recordings.

Audiometric testing was normal.

Question 3: Based upon the patient's history, physical examination, and laboratory test results, what are the most likely diagnostic considerations?

Answer 3: The patient' s laboratory test results suggest that in addition to having benign paroxysmal positional vertigo, a disorder that affects the posterior semicircular canal, the patient has a mild reduction in the function of the left horizontal semicircular canal. Moreover, the patient' s rotational test result suggests an ongoing VOR asymmetry. The patient's square-wave jerks are nonspecific and possibly are related to anxiety. Thus, the diagnoses of benign paroxysmal positional vertigo and panic disorder seem most likely. Moreover, the patient appears to have a more widespread vestibular abnormality based upon caloric and rotational testing. Note that attempting to assign a single diagnosis for this patient precludes accurate diagnosis of both the neurotologic and psychiatric disorders.

DIAGNOSIS/DIFFERENTIAL DIAGNOSIS

The patient was given the diagnoses of benign paroxysmal positional vertigo and an anxiety disorder.

Question 4: What diagnostic problems, if any, must be considered in a patient who presents with the combination of benign paroxysmal positional vertigo and anxiety?

Answer 4: As with all patients who present with two diagnoses, the issues of overlap between signs and symptoms, the sequence of onset, and the interrelationship between the disorders must be considered. For patients with benign paroxysmal positional vertigo and anxiety, there is little difficulty discerning one condition from the other. Although dizziness and vertigo occur in both disorders, the symptoms of benign paroxysmal positional vertigo are clearly position related. Panic attacks are associated with fear and a sense of impending doom not seen with uncomplicated benign paroxysmal positional vertigo. The sequence of onset and the interrelationship between benign paroxysmal positional vertigo and anxiety can be understood in the context of the relationship between balance disorders and anxiety disorders, which is discussed in Chapter 7. In this patient, benign paroxysmal positional vertigo appears to be triggering the patient's anxiety.[1] Thus, a somatopsychic mechanism seems most likely. The alternative possibilities of chance co-occurrence, psychosomatic mechanisms, and neurologic linkage are all unlikely.

TREATMENT

Question 5: How should a patient with both benign paroxysmal positional vertigo and panic disorder be treated?

Answer 5: In general, patients with two diagnoses should be treated for both disorders. This holds true especially for patients with both a neurotologic disorder and a psychiatric disorder. However, the issue of which treatment to institute first must be considered. In this patient, because benign paroxysmal positional vertigo is clearly acting as a trigger for panic attacks, the vertigo should be treated first. The panic attack induced by Dix-Hallpike testing suggests that treatment with particle repositioning may be challenging. Pretreatment with a benzodiazepine may be necessary.

The patient was treated with a particle repositioning maneuver following the ingestion of 5 mg of diazepam. Also, because of the patient's more widespread vestibular abnormalities, he was enrolled in a course of vestibular rehabilitation.

FOLLOW-UP

Following particle repositioning, the patient was much improved. He no longer suffered from positional vertigo. Also, panic attacks ceased. However, the patient still experienced mild nonspecific dizziness and a sense of imbalance. Moreover, he experienced discomfort in shopping malls and grocery stores but did not avoid them.

SUMMARY

A 39-year-old man presented with symptoms typical of benign paroxysmal positional vertigo. He also complained of disequilibrium, panic attacks, and discomfort in certain environments, such as shopping malls, grocery stores, and congested traffic. Physical examination confirmed a diagnosis of right-sided benign paroxysmal positional vertigo. The patient had a panic attack during Dix-Hallpike testing. Laboratory testing revealed a right reduced vestibular response on caloric testing and a mild left directional preponderance on rotational testing. The patient was given the diagnoses of benign paroxysmal positional vertigo and panic disorder. He was treated with a particle repositioning maneuver following pretreatment with 5 mg diazepam and was enrolled in a course of vestibular rehabilitation.

Following particle repositioning, the patient was much improved, with a resolution of his positional vertigo and panic attacks. He continued to experience discomfort in shopping malls and grocery stores but did not avoid them.

TEACHING POINTS

1. **When patients present with both benign paroxysmal positional vertigo and anxiety, there is little difficulty in distinguishing one condition from the other.** Although dizziness and vertigo occur in both disorders, the symptoms of benign paroxysmal positional vertigo are clearly position related. Panic attacks are associated with fear and a sense of impending doom not seen with uncomplicated benign paroxysmal positional vertigo.

2. **Attempting to assign a single diagnosis to a patient with both a neurotologic disorder and a psychiatric disorder precludes accurate diagnosis of both disorders and may lead to suboptimal management.**

3. **When benign paroxysmal positional vertigo is clearly triggering panic attacks, the vertigo should be treated first.**

4. **Patients with benign paroxysmal positional vertigo and an anxiety disorder may require pretreatment with a benzodiazepine prior to performing a particle repositioning maneuver.**

REFERENCES

1. Lilienfeld SO: Vestibular dysfunction followed by panic disorder with agoraphobia. J Nerv Ment Dis 177:700–701, 1989.

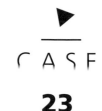

Head Trauma: Combined Central Nervous System, Labyrinthine, and Cervical Injury

HISTORY

A 50-year-old man construction worker complained of dizziness for 4 months. The patient dated the onset of his symptoms to a motor vehicle accident in which the vehicle that he was driving was struck from behind. He was not wearing a restraint device and struck his head against the steering wheel. There was a brief loss of consciousness at the time of the accident. The patient was evaluated at a local emergency room, where a CT scan of the brain was reportedly negative. Although the patient was released from the emergency room, he experienced dizziness and neck pain immediately following the accident and visited his primary care physician the next day. He was prescribed meclizine, which provided some but inadequate relief of his dizziness. Subsequently, the patient returned to his primary care physician with complaints of headache, neck pain, and imbalance. He was referred to a physical therapist for his neck pain and was advised to wear a soft cervical collar on an as-needed basis. These measures provided some additional relief, but the patient was dissatisfied.

Question 1: Based on the patient's history, what is his differential diagnosis?

Answer 1: This patient's history suggests a vestibular system disorder that may have been caused by a labyrinthine concussion, a neck injury, or possible brainstem concussion. Labyrinthine concussion (see Case 11) is most likely because the patient struck his head and experienced dizziness immediately following head trauma. Cervicogenic dizziness (see Case 53) is a possibility because of the patient's neck pain following a presumed *whiplash* (i.e., flexion-extension) injury. A brainstem or cerebellar concussion is possible given the patient's history of head trauma followed by headache and his persistent symptoms that suggest impaired vestibular compensation.

ADDITIONAL HISTORY

The patient noted exacerbation of dizziness with rapid head movements but not when turning in bed. Also, symptoms were not exacerbated by Valsalva maneuvers. He did not complain of hearing loss or tinnitus. The patient had no prior complaints of dizziness and no significant past medical history.

PHYSICAL EXAMINATION

On general examination, the patient exhibited limited head movement but was otherwise normal. Neurologic and otologic examinations were normal. Neurotologic examination using infrared goggles revealed no spontaneous nystagmus, an abnormal head thrust to the right, a low-amplitude left-beating nystagmus following head shake, negative Dix-Hallpike maneuvers, an inability to stand on a compliant foam pad with the eyes closed, a positive stepping test with abnormal rotation to the right, no pastpointing, and no nystagmus during hyperventilation, tragal stimulation, Valsalva maneuver, and pneumatic otoscopy. Cervico-ocular testing could not be performed because of the patient's limited range of motion of the head on the trunk.

Question 2: Based upon the additional information, what is this patient's likely diagnosis?

Answer 2: Based upon the patient's history and physical examination, he appears to have suffered from a labyrinthine concussion on the right and incomplete vestibular compensation. The patient's abnormal head thrust suggests a peripheral vestibular injury on the right and is consistent with a labyrinthine concussion. Incomplete vestibular compensation is suggested by the persistence of posthead-shake nystagmus, an abnormal stepping test, and inability to stand on a compliant foam pad with the eyes closed. The patient's incomplete compensation may be based upon the nature of his labyrinthine injury (i.e., aberrant vestibular function), an associated traumatic brainstem or cerebellar injury (i.e., a concussion), or his neck injury. Thus, the patient may be suffering from a combined labyrinthine, central nervous system, and cervical injury. There is no evidence of benign paroxysmal positional vertigo or perilymphatic fistula.

LABORATORY TESTING

Videonystagmography: Ocular motor testing revealed symmetrically impaired ocular pursuit and optokinetic nystagmus. A spontaneous nystagmus of 3 degrees per second using infrared goggles was noted. There was no positional nystagmus. Caloric irrigation revealed an absent response to warm and cool irrigation in the right ear. A minimal response was elicited with ice-water irrigation of the right ear.

Rotational testing revealed a mild to moderate left directional preponderance. Posturography indicated excessive sway on conditions 5 and 6.

Audiometric testing revealed a bilateral high-frequency sensorineural hearing loss. Word recognition was normal bilaterally.

A CT scan of the brain, ordered by the patient's primary care physician, was normal.

Question 3: Based upon the patient's laboratory tests, what is the most likely diagnosis?

Answer 3: The patient's laboratory tests further support the idea that the patient has suffered a labyrinthine concussion (see Case 11) on the right with impaired vestibular compensation (see Case 3). Also, the patient's abnormal ocular motor testing suggests the possibility of a brainstem or cerebellar concussion.

DIAGNOSIS/DIFFERENTIAL DIAGNOSIS

The patient was given the diagnosis of a combined labyrinthine concussion and brainstem/cerebellar concussion with possible cervicogenic dizziness.

Question 4: What are the implications of a combined injury to the ear, brain, and neck?

Answer 4: With combined injuries, there is increased diagnostic uncertainty. Moreover, a combination of injury to the ear, brain, and neck increases the likelihood that the patient will experience impaired compensation because of damage to central nervous system structures important for compensation and because of the probable role of neck afferents. Moreover, abnormal vestibular function is likely to cause abnormal neck muscle activity, which in turn can lead to increased pain and abnormal neck afferent activity, resulting in ongoing exacerbation of dizziness and neck discomfort. Also, the patient's decreased range of motion of the head on the trunk may itself interfere with vestibular compensation and provide an additional challenge for vestibular rehabilitation.

TREATMENT/MANAGEMENT

Question 5: Based upon the patient's tentative diagnoses, what are the treatment options?

Answer 5: The treatment modality most likely to be helpful is vestibular rehabilitation focused on the patient's vestibular loss, impaired compensation, decreased range of motion of the head, and neck pain. The use of pharmacotherapy is challenging because vestibular-suppressant medications and muscle relaxants may interfere with the process of vestibular compensation.

The patient was treated with a combination of vestibular rehabilitation and diazepam, 1 mg twice daily, on an as-needed basis. Meclizine was discontinued. The patient was advised to continue physical therapy for his neck.

FOLLOW-UP

The patient's symptoms gradually decreased, but he was unable to return to his occupation as a construction worker because of continued imbalance.

Question 6: What are the implications for prognosis for patients with combined injuries of the ear, brain, and neck?

Answer 6: Patients with combined injuries of the ear, brain, and neck have a poorer prognosis than patients with isolated injuries.[1] In particular, such patients require a longer period of time for recovery, require more therapy sessions, and are likely to have a persistent disability.

SUMMARY

A 50-year-old man complained of 4 months of dizziness that began following a motor vehicle accident in which he struck his head against the steering wheel and experienced brief loss of consciousness. The patient's history, physical examination, and laboratory tests suggested a combined labyrinthine, central nervous system, and cervical injury. Treatment consisted of vestibular rehabilitation, physical therapy for his neck, and diazepam on an as-needed basis.

TEACHING POINTS

1. **Head trauma, especially that caused by motor vehicle accidents, can lead to combined injury of the labyrinth, central nervous system, and neck.**
2. **Combined injury of the labyrinth, central nervous system, and neck can cause impaired vestibular compensation.** Combined injury can also lead to increased symptoms, particularly related to the neck, as compared to isolated abnormalities.
3. **Treatment of patients with combined labyrinth, central nervous system, and neck abnormalities should address the cervical and labyrinthine components of the problem.** Vestibular rehabilitation is the primary therapy. Pharmacotherapy should be tailored to maximize symptom reduction and minimize interference with vestibular compensation.
4. **The prognosis for patients with combined labyrinth, central nervous system, and neck abnormalities is less favorable than that of patients with isolated abnormalities.**

REFERENCES

1. Cass SP, Borello-France D, Furman JF: Functional outcome of vestibular rehabilitation in patients with abnormal sensory-organization testing. Am J Otol 4:581–594, 1996.

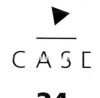

Migraine-Related Dizziness and Anxiety Disorder

HISTORY

A 56-year-old woman presented with a 3-month complaint of dizziness and disequilibrium. She stated that during the preceding 3 months she had three discrete episodes of the sudden onset of vertigo, rapid heartbeat, faintness, cold sweating, anxiety, and seeing visual spots. These episodes lasted for about 5 minutes and were followed by a sensation of swimming in her head, unsteadiness, and nausea. The patient's other complaints, which did not occur in discrete episodes, included fluctuating bilateral tinnitus and bilateral ear fullness. Complaints also included headaches characterized by head pressure and an electric-like shock sensation in her scalp. During the headaches, she complained of seeing spots, photophobia, and phonophobia. Additional complaints included occasional circumoral paresthesias and poor balance. The patient related that she had been avoiding shopping malls and grocery stores for the previous 6 weeks. Her past medical history was significant for fibromyalgia and irritable bowel syndrome. The patient's family history was significant; her father and brother had migraine headaches.

Question 1: Based upon the patient's history, what are the diagnostic considerations?

Answer 1: The patient's history is consistent with migraine-related dizziness (Case 8), an anxiety disorder (Case 5), and possibly a peripheral vestibulopathy. The diagnosis of migraine-related dizziness is supported by the episodic nature of the patient's dizziness, the type of headaches from which the patient suffers, and the patient's positive family history of migraine. The diagnosis of an anxiety disorder is supported by the patient's complaints of anxiety during her dizziness episodes, circumoral paresthesias, and space and motion discomfort.

PHYSICAL EXAMINATION

Neurologic and otologic examinations were normal. Neurotologic examination showed no spontaneous nystagmus and a normal head thrust. There was no positional nystagmus, and the Dix-Hallpike test was negative. The patient had increased sway while standing on a compliant foam pad with the eyes closed. The stepping test was normal.

Question 2: Based upon the patient's history and physical examination, what are the diagnostic considerations?

Answer 2: The patient's physical examination does not change the diagnostic considerations except to reduce the likelihood of a peripheral vestibular ailment. Thus, migraine-related dizziness and anxiety remain the most likely diagnoses.

LABORATORY TESTING

Videonystagmography revealed a normal ocular motor test and no positional nystagmus. Shortly after the first caloric irrigation, the patient discontinued caloric testing. Similarly, shortly after the start of rotational testing, the patient discontinued rotational testing. Posturography revealed increased sway in a nonspecific pattern.

Audiometric testing was normal.

Several months earlier, the patient had undergone MRI of the brain, which was normal.

Question 3: Based upon the patient's history, physical examination, and laboratory tests, what are the most likely diagnoses?

Answer 3: The patient's laboratory tests provide little additional information because the patient discontinued caloric and rotational testing. Patients with anxiety often discontinue vestibular laboratory tests because of the aversive nature of the stimulus. Posturography testing suggests a balance disorder but does not provide diagnostic information. Thus, the patient is most likely suffering from a combination of migraine-related dizziness and anxiety. The patient's anxiety may, in part, be induced by her dizziness. Alternatively, some of the patient's dizziness is directly related to her anxiety.

Question 4: Do symptoms of migraine-related dizziness and anxiety overlap with one another and thus interfere with an accurate diagnosis of these conditions?

Answer 4: Migraine-related dizziness is essentially a diagnosis of exclusion. However, recent diagnostic criteria suggested by Neuhauser et al.[1] include episodic vestibular symptoms. Some of these symptoms migraine-related dizziness overlap with symptoms attributable to panic attacks, namely, episodic vertigo and dizziness. Also, both migraine and anxiety occur in episodes that can be triggered, although for many episodes, a specific trigger cannot be identified. In this patient, the diagnosis of migraine-related dizziness is supported by the association of dizziness with headache, the positive family history of migraine, and the absence of another identifiable neurotologic syndrome. The diagnosis of anxiety disorder is supported by the patient's complaints of presyncope, anxiety, and circumoral paresthesias. Despite these distinct diagnostic aspects, the etiology of the three discrete episodes is uncertain. They may have been migraine-related dizziness, panic attacks, or a combination of both. That is, they may have begun as migraine-related or anxiety-related symptoms and then evolved into a combined migrainous and anxiety-related episode. Moreover, the patient's space and motion discomfort could be related to either her migraine-related dizziness, her anxiety, or both.

DIAGNOSIS/DIFFERENTIAL DIAGNOSIS

This patient was given a tentative diagnosis of combined migraine-related dizziness and an anxiety disorder.

Question 5: What treatment should be considered for a patient with both migraine-related dizziness and an anxiety disorder?

Answer 5: Patients with migraine-related dizziness and anxiety should be treated for both conditions. The optimal treatment for migraine-related dizziness is not known. However, such patients are typically treated with the same medications that are used to treat migraine headache, which include antidepressants. They may also benefit from low-dose benzodiazepines for symptomatic relief. Pharmacotherapy for anxiety includes benzodiazepines and antidepressants. Thus, a combination of a benzodiazepine and an antidepressant is particularly warranted in patients with both migraine-related dizziness and anxiety. Also, two recent studies suggest that vestibular rehabilitation may benefit both patients with migraine-related dizziness[2] and patients with anxiety-related dizziness.[3] Thus, vestibular rehabilitation also seems particularly appropriate for patients with both disorders.

TREATMENT

The patient was treated with a combination of clonazepam, orally twice a day, 0.25 mg and imipramine, 25 mg orally at hour of sleep. The patient was also referred for vestibular rehabilitation.

FOLLOW-UP

The patient improved markedly and no longer experienced episodic dizziness. However, she continued to experience nonlateralized tinnitus, ear fullness, and visual motion sensitivity.

Question 6: Are migraine-related dizziness and anxiety interrelated?

Answer 6: A recent study by Breslau et al.[4] indicates that migraine is more likely to occur in patients with panic disorder and panic disorder is more likely to occur in patients with migraine. Further support for a relationship other than chance

Table Case 24–1 Association Between Migraine and Anxiety: Community Studies

| Reference | N | ODDS RATIO | | | |
		Panic	Phobia	GAD	Any Anxiety
Stewart et al.[6]	10,169	5.3	—	—	—
Merikangas et al.[7]	457	3.3	2.4	5.3	2.7
Breslau et al.[8]	1,007	6.0	1.9	5.3	1.9

Source: With permission from Merikangas KR, Stevens DE: Comborbidity of migraine and psychiatric disorders. Neurol Clin 15(1):115–123, 1997.[5]

co-occurrence is given in Table Case 24–1, in which the odds ratio for anxiety disorders is clearly higher in patients with migraine. Merikangas and Stevens[5] suggest that the co-occurrence of panic disorder and migraine is complex and bidirectional rather than one condition simply increasing the risk of the other. They suggest that shared environmental or genetic factors or overlapping neurotransmitter systems may explain the co-occurrence of migraine and panic disorder.

Question 7: What psychiatric disorders have been associated with migraine?

Answer 7: Although no information is available specifically regarding migraine-related dizziness, there is an increased incidence of anxiety, depression, and social fears in patients with migraine headache.[5]

SUMMARY

A 56 year old woman presented with a 3-month complaint of dizziness and disequilibrium. She had three discrete episodes of vertigo, rapid heartbeat, faintness, cold sweating, anxiety, and seeing visual spots lasting for 5 minutes followed by a sensation of swimming in her head, unsteadiness, and nausea. She also complained of fluctuating bilateral tinnitus and ear fullness. Other complaints included headaches, head pressure, an electric-like shock sensation in her scalp, seeing spots, photophobia, phonophobia, circumoral paresthesias, and poor balance. The patient's family history was significant for migraine headache. Physical examination was normal, with the exception of increased sway while standing on a compliant foam pad. Laboratory testing was incomplete because the patient discontinued caloric and rotational testing. Posturography revealed increased sway in a nonspecific pattern. She was given a diagnosis of combined migraine-related dizziness and an anxiety disorder. The patient was treated with a combination of clonazepam, imipramine, and vestibular rehabilitation. The patient no longer experienced episodic dizziness but continued to experience nonlateralized tinnitus, ear fullness, and visual motion sensitivity.

TEACHING POINTS

1. **Patients with anxiety often discontinue vestibular laboratory testing because of the aversive nature of the stimulus.**

2. **Symptoms of migraine-related dizziness and of anxiety may overlap, creating diagnostic uncertainty.**
3. **Patients with migraine-related dizziness and anxiety should be treated for both conditions.** A combination of benzodiazepines and antidepressants should be considered, as should vestibular rehabilitation.
4. **Migraine is more likely to occur in patients with panic disorder, and panic disorder is more likely to occur in patients with migraine.** This relationship may be based upon shared environmental or genetic factors or overlapping neurotransmitter systems.
5. **There is an increased incidence of anxiety, depression, and social fears in patients with migraine.**

REFERENCES

1. Neuhauser H, Leopold M, von Brevern M, Arnold G, Lempert T: The interrelations of migraine, vertigo, and migrainous vertigo. Neurology 56(4):436–441, 2001.
2. Whitney SL, Wrisley DM, Brown KD, Furman JM: Physical therapy for migraine-related vestibulopathy and vestibular dysfunction with history of migraine. Laryngoscope 110(9):1528–1534, 2000.
3. Jacob RG, Whitney SL, Setweiler-Shostak G, Furman JM: Vestibular rehabilitation for patients with agoraphobia and vestibular dysfunction: A pilot study. J Anxiety Disorders 15(1-2):131–146, 2000.
4. Breslau N, Schultz LR, Stewart WF, Lipton R, Welch KMA: Headache types and panic disorder: Directionality and specificity. Neurology 56:350–354, 2001.
5. Merikangas KR, Stevens DE: Comorbidity of migraine and psychiatric disorders. Neurol Clin 15(1):115–123, 1997.
6. Stewart WF, Linet MS, Celentano DD: Migraine headaches and panic attacks. Physcosom Med 51:559–569, 1989.
7. Merikangas KR, Angst J, Isler H: Migraine and psychopathology: Results of the Zurich cohort study of young adults. Arch Gen Psychiatry 47:849–853, 1990.
8. Breslau N, Davis GC, Andreski P: Migraine, psychiatric disorders, and suicide attempts. An epidemiologic study of young adults. Psychiatry Res 37:11–23, 1991.

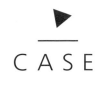

Meniere's Disease and Benign Paroxysmal Positional Vertigo

HISTORY

A 63-year-old woman presented with the chief complaint of dizziness when rolling over in bed. The patient noted that this type of dizziness began several months earlier and lasted for only about 1 minute when turning toward the right while lying in bed. Symptoms were also noticeable when looking up and occasionally when leaning forward. The patient was being treated for Meniere's disease affecting the right ear. Several years previously, she began experiencing weekly episodes of vertigo, right-sided hearing loss, right-sided tinnitus, right-sided ear fullness, nausea, and occasional vomiting. These episodes were spontaneous and typically were not associated with any particular activity. They lasted for about 30 minutes but were occasionally brief (i.e., only a few minutes) or more prolonged (i.e., several hours). The patient had been evaluated by an otolaryngologist, who diagnosed Meniere's disease and prescribed a diuretic and sodium restriction. The patient responded well to this treatment, experiencing only brief (several minutes long) episodes every few months. Then the patient began to experience positional vertigo. Her patient's past medical history was otherwise negative. Her only medication was a combination of hydrochlorothiazide and triamterene prescribed by her otolaryngologist. The family history was noncontributory.

Question 1: Based upon the patient's history, what is her diagnosis?

Answer 1: The patient's history strongly suggests the combination of Meniere's disease and, more recently, benign paroxysmal positional vertigo. It is possible that the patient's positional symptoms are in some way related to her Meniere's disease, manifesting as *pseudo–benign paroxysmal positional vertigo*, that is, benign paroxysmal positional vertigo–type postural nystagmus and vertigo caused by disorders other than benign paroxysmal positional vertigo.

PHYSICAL EXAMINATION

Neurologic examination was normal. Otologic examination revealed that on Weber's test the patient lateralized to the left. Neurotologic examination revealed no spontaneous nystagmus, a normal head thrust, and normal sway on a compliant foam surface even with the eyes closed. On Dix-Hallpike testing, the patient had no signs or symptoms with the left ear down. However, with the right ear down, the patient manifested typical signs and symptoms of benign paroxysmal positional vertigo.

Question 2: Based upon the physical examination, what is this patient's likely diagnosis?

Answer 2: The patient's physical examination confirms the diagnosis of benign paroxysmal positional vertigo affecting the right ear. Additionally, the abnormal Weber test suggests a sensorineural hearing loss in the right ear, supporting a diagnosis of Meniere's disease. There were no central nervous system abnormalities to suggest a neurologic diagnosis. The patient's excessive sway while standing on a compliant foam surface indicates a nonspecific abnormality.

LABORATORY TESTING

Videonystagmography revealed normal ocular motor function, no persistent positional nystagmus, and a right reduced vestibular response on caloric testing of 50%. Rotational and posturography tests were normal.

Audiometric testing revealed a low-frequency sensorineural hearing loss on the right. Hearing was normal on the left. Word recognition was excellent bilaterally.

Question 3: Based upon the patient's history, physical examination, and laboratory tests, what are the likely diagnoses?

Answer 3: Laboratory testing indicates a reduced vestibular response and a low-frequency sensorineural hearing loss on the right. These findings support a diagnosis of right-sided Meniere's disease. Although laboratory testing is not typically used to diagnose benign paroxysmal positional vertigo, a reduced caloric response is commonly seen in patients with this condition.

DIAGNOSIS/DIFFERENTIAL DIAGNOSIS

The patient was given the diagnoses of Meniere's disease and benign paroxysmal positional vertigo.

Question 4: What diagnostic problems, if any, are caused by the co-occurrence of Meniere's disease and benign paroxysmal positional vertigo?

Answer 4: Meniere's disease and benign paroxysmal positional vertigo generally have different symptoms and signs. Meniere's disease is characterized by spontaneous episodes, whereas specific head movements trigger benign paroxysmal positional vertigo. Meniere's disease generally lasts for minutes to hours, whereas benign paroxysmal positional vertigo generally lasts less than 1 minute. Meniere's disease is accompanied by unilateral hearing loss and tinnitus, whereas benign paroxysmal positional vertigo is not associated with abnormalities of hearing. The onset of Meniere's disease frequently precedes the onset of benign paroxysmal positional vertigo.[2]

TREATMENT

Question 5: Should the treatment of a patient with benign paroxysmal positional vertigo with coexisting Meniere's disease be different from that of a patient without coexisting Meniere's disease? Should the treatment of a patient with Meniere's disease with coexisting benign paroxysmal positional vertigo be different from that of a patients without coexisting benign paroxysmal positional vertigo?

Answer 5: Coexisting Meniere's disease should not affect the use of particle repositioning to treat benign paroxysmal positional vertigo. However, treatment of recurrent benign paroxysmal positional vertigo by surgical semicircular canal plugging may be more likely to cause hearing loss in an ear affected by Meniere's disease. Also, coexisting benign paroxysmal positional vertigo should not affect the choice of treatment for a patient with Meniere's disease.

The patient was treated with a particle repositioning maneuver (see Case 7) and was asymptomatic on second Dix-Hallpike testing following the therapeutic maneuver. The patient was advised to continue her treatment for Meniere's disease.

FOLLOW-UP

One week following particle repositioning, the patient returned with continued positional vertigo. Another particle repositioning maneuver was repeated and was apparently successful. However, the patient returned 2 weeks later with continued positional complaints.

Question 6: How might Meniere's disease predispose a patient to develop benign paroxysmal positional vertigo?

Answer 6: Gross et al.[2] hypothesized that Meniere's disease may damage the otolith organs, thereby releasing utricular otoconia into the endolymph.

Question 7: Is the patient's recalcitrance to treatment in some way related to her Meniere's disease?

Answer 7: Gross et al.[2] have noted that benign paroxysmal positional vertigo associated with Meniere's disease may be more difficult to treat than idiopathic benign paroxysmal positional vertigo. Intractable benign paroxysmal positional vertigo has been attributed, in some patients, to obstruction within the membranous ducts of the posterior semicircular canal.[3] The mechanism of such an obstruction is unknown, but in patients with associated Meniere's disease, partial obstruction of the posterior semicircular canal may be caused by a dilated saccule or a stricture of the membranous labyrinth.[2,3]

SUMMARY

A 63-year-old woman presented with the chief complaint of dizziness when rolling over in bed that is typical of benign paroxysmal positional vertigo. The patient was also being treated for Meniere's disease affecting the right ear. Physical examination confirmed the diagnosis of benign paroxysmal positional vertigo affecting the right ear. Laboratory testing supported a diagnosis of right-sided Meniere's disease. The patient was treated with a particle repositioning maneuver and was advised to continue her treatment for Meniere's disease. She returned with continued positional complaints that were difficult to manage.

TEACHING POINTS

1. **Some patients suffer from Meniere's disease and benign paroxysmal positional vertigo simultaneously.** Generally, the onset of Meniere's disease precedes the onset of the vertigo.
2. **Coexisting Meniere's disease does not affect the use of particle repositioning to treat benign paroxysmal positional vertigo.** Also, coexisting benign paroxysmal positional vertigo does not affect the treatment for a patient with Meniere's disease
3. **Meniere's disease may damage the otolith organs, thereby releasing utricular otoconia into the endolymph, leading to benign paroxysmal positional vertigo.**
4. **Benign paroxysmal positional vertigo associated with Meniere's disease may be more difficult to treat than idiopathic benign paroxysmal positional vertigo.** Intractable benign paroxysmal positional vertigo has been attributed, in some patients, to obstruction within the membranous ducts of the posterior semicircular canal.[3]

REFERENCES

1. Hughes CA, Proctor L: Benign paroxysmal positional vertigo. Laryngoscope 107:607–613, 1997.
2. Gross EM, Bradford BD, Viirre ES, Nelson JR, Harris JP: Intractable benign paroxysmal positional vertigo in patients with Meniere's disease. Laryngoscope 110:655–659, 2000.
3. Parnes LS, Price-Jones R: Particle repositioning maneuver for benign paroxysmal positional vertigo. Ann Otol Rhinol Laryngol 102:325–331, 1993.

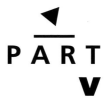

Unusual Disease Case Studies

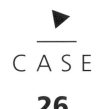

Mal de Débarquement Syndrome

HISTORY

A 45-year-old female molecular biologist complained of persistent dizziness after a 1-week pleasure cruise in the Caribbean 6 weeks before evaluation. The patient had no prior history of dizziness or disequilibrium and used no medications. During her vacation, she had a sense of malaise and motion sickness while on board ship. These symptoms were mild, not associated with vomiting, and treated successfully by the ship's doctor with medication that she wore as a patch behind her ear (most likely scopolamine). The patient noted that while returning home, she was bothered by motion sickness during air travel. She had not experienced air sickness previously. Following her arrival home, the patient noted a persistent rocking sensation. She had no complaints of hearing loss, tinnitus, or fullness in the ears. The patient had no significant family history. Meclizine had been prescribed but was not helpful. An MRI scan, requested by the patient's primary care physician, was normal.

Question 1: Based on the patient's history, what are the diagnostic considerations?

Answer 1: This patient has persistent complaints referable to the vestibular system following a sea voyage. Diagnostic considerations include a vestibulopathy or some other balance disorder that coincidentally began during the patient's travel or an unusual syndrome known as *mal de deabarquement*. Mal de débarquement syndrome has been defined as "sensations of motion experienced on return to stable land after adaptation to motion lasting from hours to days for normal individuals."[1]

PHYSICAL EXAMINATION

The general, neurologic, otologic, and neurotologic examinations were normal.

LABORATORY TESTING

Videonystagmography: Ocular motor, positional, and caloric tests were normal.
Rotational test was normal.
Posturography was normal.
An MRI scan of the brain, which the patient underwent prior to evaluation, was normal.

DIAGNOSIS/DIFFERENTIAL DIAGNOSIS

This patient was given the diagnosis of mal de débarquement syndrome.

Question 2: What is the pathophysiologic basis of mal de débarquement syndrome?

Answer 2: Mal de débarquement syndrome probably results from the ability of the vestibular system to adapt to various motion environments that include combinations of vestibular and visual stimuli. Animal studies have suggested that even vestibular-induced nystagmus can continue beyond the cessation of a repetitive stimulus.[2] The existence of a rare ocular motor disorder known as *periodic alternating nystagmus*[3] suggests that the human vestibular system can oscillate indefinitely. Possibly, patients with mal de débarquement syndrome have adapted to an environment that is no longer present and cannot "unadapt." That is, they have adapted to the environment on board ship, and this is no longer appropriate for dry land. The precise origin of mal de débarquement syndrome is uncertain. Such factors as the otolith organs, hormonal factors, and central nervous system abnormalities have been postulated but not proven to be related to the syndrome.[4]

TREATMENT/MANAGEMENT

Question 3: What treatments should be considered for mal de débarquement syndrome?

Answer 3: Considerations for treatment of mal de débarquement syndrome include vestibular suppressants such as meclizine and promethazine, anxiolytics such as diazepam and clonazepam, antidepressants such as amitriptyline, and the carbonic anhydrase inhibitor acetazolamide.[4]

Before evaluation, the patient failed treatment with meclizine. Low-dose diazepam, 2 mg orally twice a day, was prescribed, with some benefit. The patient was also enrolled in a course of vestibular rehabilitation therapy. She was advised to avoid further prolonged exposure to motion environments. Over the next 3 to 6 months, her symptoms gradually declined.

SUMMARY

A 45-year-old woman presented with the complaint of 6 weeks of persistent dizziness and disequilibrium characterized by a sense of rocking and imbalance that began following a 1-week sea voyage. The patient did not gain relief from meclizine. Physical examination, brain imaging findings, and vestibular laboratory tests were all normal. She was given a diagnosis of mal de débarquement syndrome. Low-dose diazepam and a vestibular rehabilitation therapy provided some relief. The patient's symptoms gradually declined over 3 to 6 months.

TEACHING POINTS

1. **Mal de débarquement syndrome is an unusual disorder defined as a sensation of motion experienced on return to stable land after adaptation to motion, lasting from hours to days for normal individuals.**[1]
2. **The pathophysiology of mal de débarquement syndrome is probably related to the ability of the vestibular system to adapt to various motion environments that include combinations of vestibular and visual stimuli.**
3. **Treatments for mal de débarquement syndrome include vestibular suppressants anxiolytics, antidepressants, and acetazolamide.** Most cases of mal de débarquement syndrome resolve spontaneously within weeks to months.

REFERENCES

1. Brown JJ, Baloh RW: Persistent mal de débarquement syndrome: A motion-induced subjective disorder of balance. Acta Otolaryngol 8:219–222, 1987.
2. Von Baumgarten RJ: Plasticity in the nervous system at the unitary level. In: Schmitt FO (ed). The Neurosciences: Second Study Program. New York: Rockefeller University, 1970, pp 260–271.
3. Leigh RJ, Zee DS: The Neurology of Eye Movements, ed 3. New York: Oxford University Press, 1999.
4. Murphy TP: Mal de débarquement syndrome: A forgotten entity? Otolaryngol Head Neck Surg 109:10–13, 1993.

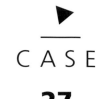

Autoimmune Inner Ear Disease

HISTORY

A 33-year-old woman who worked in a day-care center presented with a chief complaint of hearing loss and disequilibrium that had gradually worsened over 14 months. The patient noted that her symptoms were more or less constant, with periodic exacerbations. Her dizziness was characterized by lightheadedness and a sense of disequilibrium exacerbated by rapid head movements and ambulation. She also noted that her hearing in both ears was impaired and periodically worsened, improving subsequently, but sometimes not to her baseline. The patient had no significant past medical history. There were no complaints of abnormal strength or sensation. Aside from some blurred vision during episodes of extreme dizziness, there were no visual complaints. The family history was negative. Meclizine had been prescribed, with no benefit.

Question 1: Based on the patient's history, what are the diagnostic considerations?

Answer 1: This patient has a history consistent with a peripheral vestibulopathy. Based on the complaints of bilateral hearing loss, the patient may be suffering from bilateral otologic disease. Given the information available from the history, the differential diagnosis for the patient's condition is broad. However, the progressive nature of the illness and the associated complaints of bilateral hearing loss render some diagnoses more likely than others. Meniere's disease (see Cases 9, 16, 21, 25), ototoxicity (see Case 4), neurosyphilis, HIV infection, Lyme disease, autoimmune inner ear disease, Cogan's syndrome,[1] bilateral acoustic neuroma associated with neurofibromatosis, and otosclerosis (see Case 43) are all possible.

PHYSICAL EXAMINATION

Neurologic examination revealed a left-beating nystagmus on left gaze. There were no other abnormalities of cranial nerves. Motor examination, sensation, and coordination were normal. The patient had a very wide-based and unsteady gait. Romberg's test was negative. Otoscopy was normal. She demonstrated some difficulty understanding speech during the interview, especially when lipreading was prevented. Weber's test was midline, and the Rinne test was positive bilaterally. Neurotologic examination revealed left-beating nystagmus with infrared glasses in the primary position that was worsened by left lateral gaze. There was a left-beating post-head-shake nystagmus. The head thrust test was abnormal toward the left and normal toward the right. The patient was unable to stand on a compliant surface even with her eyes open.

Question 2: Does the physical examination help to establish a diagnosis? What laboratory tests should be ordered to rule out other diagnostic possibilities?

Answer 2: The presence of spontaneous nystagmus and abnormal postural control on physical examination indicates a vestibular imbalance, and the patient notes a bilateral hearing impairment. These findings support the idea of bilateral otologic disease. Laboratory testing should be performed to document the extent of hearing loss and the extent of vestibular involvement. An MRI scan should be performed, with special attention to the internal auditory canals. Blood studies should include rheumatologic studies, a serum fluorescent treponemal antibody absorption test (FTA-ABS), and HIV and Borrelia burgdorferi (Lyme) titer.

LABORATORY TESTING

Videonystagmography: Ocular motor function was normal, with the exception of a left-beating spontaneous vestibular nystagmus. There was a direction-fixed left-beating positional nystagmus. Alternate binaural bithermal caloric responses were absent bilaterally. A minimal response to ice-water irrigation was apparent on the right, and responses were absent on the left.

Rotational testing revealed markedly reduced responses and a left-directional preponderance.

Posturography indicated excessive sway on conditions 4, 5, and 6, that is, a surface dependence pattern.

Audiometric testing revealed a bilateral flat sensorineural hearing loss of moderate to severe degree. The word recognition score was 60% in the right ear and 80% in the left ear (Fig. Case 27–1).

An MRI scan of the brain was normal.

Serum FTA-ABS, HIV, and Borrelia burgdorferi (Lyme) titers were all negative. The erythrocyte sedimentation rate was slightly elevated; serum immunoglobulin levels, antinuclear antibody, rheumatoid factor, circulating immune complexes, and C3 and C4 levels were all normal.

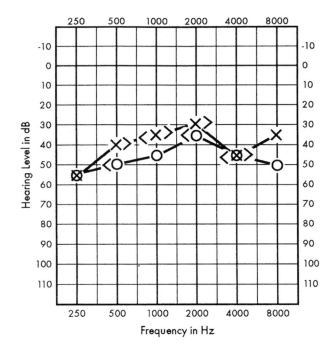

Word Recognition Score	Air	unmasked masked	Right ⊶ △—△	Left ✕—✕ ▫—▫
Right : 60% Left : 80%	Bone	unmasked masked	◄- - -< E- - -[	>- - -► }- - -]

Figure Case 27–1 Audiogram.

DIAGNOSIS/DIFFERENTIAL DIAGNOSIS

Question 3: Based on the history, physical examination, and laboratory test results, what is the most likely diagnosis?

Answer 3: This patient's diagnosis is uncertain. She clearly has bilateral otologic disease impairing both cochlear and vestibular function. Autoimmune inner ear disease is an appropriate provisional diagnosis because there is no evidence of ototoxic drug exposure, little evidence of an infectious process, and no family history or imaging evidence of neurofibromatosis.

Question 4: What is autoimmune inner ear disease? What are its manifestations? Are there any diagnostic tests that can confirm the diagnosis of autoimmune inner ear disease?

Answer 4: Autoimmune inner ear disease is a disorder characterized by auditory and vestibular dysfunction that most often is bilateral and is thought to be produced by damage mediated by both cellular and humoral immune mechanisms.[2,3] Autoimmune inner ear disease is usually bilateral, but it can begin unilaterally and rapidly progress to involve both sides. In its early stages, autoimmune disease may present in a fashion similar to endolymphatic hydrops. The typical patient is a middle-aged woman.[3]

There are currently no well-accepted diagnostic tests that can confirm the diagnosis of autoimmune inner ear disease, although a positive rheumatologic battery or an elevated erythrocyte sedimentation rate may be suggestive. The diagnosis is usually one of exclusion and rests on clinical criteria and response to treatment (see later text). Several experimental tests are being studied, including testing patients' serum against inner ear antigens using Western blot analysis, the lymphocyte transformation test, and the migration inhibition test. These tests show some promise of detecting an autoimmune inner ear disorder. A positive test result is thought to predict a positive response to steroid treatment. Development of more antigen-specific tests is likely to increase the sensitivity and specificity of blood testing for autoimmune inner ear disease.[4–6] For example, Yoo[7] has reported the detection of autoantibodies to type II collagen in autoimmune inner ear disease, and animal studies have furthered the current concepts of autoimmune inner ear disease.[8–10] Thus, patients with suspected autoimmune disease of the ear should undergo blood tests similar to those used for the evaluation of systemic rheumatologic disease. Moreover, because autoimmune inner ear disease is a feature of Cogan's syndrome, which is characterized by autoimmune inner ear disease and nonsyphilitic interstitial keratitis, slit lamp evaluation to search for interstitial keratitis should be undertaken.

Question 5: What are the cochleovestibular manifestations of systemic rheumatologic disease?

Answer 5: Several rheumatologic diseases have been associated with cochleovestibular dysfunction. The nature of this dysfunction is not well characterized but may include both unilateral and bilateral disease. Hearing loss is better documented than vestibular involvement. Table Case 27–1 lists the disorders in which cochleovestibular findings have been reported.

Question 6: What treatments have been advocated for autoimmune inner ear disease?

Answer 6: The most widely accepted treatment of autoimmune inner ear disease includes corticosteroids such as prednisolone, 1 mg/kg per day for 1 to 2 weeks, followed by a tapering dose. Cytotoxic agents such as azathioprine, methotrexate, and cyclophosphamide have also been advocated as an adjunct to steroid

Table Case 27–1
Systemic Autoimmune Diseases Associated with Inner Ear Manifestations

Systemic lupus erythematosus
Rheumatoid arthritis
Vasculitides
  Polyarteritis nodosa
  Wegener's granulomatosis
  Cogan's syndrome
  Behcet's disease
Ulcerative colitis

Source: Adapted with permission from Barna GB, Hughes BP: Autoimmunity and otologic disease: Clinical and experimental aspects. Clin Lab Med 8:389, 1988.[13]

therapy.[11] Lastly, plasmapheresis has been proposed.[12] Each of these treatments is variably successful. Often, patients require long-term treatment to prevent relapse.

The patient was given the diagnosis of autoimmune inner ear disease.

TREATMENT/MANAGEMENT

The patient was treated with steroids in the form of oral prednisolone, 60 mg daily for 2 weeks. During this time, she experienced a slight improvement in hearing, especially in her ability to understand speech, and a slight improvement in balance. After the 2-week course of high-dose steroids, the dose was slowly tapered. When it reached 5 mg daily, the patient noticed worsening of her hearing and balance. The dose was then increased to 20 mg every other day, after which her hearing stabilized. The patient was enrolled in a vestibular rehabilitation program and noticed gradual improvement of balance.

SUMMARY

A 33-year-old woman presented with bilateral hearing loss and disequilibrium that had both gradually worsened over 14 months. On examination, the patient was found to be have bilateral hearing loss and spontaneous vestibular nystagmus. Laboratory testing revealed bilateral sensorineural hearing loss, bilateral vestibular loss with a vestibular asymmetry, and a normal MRI scan. Blood studies did not show evidence of an infectious process. Rheumatologic parameters were normal, with the exception of a mildly elevated erythrocyte sedimentation rate. On the basis of the patient's clinical presentation and positive response to a trial of steroids, the diagnosis of autoimmune inner ear disease was made. Treatment consisted of high-dose corticosteroids and vestibular rehabilitation. The patient's hearing loss and vestibular symptoms stabilized.

TEACHING POINTS

1. **Bilateral otologic disease can cause dizziness symptoms consistent with peripheral vestibular dysfunction in conjunction with bilateral hearing loss.** The differential diagnosis for this clinical situation includes bilateral Meniere's disease, ototoxicity, neurosyphilis, HIV infection, Lyme disease, autoimmune inner ear disease, bilateral acoustic neuroma associated with neurofibromatosis, and otosclerosis.
2. **Autoimmune inner ear disease is a disorder characterized by auditory and vestibular dysfunction that most often is bilateral and is thought to be produced by damage mediated by both cellular and humoral immune mechanisms.** Autoimmune inner ear disease is usually bilateral but may begin unilaterally and progress rapidly to involve both sides.
3. **A diagnosis of autoimmune inner ear disease is difficult to confirm. A positive rheumatologic battery or an elevated erythrocyte sedimentation rate may be suggestive.** Thus, patients with suspected au-

toimmune inner ear disease should undergo blood tests similar to those used for the evaluation of systemic rheumatologic disease. Also, slit lamp evaluation to search for interstitial keratitis, a component of Cogan's syndrome, should be undertaken. Autoimmune inner ear disease is often a diagnosis of exclusion and frequently depends on clinical criteria and the response to a trial of corticosteroid therapy.

4. **Rheumatologic diseases can be associated with cochleovestibular dysfunction.** Case Table 27–1 lists the systemic autoimmune diseases in which cochleovestibular findings have been reported.

5. **Treatment of autoimmune inner ear disease usually includes corticosteroids, such as prednisolone, 1 mg/kg per day for 1 to 2 weeks, followed by a tapering dose and a maintenance dose if a positive response has occurred.** Cytotoxic agents such as azathioprine and cyclophosphamide have also been advocated as an adjunct if the disease stops responding to steroid therapy. Plasmapheresis may be effective.

REFERENCES

1. Cogan DS: Syndrome of nonsyphilitic interstitial keratitis and vestibuloauditory symptoms. Arch Ophthalmol 33:144, 1945.
2. Veldman JE, Roord JJ, O'Connor AF, Shea JJ: Autoimmunity and inner ear disorders: An immune-complex mediated sensorineural hearing loss. Laryngoscope 94:501, 1984.
3. Griffith AJ: Biological and clinical aspects of autoimmune inner ear disease. Yale J Biol Med 65:17–28, 1992.
4. Moscicki RA, San Martin JE, Quintero CH, Rauch SD, Nadol JB Jr, Bloch KJ: Serum antibody to inner ear proteins in patients with progressive hearing loss. JAMA 272:611–616, 1994.
5. Yamanobe S, Harris JP: Inner ear-specific antibodies. Laryngoscope 103:319–326, 1993.
6. Hughes GB, Barna BP, Kinney SE, Calabrese LH, Nalepa NL: Predictive value of laboratory tests in "autoimmune" inner ear disease: Preliminary report. Laryngoscope 96:502–505, 1986.
7. Yoo TJ: Etiopathogenesis of Meniere's disease: A hypothesis. Ann Otol Rhinol Laryngol 93(Suppl 113):6–12, 1984.
8. Soliman AM: Experimental autoimmune inner ear disease. Laryngoscope 99:188–194, 1989.
9. Yoo TJ, Yazawa Y, Tomoda K, Floyd R: Type II collagen-induced autoimmune endolymphatic hydrops in guinea pig. Science 222:65–67, 1983.
10. Harris JP: Immunologic mechanisms in disorders of the inner ear. Otolaryngol Head Neck Surg, Update 1 380–395, 1989.
11. McCabe BF: Autoimmune inner ear disease: Therapy. Am J Otolaryngol 10:196–197, 1989.
12. Luetje CM: Theoretical and practical implications for plasmapheresis in autoimmune inner ear disease. Laryngoscope 99:1137–1146, 1989.
13. Barna GB, Hughes BP: Autoimmunity and otologic disease: Clinical and experimental aspects. Clin Lab Med 8:389, 1988.

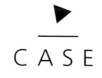

CASE

28

Orthostatic Hypotension

HISTORY

A 50-year-old man who worked as an electronics repairman complained of constant dizziness and lightheadedness that had gradually worsened over several years. He rarely experienced vertigo. The patient's symptoms included a sense of disequilibrium and a feeling of generalized weakness and faintness. These symptoms were especially noticeable on first arising and on standing for more than several minutes in one place. The patient had no complaint of hearing loss, tinnitus, paresthesias, air hunger, palpitations, fear, or anxiety. The family history was positive for adult-onset diabetes mellitus and negative for neurologic or otologic disease. The patient stated that he had recently been tested for blood sugar level and that this was normal. He was not using medications.

Question 1: What are the diagnostic considerations in this case? What additional history should be obtained? What special maneuvers, if any, should be performed during physical examination?

Answer 1: This patient's history provides little information for establishing a definitive diagnosis of a peripheral or central vestibular disorder. In fact, the symptoms of faintness and generalized weekness suggest a nonvestibular cause for the patient's dizziness. Disorders to be considered include hypotension, especially orthostatic hypotension, intermittent hyperventilation associated with anxiety and/or a chronic anxiety state, hypoglycemia, anemia, hyperthyroidism or hypothyroidism, and medication side effects.

    The patient also has little to suggest an anxiety disorder. He indicated that he had been checked for hypoglycemia and that this was negative. The patient should be asked whether he had undergone blood studies for anemia and hy-

228

pothyroidism. During physical examination, blood pressure and pulse should be measured with the patient seated and at 1, 3, and 5 minutes after standing.

ADDITIONAL HISTORY

The patient indicated that a complete blood count, thyroid and adrenocortical steroid function tests, and a screening electrolyte battery were normal.

PHYSICAL EXAMINATION

The patient's examination revealed a blood pressure of 130/85 while he was seated, with a pulse of 70. After 1 minute of standing, his blood pressure was 90/60 and his pulse was 90. The patient stated that he was experiencing his typical symptoms of faintness and asked to sit down. He felt less symptomatic almost immediately on sitting. The remainder of the neurologic examination was normal, except that the patient had a somewhat wide-based gait. During Romberg's test, the patient complained of feeling lightheaded, but he did not fall with his eyes closed and was able to stand on a compliant foam surface without difficulty. The neurotologic and otologic examinations were normal.

DIAGNOSIS/DIFFERENTIAL DIAGNOSIS

Question 2: Based on the patient's history and physical examination, what is the probable diagnosis?

Answer 2: This patient has orthostatic hypotension. Patients with this condition become and remain dizzy when they move from a recumbent to an upright position. Examination before and after this movement reveals a significant (>10 mm Hg) drop in mean blood pressure when standing, often with a concomitant increase (>10 beats per minute) in heart rate. Nonneurogenic causes are associated with an increase in heart rate of more than 15 beats per minute. Absence of an increase in heart rate suggests a neurogenic cause. Blood pressure and heart rate should be measured with the patient seated and after standing for 2 minutes. This allows for differentiation between transient symptoms due to a sluggish baroreceptor response (common in the elderly) and true orthostatic hypotension. The physical examination in this patient provided no evidence of vestibular system disease. Blood studies ruled out several other diagnostic possibilities.

LABORATORY TESTING

Question 3: What are the characteristics of nonvestibular dizziness, and how do they differ from the symptoms of vestibular-induced dizziness?

Answer 3: Patients with vestibular dizziness often complain of vertigo that may include spinning or tilting and a sense of being off balance, whereas patients with nonvestibular dizziness often complain of lightheadedness, a floating sensation, a swimming sensation, or giddiness. Vestibular dizziness is often episodic, whereas nonvestibular dizziness is often constant. Vestibular dizziness is often produced or exacerbated by rapid head movements and certain changes in position, such as rolling over in bed. Symptoms associated with vestibular disorders can include nausea, vomiting, unsteadiness, tinnitus, hearing loss, impaired vision, and oscillopsia, whereas nonvestibular dizziness may be associated with perspiration, palpitations, paresthesias, syncope or presyncope, difficulty concentrating, and malaise.[1] Unfortunately, there is much overlap between vestibular and nonvestibular symptoms, so that it is difficult to make such a distinction from the history alone.

This patient was given the diagnosis of idiopathic orthostatic hypotension.

Question 4: What are the possible causes of orthostatic hypotension?

Answer 4: Orthostatic hypotension is not a specific disease but rather a manifestation of abnormal blood pressure regulation, which may be due to many different causes. The most common cause is hypovolemia due to excessive use of diuretic agents or other medications, including vasodilator agents (nitrate preparations and calcium antagonists) and agents that impair autonomic reflex mechanisms (certain antihypertensive drugs, monoamine oxidase inhibitors, antidepressants, phenothiazine antipsychotic drugs, quinine, L-dopa, barbiturates, alcohol, and vincristine). Orthostatic hypotension after prolonged bed rest may be due to decreased baroreceptor responsiveness. Hypotension also may be a sign of underlying autonomic system insufficiency, which can occur in several neurologic disorders. Signs and symptoms of autonomic dysfunction include impotence, fecal and urinary incontinence, iris atrophy, decreased sweating, decreased tearing, and decreased salivation. When symptoms are confined to the autonomic nervous system, the syndrome is referred to as *pure autonomic failure.* When other neurologic abnormalities are present, the syndrome is called *multiple system atrophy.* In the latter syndrome, there may be signs of cerebellar disease, parkinsonism, and corticobulbar tract dysfunction. Several other disorders that can cause orthostatic hypotension include diabetic neuropathy, amyloidosis, tabes dorsalis, syringomyelia, pernicious anemia, alcoholic neuropathy, vasospastic disorders, and peripheral vascular insufficiency.

Question 5: What is the physiologic basis for the nausea and malaise associated with vestibular system ailments?

Answer 5: The vestibular system has powerful influences on the autonomic nervous system, particularly the sympathetic nervous system, and on respiration.[2–4] Vestibular activity can alter blood pressure and heart rate and can influence the baroreflex. Vestibular inputs that are excessive or in conflict with other sensory inputs can produce motion sickness,[5] wherein individuals have a sense of malaise associated with nausea, diaphoresis, and sometimes vomiting.

The mechanism whereby vestibular abnormalities and excessive vestibular stimulation induce motion sickness is unknown. Moreover, the purpose of motion sickness is unknown. It is interesting that symptoms of postural hypotension mimic some of the symptoms of vestibular system dysfunction. Possibly, the vestibuloautonomic pathways are responsible for this overlap in symptoms.

TREATMENT/MANAGEMENT

This patient was treated with support stockings, increased dietary sodium intake, and fludrocortisone, 0.1 mg twice daily. He was also advised that when changing from a seated to a standing position he should do so slowly and, once upright, he should begin ambulation as soon as possible to avoid standing in one place for more than a very brief time.

The patient responded favorably to this treatment but still experienced some dizziness and lightheadedness when standing.

SUMMARY

A 50-year-old man presented with the chief complaint of dizziness, especially when standing, associated with a sense of faintness and lower-extremity weakness. The patient's examination revealed postural hypotension without evidence of vestibular system abnormality. The patient was treated with support stockings, increased dietary sodium, and fludrocortisone and experienced a reduction in symptoms.

TEACHING POINTS

1. **Dizziness of vestibular origin and dizziness of nonvestibular origin cannot be distinguished easily from one another.**
2. **Patients with dizziness of vestibular origin often complain of episodic vertigo that may include spinning or tilting and a sense of being off balance, whereas patients with nonvestibular dizziness often complain of constant lightheadedness, a floating sensation, a swimming sensation, or giddiness.** Dizziness of vestibular origin is often produced or exacerbated by rapid head movements and certain changes in position such as rolling over in bed.
3. **Symptoms associated with vestibular disorders include nausea, vomiting, unsteadiness, tinnitus, hearing loss, impaired vision, and oscillopsia, whereas nonvestibular dizziness is more likely to be associated with perspiration, palpitations, paresthesias, syncope or presyncope, difficulty concentrating, and malaise.**
4. **Symptoms of faintness and presyncope should suggest a nonvestibular cause for a patient's dizziness, such as postural hypotension, intermittent hyperventilation associated with anxiety, hypoglycemia, anemia, hypothyroidism, or medication side effects.**
5. **Vestibuloautonomic pathway may underlie the mechanism whereby vestibular abnormalities cause malaise, nausea, and vomiting.** These pathways are thought to underlie the ability of vestibular activity to alter blood pressure and heart rate.
6. **Patients with orthostatic hypotension become dizzy when they move from a recumbent to an upright position.** Blood pressure and heart rate should be measured with the patient seated and after standing for 2 minutes. This allows differentiation between transient symptoms due to a sluggish baroreceptor response (common in the elderly) and true orthostatic hypotension. Sustained decrease in systolic BP of more than 20 mm Hg or diastolic BP of more than 10 mm Hg while standing is diagnostic of orthostatic hypotension.
7. **Orthostatic hypotension, which is a manifestation of abnormal blood pressure regulation, has many different causes.** The most common

causes are hypovolemia due to excessive use of diuretic agents or other medications, impaired autonomic reflex mechanisms due to use of certain medications, multiple system atrophy, diabetic neuropathy, other disorders associated with autonomic insufficiency, and peripheral vascular insufficiency.

REFERENCES

1. Baloh RW, Honrubia V: Clinical Neurophysiology of the Vestibular System, ed. 3. New York: Oxford University Press, 2001.
2. Yates BJ: Vestibular influences on the sympathetic nervous system. Brain Res Rev 17:51–59, 1992.
3. Yates B, Jakus J, Miller A: Vestibular effects on respiratory outflow in the decerebrate cat. Brain Res 629:209–217, 1993.
4. Yates BJ, Miller AD (eds): Vestibular Autonomic Regulation. Boca Raton: CRC Press, 1996.
5. Crampton, GH (ed): Motion and Space Sickness. Boca Raton: CRC Press, 1990.

Wallenberg's Syndrome— Posterior Inferior Cerebellar Artery Infarction

HISTORY

A 55-year-old male high school teacher presented with an acute onset of severe disequilibrium 1 week before evaluation that was characterized by a sensation of being pushed to the ground from the left. The patient also complained of vertigo, nausea, blurred vision, and an inability to stand without assistance. His symptoms were constant. There was no associated hearing loss or tinnitus. His past medical history was significant for hypertension. The family history was significant for cerebral vascular disease.

Question 1: Based on the patient's history, what is the likely diagnosis?

Answer 1: The patient's history suggests a vestibular system abnormality. The presence of an illusionary sensation of movement, visual impairment, and postural instability suggests a vestibular system problem but does not allow localization to either the central or peripheral vestibular system.

The patient's complaint of feeling pushed to the ground, so-called lateropulsion, and persistent symptoms for 1 week suggest a central rather than peripheral vestibular abnormality. Moreover, the patient's history of hypertension suggests that he may have cerebral vascular disease. Thus, the most likely diagnosis is an acute vascular insult involving central vestibular structures. However, the differential diagnosis is very broad and includes both peripheral and central vestibular disorders.

PHYSICAL EXAMINATION

The patient had a normal general examination except for mildly elevated blood pressure. He was awake and alert. A right gaze preference was observed when

233

the patient was distracted, but when he was encouraged to look straight ahead or to the left, he could do so. When asked to look from side to side, the patient exhibited saccadic lateropulsion, a condition characterized by excessively large saccades in one direction (known as *overshoot dysmetria* or *saccadic hypermetria*) and excessively small saccades in the other direction (known as *undershoot dysmetria* or *saccadic hypometria*). In this patient's case, the saccadic overshoots were seen when looking from left to right, and the undershoots were seen when looking from right to left. The patient had asymmetrically impaired ocular pursuit: there was more difficulty pursuing targets moving to the left. With his eyes open in the light, he had a low-amplitude primary-position left-beating nystagmus that increased on left gaze. On right gaze, however, the nystagmus became right-beating and was coarse, that is, low frequency with a large position amplitude. It was clearly different from the nystagmus seen in the primary position, which was fine, that is, high frequency with a small position amplitude. The patient was noted to have diminished sensation on the right side of the face. He had no asymmetry of facial movement. The gag reflex was diminished. Strength was normal. Dysmetria was seen in the right upper extremity on finger-to-nose testing. Sensation to pain and temperature was diminished on the left side of the body, including the left arm and left leg. The patient was unable to stand without assistance, and when walking, which he could do only with assistance, he had a wide-based gait. Otologic examination was normal.

Question 2: Based on the patient's physical examination, what physiologic mechanisms have been disrupted, and what is the most likely localization of this patient's lesion?

Answer 2: The patient's right gaze preference suggests that tonic drive to the medial and lateral rectus muscles is unequal. Such an imbalance could be the result of an acute lesion affecting mechanisms that drive the eyes to the left, for example, an abnormality in the right *frontal eye fields*, or in the left pontine *gaze center*, which includes the paramedian pontine reticular formation. The saccadic lateropulsion suggests an interruption of cerebellar pathways that control saccadic accuracy.[1] This patient's history and physical examination suggest a brainstem abnormality because of the combination of a dissociated sensory loss, that is, a loss of pain and temperature sensation with preservation of touch and position sensation; incoordination; abnormal eye movements; and subjective as well as objective lateropulsion. The patient's left-beating primary-position nystagmus, which increased on left lateral gaze, suggests a vestibular system abnormality characterized by diminution of the drive coming from the right vestibular system.[2] The patient's coarse nystagmus on right gaze is probably gaze-evoked nystagmus resulting from brainstem or cerebellar system involvement. Given the other features of this patient's condition, it is likely that central vestibular structures, including the vestibular nuclei in the right medulla, have been damaged.

Question 3: How can this patient's signs and symptoms be explained by damage to central vestibular pathways?

Answer 3: This patient's right gaze preference suggests that the tonic balance between the left and right vestibular nuclei has been disrupted so that the eyes are being driven slowly to the right. The left-beating nystagmus is a result of this tonic imbalance interrupted by rapid eye movements (quick components of nystagmus) to the left. An acute vestibular imbalance with resulting vestibulospinal difficulties also accounts for the patient's inability to stand or walk without assistance. The patient's complaints of nausea are probably related to a vestibuloautonomic imbalance. The complaint of feeling pushed to the ground may be related to erroneous signals to the cerebral cortex via vestibulocortical projections.

LABORATORY TESTING

An MRI scan of the brain revealed increased T2 signal intensity in the right lateral medulla, with no other abnormality seen.

DIAGNOSIS/DIFFERENTIAL DIAGNOSIS

Question 4: What is this patient's diagnosis? What other lesions present similarly?

Answer 4: It is likely that this patient suffered an ischemic infarction in the territory of the posterior inferior cerebellar artery, that is, a lateral medullary infarction, also known as *Wallenberg's syndrome*. Other conditions that can present similarly include the anterior inferior cerebellar artery syndrome (see Case 30). Distinguishing between the lateral medullary syndrome and the syndrome of the anterior inferior cerebellar artery can be difficult. However, the character of the patient's nystagmus, the lack of hearing loss, and the location of the abnormality as seen on MRI make lateral medullary syndrome the most likely diagnosis.[3] Although other lesions such as demyelination and neoplasia can rarely present with a syndrome similar to Wallenberg's syndrome, these diagnoses are most unlikely because of the acute onset of this patient's symptoms and signs and the findings on the MRI scan.

The patient was diagnosed as having Wallenberg's syndrome caused by an infarction in the territory of the posterior inferior cerebellar artery.

TREATMENT/MANAGEMENT

This patient was treated with antihypertensive agents and aspirin, one tablet per day.

SUMMARY

A 55-year-old hypertensive man presented with the acute onset of vertigo, nausea, disequilibrium, and blurred vision. Examination revealed signs characteristic of the lateral medullary syndrome, including nystagmus, limb dysmetria, and contralateral impairment of pain and temperature. An MRI scan confirmed a lateral medullary infarction. Treatment consisted of blood pressure control and an antiplatelet agent.

TEACHING POINTS

1. **The central vestibular system is composed of several structures and pathways.** These include the vestibular nuclei, vestibulo-ocular pathways, vestibulospinal pathways, vestibuloautonomic pathways,

vestibulocortical pathways, vestibulocerebellum, and other associated structures, such as the perihypoglossal nuclei.

2. **Lateropulsion, a feeling of being pushed or pulled to the ground, suggests a central vestibular abnormality.**

3. **An acute central vestibular imbalance can mimic an acute peripheral vestibular ailment.** Signs and symptoms may include (*1*) nystagmus, because of an abnormal vestibulo-ocular reflex; (*2*) an inability to stand or walk without assistance because of vestibulospinal difficulties; (*3*) nausea, because of vestibuloautonomic imbalance; and (*4*) vertigo, for example, the sensation of being pushed to the ground, because of erroneous signals in vestibulocortical projections.

4. **Wallenberg's syndrome is caused by a lesion in the lateral medulla, usually an infarction in the territory of the posterior inferior cerebellar artery.** Patients typically present with the acute onset of a vestibular imbalance in the presence of unequivocal central nervous system symptoms or signs suggestive of lateral medullary infarction.

REFERENCES

1. Leigh RJ, Zee DS: The Neurology of Eye Movements, ed 3. New York: Oxford University Press, 1999.
2. Baloh RW, Yee RD, Honrubia V: Eye movements in patients with Wallenberg's syndrome. Ann NY Acad Sci 374:600–614, 1981.
3. Amarenco P, Rosengart A, DeWitt LD, Pessin MS, Caplan LR: Anterior inferior cerebellar artery infarcts. Arch Neurol 50:154–161, 1993.

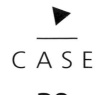

Anterior Inferior Cerebellar Artery Infarction

HISTORY

A 60-year-old man who worked as a building custodian presented with the acute onset of vertigo, hearing loss, and tinnitus in the left ear, left facial weakness, and disequilibrium. The patient experienced blurred vision and mild nausea. There was no complaint of loss of strength, but he complained of great difficulty ambulating and noted veering to the left. His past medical history was significant for hypertension. The family history was not contributory. The patient's family rushed him to a local emergency room, where a CT scan of the head was interpreted as within normal limits.

Question 1: Based upon the patient's history, where is his lesion located and what is the differential diagnosis?

Answer 1: The patient's complaints of vertigo, hearing loss, and tinnitus suggest an acute peripheral vestibular lesion. However, the facial weakness and disequilibrium suggest a central abnormality. Diagnostic possibilities include brainstem or cerebellar infarction or hemorrhage, an infectious process, and a peripheral vestibular ailment.

PHYSICAL EXAMINATION

The patient's general examination was normal aside from an elevated blood pressure of 150/100. The cranial nerve examination revealed an inability to move his eyes to the left. He had left facial weakness affecting the entire left side of the face and decreased sensation on the left side of the face. Strength was normal. There was left upper and lower extremity dysmetria. Sensation was reduced for pain and temperature in the right arm and leg. He could not stand or walk unassisted. Otoscopy was normal. On tuning-fork testing, Weber's test showed lateralization to the right and the Rinne test was positive on the right, indicating a sensorineural hearing in the left ear. On neurotologic examination, right-beating nystagmus was seen with infrared glasses.

Question 2: Based on the history and physical examination, what is the likely diagnosis and what further diagnostic studies would be helpful?

Answer 2: This patient's examination is consistent with a lesion of the brainstem and cerebellum. However, the vertigo, tinnitus, hearing loss, and spontaneous nystagmus suggest a peripheral otologic lesion.

The most likely diagnosis is an infarction in the territory of the anterior inferior cerebellar artery, because this artery supplies the inner ear, lateral pons, and middle cerebellar peduncle.[1,2] Further diagnostic information should be obtained from an MRI scan. Audiometric and vestibulo-ocular testing would also help confirm this diagnosis.

LABORATORY TESTING

Videonystagmography: There was an inability to move the eyes to the left. A right-beating nystagmus was seen during loss of visual fixation. Caloric responses were absent on the left.

Audiometric testing revealed complete deafness on the left and normal hearing on the right.

An MRI scan of the brain showed evidence of acute infarction in the territory of the anterior inferior cerebellar artery involving the lateral pons and adjacent middle cerebellar peduncle.

DIAGNOSIS/DIFFERENTIAL DIAGNOSIS

This patient was given the diagnosis of an infarction in the territory of the anterior inferior cerebellar artery.

Question 3: What arteries supply the vestibular system, including the peripheral labyrinth, and central vestibular structures, including the vestibulocerebellum?

Answer 3: The arterial supply of the labyrinth arises from the labyrinthine artery, which arises from the anterior inferior cerebellar artery, the first branch of the basilar artery (Fig. Case 30–1A). Figure Case 30–1B and Figure Case 30–1C indicate that the vestibular nerve, the vestibular root-entry zone, and the cerebellar flocculus are all supplied by the anterior inferior cerebellar artery.[3] The vestibular nuclei, deep cerebellar nuclei, and inferior vermis are supplied by the posterior inferior cerebellar artery[4] (see Case 29).

Question 4: How does the lateral medullary syndrome differ from the anterior inferior cerebellar artery syndrome?

Answer 4: The lateral medullary syndrome (i.e. Wallenberg's syndrome) (see Case 29) results from infarction in the territory of the posterior inferior cerebellar artery,

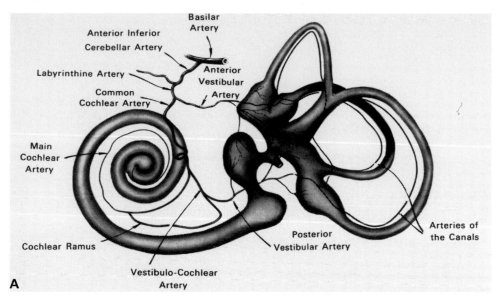

A

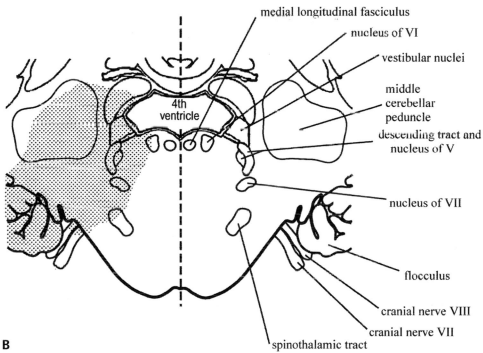

medial longitudinal fasciculus
nucleus of VI
vestibular nuclei
middle cerebellar peduncle
descending tract and nucleus of V
nucleus of VII
flocculus
cranial nerve VIII
cranial nerve VII
spinothalamic tract
4th ventricle

B

Case Figure 30–1 Vascular distribution of the anterior inferior cerebellar artery (AICA). (A) Arterial supply to the inner ear. (B) Line drawing of an axial section through the brainstem showing the major anatomic structures of the brainstem supplied by the AICA. The shaded region represents the region of the brainstem supplied by the AICA. (C) Line drawing of an anterior view of the cerebellum. Shaded areas represent regions supplied by AICA. (*Source*: (A) Modified by permission of the publisher from Schuknecht HF: Pathology of the Ear. Cambridge: Harvard University Press, Copyright 1974 by the President and Fellows of Harvard College, p 62.[5] (B) and (C) modified with permission from Oas JG, Baloh RW: Vertigo and the anterior inferior cerebellar artery syndrome. Neurology 42:2274–2279, 1992, p 2276.[1])

(*continued*)

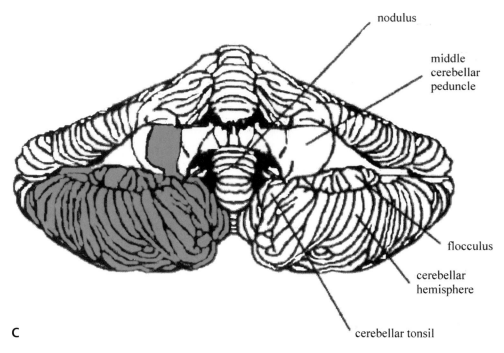

C

Case Figure 30–1 (*Continued*)

which supplies a different region of the brain than the anterior inferior cerebellar artery. Although some of the presenting symptoms and signs of the lateral medullary syndrome and the anterior inferior cerebellar artery syndrome are the same, there are distinct and significant differences. Table Case 30–1 lists these similarities and differences and their pathophysiologic origin.[1–4]

TREATMENT/MANAGEMENT

The patient was treated with supportive measures, antihypertensive agents, and aspirin as an antiplatelet agent.

SUMMARY

A 60-year-old man presented with the acute onset of vertigo, left-sided hearing loss and tinnitus, left facial weakness, and disequilibrium. His past medical history was significant for hypertension. Physical examination revealed left-sided hearing loss, an inability to move the eyes to the left, and abnormal sensation on the left side of the face and in the right arm and leg. MRI indicated infarction in the territory of the anterior inferior cerebellar artery, which was thought to account for all of the patient's symptoms. Treatment consisted of supportive measures and an antiplatelet agent.

Table Case 30-1 Comparison of Posterior Inferior Cerebellar Artery (PICA) and Anterior Inferior Cerebellar Artery (AICA) Syndromes

	Seen in Both PICA and AICA Syndromes	Typically Seen Only in PICA Syndrome	Typically Seen Only in AICA Syndrome
Symptoms	Vertigo, lateropulsion, unusual visual illusions, facial numbness, limb numbness, disequilibrium, dysphagia, and incoordination	Hoarseness	Tinnitus, hearing loss, and facial weakness
Signs	Vestibular nystagmus, decreased facial sensation ipsilaterally, sensory loss to pain and temperature contralaterally, Horner's syndrome, ipsilateral limb ataxia, and gait ataxia	Saccadic lateropulsion, i.e., saccades that are too large when looking in one direction horizontally and too small when looking in the other direction, skew deviation, and vocal cord paralysis	Hearing loss, facial weakness, and gaze palsy
Laboratory Abnormalities	Abnormal imaging, spontaneous nystagmus, and decreased hearing	Saccadic lateropulsion	Caloric reduction ipsilaterally
Pathophysiology	Damage of fifth nerve nucleus, spinothalamic tract, and vestibular nuclei	Damage of nucleus ambiguus and dorsal motor nucleus	Damage of inner ear, eighth cranial nerve, seventh cranial nerve, seventh and eighth cranial nerve root-entry zones, sixth nerve nucleus, flocculus, and middle cerebellar peduncle

TEACHING POINTS

1. **The arterial supply of the inner ear arises from the labyrinthine artery, which arises from the anterior inferior cerebellar artery, the first branch of the basilar artery.**
2. **The anterior inferior cerebellar artery supplies the inner ear, the vestibular nerve, the vestibular root-entry zone, the lateral pons, the middle cerebellar peduncle, and the cerebellar flocculus.**
3. **Infarction in the territory of the anterior inferior cerebellar artery produces a syndrome of acute vertigo, tinnitus, and hearing loss because of interruption of the vascular supply to the inner ear and its nerves.** Neurologic abnormalities including ipsilateral facial nerve paralysis, contralateral reduced pain and temperature sensation, and ipsilateral upper- and lower-extremity dysmetria are consistent with a lesion of the brainstem and cerebellum.
4. **The anterior inferior cerebellar artery syndrome shares many of the clinical features of the lateral medullary syndrome (i.e., Wallenberg's syndrome), which results from infarction in the territory of the posterior inferior cerebellar artery.** Although some of the presenting symptoms and signs of the lateral medullary syndrome and the anterior inferior cerebellar artery syndrome are the same, there are distinct and significant differences (Table Case 30–1).

REFERENCES

1. Oas JG, Baloh RW: Vertigo and the anterior inferior cerebellar artery syndrome. Neurology 42:2274–2279, 1992.
2. Amarenco P, Rosengart A, DeWitt LD, Pessin MS, Caplan LR: Anterior inferior cerebellar artery territory infarcts. Arch Neurol 50:154–161, 1993.
3. Amarenco P, Hauw J-J: Cerebellar infarction in the territory of the anterior and inferior cerebellar artery. Brain 113:139–155, 1990.
4. Gilman S, Bloedel JR, Lechtenberg R (eds): Disorders of the Cerebellum. Contemporary Neurology Series. Philadelphia: FA Davis, 1981.
5. Schuknecht HF: Pathology of the Ear. Cambridge: Harvard University Press, 1974.

Benign Paroxysmal Positional Vertigo—Surgical Management

HISTORY

A 70-year-old retired woman complained of bouts of vertigo that occurred daily for 8 months before evaluation. The patient reported that vertigo could be provoked by lying down in bed, rolling over in bed, or getting out of bed. She expressed a fear of falling and was unable to leave her home because of fear of her vertigo. The patient reported that similar vertiginous episodes had recurred intermittently for the previous 20 years.

Recently, the patient was treated using particle-repositioning maneuvers (see Cases 7 and 39). Although the maneuvers were repeated at six different office visits, she continued to suffer from positional vertigo. After the particle-repositioning maneuvers failed, the patient underwent a 3-month course of vestibular rehabilitation therapy that focused on Brandt-Daroff exercises. After physical therapy, the positional vertigo continued unabated.

Question 1: This patient reported a 20-year history of symptoms consistent with benign paroxysmal positional vertigo. Is it unusual for benign positional vertigo to persist this long?

Answer 1: A history of recurrent periods of positional vertigo spanning 20 years is not unusual. Studies of the natural history of benign paroxysmal positional vertigo show that up to 25% of patients with this condition report symptoms that have persisted for more than 1 year, and many report vertigo lasting for 5 to 20 years.[1] Most patients have symptoms intermittently, but some have positional vertigo that is always present. These individuals have learned never to sleep on the affected side, bend over, or pitch their head backward. Interestingly, by sleeping with the head turned away from the affected side, these individuals have probably inadvertently prolonged their vertigo, because the presumed free-floating endolymph particles that cause benign paroxysmal positional vertigo never have a chance to escape the posterior semicircular canal. Typically, periods of benign paroxysmal positional vertigo can last for 6 to 8 weeks and then spontaneously disappear. Recurrent episodes may occur several times each year.

Question 2: This patient presented with what appears to be typical benign paroxysmal positional vertigo. However, the vertigo was unresponsive to treatment using particle-repositioning maneuvers and physical therapy that included Brandt-Daroff exercises. Is it unusual for benign paroxysmal positional vertigo to be unresponsive to these treatments?

Answer 2: Benign paroxysmal positional vertigo that is unresponsive to particle-repositioning maneuvers or to Brandt-Daroff exercises is unusual but does occasionally occur. More commonly, the vertigo disappears either spontaneously or after treatment but recurs later. It is estimated that approximately 15% of individuals with one episode of benign paroxysmal positional vertigo will have a recurrence within 1 year.[2]

Question 3: What other conditions should be considered in patients with benign paroxysmal positional vertigo that is unresponsive to treatment?

Answer 3: Even if a patient's description is quite typical of benign paroxysmal positional vertigo, it is important to rule out (1) a central nervous system cause of apparent benign paroxysmal positional vertigo,[3–5] (2) bilateral benign paroxysmal positional vertigo, (3) horizontal semicircular canal benign paroxysmal positional vertigo (see below), and (4) an associated chronic peripheral vestibular disorder other than benign paroxysmal positional vertigo that is contributing to the patient's symptoms.

Rarely, patients with symptoms and signs identical to those characteristic of benign paroxysmal positional nystagmus and vertigo have been diagnosed as having a brainstem neoplasm or brainstem infarction.[4,5]

Bilateral benign paroxysmal positional vertigo occurs infrequently in patients with benign paroxysmal positional vertigo and can be ruled out by performing the Dix-Hallpike maneuver with the head turned both to the right and to the left. If benign paroxysmal positional vertigo is present bilaterally, sequential particle-repositioning maneuvers can be performed.

Horizontal semicircular canal benign paroxysmal positional vertigo (HCBPPV), presumably caused by debris in the horizontal rather than the posterior semicircular canal,[6] can be detected by placing the individual in the supine position and then turning the head rapidly to the head right or right lateral position and then quickly to the head left or left lateral position (see Case 39). HCBPPV produces horizontal right-beating nystagmus with the head turned to the right and left-beating nystagmus with the head turned to the left. HCBPPV can be seen in patients who have undergone a particle-repositioning maneuver for typical, that is, posterior semicircular canal benign paroxysmal positional vertigo. Presumably, these patients have debris that moved from the posterior to the horizontal semicircular canal. HCBPPV can be treated using a modified particle-repositioning maneuver (see Case 39).[7]

A peripheral vestibulopathy associated with benign paroxysmal positional vertigo is not unusual,[6] especially if the vertigo follows an acute labyrinthine disorder. Presumably, an acute vestibulopathy, whether viral, traumatic, or other, can produce degeneration within the inner ear, resulting in the formation of free-floating endolymphatic debris that causes benign paroxysmal positional vertigo (see Case 7). Thus, in a patient with symptoms that persist despite treatment for benign paroxysmal positional vertigo, the symptoms may actually be due to the prior peripheral labyrinthine injury. The patient may not have fully compensated for a peripheral disorder, or the peripheral disorder may be fluctuating, producing intermittent symptoms. Such symptoms should be easily distinguished from those of typical benign paroxysmal positional vertigo.

Although benign paroxysmal positional vertigo is usually caused by free-floating endolymph particles, it has been postulated that occasionally a fixed cupular density may occur. In this situation, particle repositioning or exercises may not cause dispersion of the cupular density. This situation is called *cupulolithiasis* rather than *canalithiasis*. The direction of typical positional nystagmus and its fatigability, when present, are difficult to explain physiologically using the cupulolithiasis theory. As a result, even the existence of cupulolithiasis is now controversial.

PHYSICAL EXAMINATION

The patient's neurologic and otologic examinations were normal. On neurotologic examination, performance of the Dix-Hallpike test with the head turned to the right provoked a torsional-upbeat nystagmus typical of benign paroxysmal positional vertigo. The patient experienced vertigo. The nystagmus and vertigo began approximately 5 seconds following positioning and lasted for approximately 30 seconds. A particle-repositioning maneuver was performed (see Case 7), but upon repeat Dix-Hallpike testing, nystagmus and vertigo, although decreased in intensity, remained present. The Dix-Hallpike test with the head turned to the left produced no vertigo or nystagmus. Testing for HCBPPV (see Case 39) by rapidly shifting the patient to the head-left or head-right position from the supine position was negative.

LABORATORY TESTING

Videonystagmography: Ocular motor and static positional tests were normal. However, Dix-Hallpike tests produced vertigo and upbeating nystagmus typical of benign paroxysmal positional vertigo in the head-hanging right position. The caloric test was normal.

An MRI scan of the brain was performed and was normal.

Question 4: Based on the additional information from physical examination and laboratory testing, what are the diagnostic considerations?

Answer 4: This patient appears to have typical benign paroxysmal positional vertigo that is refractory to conventional treatments. Examination and laboratory testing have ruled out bilateral benign paroxysmal positional vertigo, HCBPPV, and a posterior fossa lesion. An associated vestibulopathy is also unlikely.

Question 5: What surgical procedures are available for treatment of patients with benign paroxysmal positional vertigo that has been unresponsive to treatment with physical maneuvers?

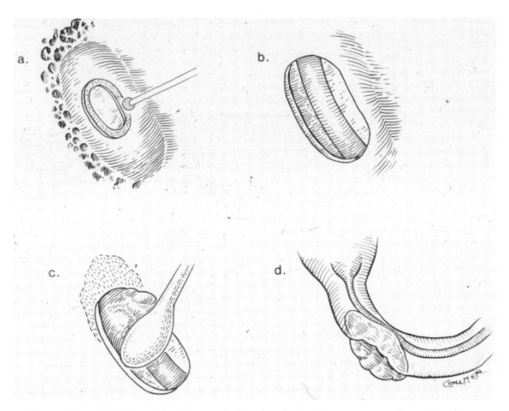

Figure Case 31–1 Semicircular canal plugging for benign paroxysmal positional vertigo. (a) The posterior semicircular canal is exposed within the mastoid cavity, and a small oval island of bone is drilled free. (b) The island of bone is removed with a pick, revealing the perilymphatic and endolymphatic compartments within the bony semicircular canal. (c) Bone wax or bone pâte is then inserted into the opening in the semicircular canal. (d) Plugging of the bony canal results in compression and occlusion of the endolymphatic compartment, which physiologically inactivates the posterior semicircular canal. (*Source*: With permission from Hirsch BE et al: Translabyrinthine approach to skull base tumors with hearing preservation. Am J Otol 14(6):533–543, 1993.[11])

Answer 5: Three surgical procedures have been performed for patients with benign paroxysmal positional vertigo refractory to other nonsurgical treatments: (1) singular neurectomy,[8] (2) posterior semicircular canal "plugging" (occlusion)[9] (Fig. Case 31–1), and (3) vestibular nerve section.[10] Because the singular nerve is composed of only eighth nerve afferent fibers that innervate the ampulla of the posterior semicircular canal, singular neurectomy, a procedure in which the singular nerve is selectively sectioned, removes all afferent activity arising from the posterior semicircular canal. Posterior semicircular canal plugging is a procedure in which the bony posterior semicircular canal is opened surgically and then occluded with bone wax or a "pâte" of bone dust and fibrin glue. This procedure inactivates the posterior semicircular canal ampulla. Vestibular nerve section involves sectioning of the entire vestibular nerve (see also Case 16).

Question 6: How do these three alternative surgical procedures address the underlying pathophysiology of benign paroxysmal positional vertigo?

Answer 6: Singular neurectomy takes advantage of the fact that the posterior semicircular canal ampulla is abnormally stimulated in patients with benign paroxysmal positional vertigo. Thus, by sectioning the afferent nerve to the posterior canal ampulla, erroneous signals resulting from abnormal stimulation of the posterior semicircular canal that occurs with certain head movements are not transmitted to the central nervous system, and thus vertigo and nystagmus are prevented. Occlusion (plugging) of the posterior semicircular canal (Fig. Case 31–1) prevents the flow of endolymph in the posterior semicircular canal. When endolymph flow is prevented, the posterior semicircular canal is effectively inactivated. Thus, free-floating particles either become locked in place and cannot provoke vertigo with head movement or are no longer able to cause deflection of the posterior semicircular canal cupula because they are physically separated from the ampulla. Vestibular nerve section does not specifically address the pathophysiology of benign paroxysmal positional vertigo and is generally not indicated for patients with this form of vertigo because the procedure results in denervation of the entire vestibular portion of the inner ear. However, vestibular nerve section may be indicated in selected patients with concomitant labyrinthine dysfunction in addition to benign paroxysmal positional vertigo.

Question 7: How often is a surgical remedy required for benign paroxysmal positional vertigo?

Answer 7: We estimate that fewer than 1 in 100 cases of benign paroxysmal positional vertigo require surgical intervention. Both the natural history of this vertigo and the success of particle-repositioning maneuvers and vestibular exercises ensure that most of these patients can be cured without surgery.

DIAGNOSIS/DIFFERENTIAL DIAGNOSIS

This patient has benign paroxysmal positional vertigo recalcitrant to medical management. Causes other than a unilateral posterior semicircular canal lesion, including a central nervous system disease, bilateral benign paroxysmal positional vertigo, HCBPPV, and an associated labyrinthine injury, were ruled out.

TREATMENT/MANAGEMENT

This patient was successfully treated with surgical occlusion (plugging) of the posterior semicircular canal. In the immediate postoperative period, she had mild disequilibrium that was treated with additional physical therapy. Three months after treatment, the patient was asymptomatic.

SUMMARY

A 70-year-old retired woman with a complaint of positional vertigo was diagnosed as having benign paroxysmal positional vertigo. The patient's condition was unresponsive to physical therapy, including particle-repositioning maneuvers and Brandt-Daroff exercises. Central nervous system causes of apparent benign paroxysmal positional vertigo, associated labyrinthine dysfunction, bilateral benign paroxysmal positional vertigo, and HCBPPV were all ruled out. A semi-circular canal occlusion (plugging) procedure was performed. The patient was cured of her benign paroxysmal positional vertigo.

TEACHING POINTS

1. **Benign paroxysmal positional vertigo may be long-standing; 25% of these patients report symptoms that have persisted for more than 1 year, and many report vertigo lasting for 5 to 20 years.** Most patients have intermittent symptoms, but some have positional vertigo that is always present. Typically, periods of benign paroxysmal positional vertigo can last for 6 to 8 weeks and then spontaneously disappear.

2. **Benign paroxysmal positional vertigo may remit and then recur. It is estimated that approximately 15% of individuals with one episode of benign paroxysmal positional vertigo will have a recurrence within 1 year.** Recurrent episodes may occur several times each year.

3. **Benign paroxysmal positional vertigo that is recalcitrant to treatment may be caused by (1) a central nervous system abnormality that manifests as apparently benign paroxysmal positional vertigo, (2) bilateral benign paroxysmal positional vertigo, (3) HCBPPV, and (4) an associated chronic peripheral vestibular disorder other than benign paroxysmal positional vertigo that is contributing to the patient's symptoms.**

4. **Surgical procedures for patients with benign paroxysmal positional vertigo that is refractory to nonsurgical treatments include (1) singular (posterior semicircular canal nerve) neurectomy, (2) posterior semicircular canal plugging (occlusion), and (3) vestibular nerve section.**

REFERENCES

1. LeLiever WC: Comparative repositioning maneuvers for benign paroxysmal positional vertigo. Proceedings of the Combined Otolaryngologic Spring Meeting, Palm Beach, Florida; May 7–13, 1994.
2. Nunez RA, Cass SP, Furman JM: Short- and long-term outcomes of canalith repositioning for benign paroxysmal positional vertigo. Otolaryngol Head Neck Surg 122(5):647–653, 2000.
3. Drachman DA, Diamond ER, Hart CW: Posturally-evoked vomiting: Association with posterior fossa lesions. Ann Otol 86:97–101, 1977.
4. Watson P, Barber HO, Deck J, Terbrugge K: Positional vertigo and nystagmus of central origin. J Can Sci Neurol 8:133, 1981.
5. Watson CP, Terbrugge K: Positional nystamus of the benign paroxysmal type with posterior fossa medullobastoma. Arch Neurol 39:601–602, 1982.
6. Baloh RW, Honrubia V, Jacobson K: Benign positional vertigo: Clinical and oculographic features in 240 cases. Neurology 37:371–378, 1987.
7. Baloh RW, Jacobson K, Honrubia V: Horizontal semicircular canal variant of benign positional vertigo. Neurology 43:2542–2549, 1993.
8. Gacek RR: Singular neurectomy update II: Review of 102 cases. Laryngoscope 101:855–862, 1991.
9. Parnes LS, McClure JA: Posterior semicircular canal occlusion for intractable benign paroxysmal positional vertigo. Ann Otol Rhinol Laryngol 99:330–334, 1990.
10. Cass SP, Kartush JM, Graham MD: Patterns of vestibular function following vestibular nerve section. Laryngoscope 102:388–394, 1992.
11. Hirsch BE, Cass SP, Sekhar LN, Wright DC: Translabyrinthine approach to skull base tumors with hearing preservation. Am J Otol 14(6):533–543, 1993.

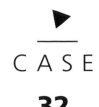

CASE

32

Lithium-Induced Dizziness

HISTORY

A 40-year-old female administrative assistant presented with constant dizziness and disequilibrium for the last several months. The patient noted minimal day-to-day fluctuation of symptoms. She complained of unsteadiness, jumping of her vision, difficulty breathing, and difficulty driving. She denied having spontaneous episodes of vertigo and reported no positionally provoked vertigo. The patient's past medical history was significant for a bipolar affective disorder that had been treated with lithium for 20 years. There was no prior history of dizziness or disequilibrium. The family history was significant for depression.

Question 1: Based on the patient's history, what diagnoses should be considered?

Answer 1: The absence of vertigo suggests that a peripheral vestibular disorder is unlikely. A possible central nervous system disorder is suggested by the nonfluctuating visual difficulties and constant unsteadiness. Considerations include anxiety-related dizziness, migraine-related dizziness, medication side effect, chronic fatigue syndrome, a posterior fossa mass lesion, and cerebellar degeneration. Based upon the patient's history of bipolar affective disorder and long-term use of lithium, a medication side effect should be strongly considered.[1–4]

PHYSICAL EXAMINATION

General examination was normal. Neurologic examination revealed downbeating nystagmus in the center gaze and impaired tandem walking. The remainder of the neurologic examination was normal. Neurotologic examination revealed no spontaneous nystagmus, a normal head thrust test, a negative Dix-Hallpike test except for a continuous downbeating nystagmus, and difficulty maintaining stability on a foam pad with the eyes closed.

Question 2: What is the significance of this patient's abnormal physical examination?

Answer 2: The downbeating nystagmus observed during fixation with the patient seated and during positioning testing suggests a central nervous system disorder. The pathophysiology of downbeating nystagmus (see Case 40) includes an imbalance of up versus down ocular motor drive, which can occur as a result of a central vestibular imbalance or an imbalance related to down versus up ocular pursuit.[5] The localization for downbeating nystagmus includes the caudal midline cerebellum.

Question 3: Would laboratory testing be helpful in establishing a diagnosis?

Answer 3: Vestibular laboratory testing would provide additional information regarding possible coexisting labyrinthine dysfunction and the vestibulo-ocular reflex. This information may be helpful in determining the basis for the patient's symptoms.

LABORATORY TESTING

Videonystagography: Ocular motor testing revealed downbeating nystagmus without other abnormalities. Caloric and rotation responses were normal.
   Audiometry was normal.
   MRI scan of the brain was normal. The blood magnesium level was normal.

Question 4: What is the significance of this patient's vestibular laboratory test results?

Answer 4: Laboratory testing indicated that there was no peripheral vestibular dysfunction and no abnormality of the horizontal VOR. Brain imaging and blood testing did not disclose a cause for the patient's downbeating nystagmus.

DIAGNOSES/DIFFERENTIAL DIAGNOSIS

Question 5: Based upon the information available, what is the most likely diagnosis?

Answer 5: The patient's history, physical examination, and laboratory test results suggest a central nervous system disorder related to vertical ocular motor tone. Additionally, based upon the patient's complaint of imbalance, it is likely that she is suffering from a central vestibular disorder affecting the vestibular spinal system, although her vertical nystagmus may be impairing her vision and thereby interfering with her upright balance. The most likely cause of this patient's complaints is a side effect of lithium, which is noted to cause downbeating nystagmus.[1-4]

Question 6: What types of medication can cause dizziness affecting the central nervous system?

Answer 6: Many types of medication can cause dizziness and disequilibrium including anticonvulsants, antiarrhythmic medications, antihypertensive medications, psychoactive medications, and even medications that are prescribed specifically for dizziness (see Case 17).[6-7] Examples of anticonvulsants that may cause dizziness or disequilibrium include diphenylhydantoin, phenobarbital, carbamazepine, primidone, and benzodiazepines. Antihypertensive agents that may cause dizziness include beta blockers, possibly as a result of orthostatic hypotension (see Case 28). The side effects of these medications can be additive and particularly problematic in older patients.

Question 7: What medications, when discontinued, can cause dizziness and disequilibrium?

Answer 7: In our experience, discontinuation of selective serotonin reuptake inhibitors and benzodiazepine derivatives is associated with a withdrawal syndrome characterized, in part, by dizziness and disequilibrium. Discontinuation of scopolamine, which is frequently prescribed for motion sickness, may be associated with extreme dizziness.

This patient was given the diagnosis of lithium-induced dizziness, disequilibrium, and downbeating nystagmus.

TREATMENT/MANAGEMENT

After consulting with the patient's psychiatrist, lithium was discontinued and valproic acid was started. At a follow-up evaluation 3 months later, the patient's downbeating nystagmus and had diminished to some extent, as had her dizziness and disequilibrium, although she was still symptomatic. The patient was given a trial of gabapentin, without benefit.

SUMMARY

A 40-year-old woman with a history of bipolar affective disorder treated with lithium presented with constant symptoms of dizziness and disequilibrium. The patient was found to have downbeating nystagmus and no evidence of peripheral vestibular dysfunction on vestibular laboratory. She was given a diagnosis of lithium-induced dizziness. Discontinuation of lithium provided incomplete relief, and the downbeating nystagmus persisted. A trial of gabapentin was unsuccessful.

TEACHING POINTS

1. **Side effects of medications should always be considered as a possible cause of dizziness or disequilibrium.** The most common medications to consider are anticonvulsant, antihypertensive, antiarrhythmic, and psychoactive medications.
2. **Long-term use of lithium can cause downbeating nystagmus.** The onset of this disorder is often insidious even if therapeutic levels of the medication are maintained. Discontinuation of lithium may or may not be associated with a reduction of symptoms and signs.

3. **The discontinuation of certain medications can be associated with dizziness and disequilibrium.** Examples include medications that are successfully controlling dizziness, selective serotonin reuptake inhibitors, and scopolamine.
4. **Dizziness caused by the side effect of a medication can be additive with dizziness caused by other medications or other medical conditions, especially in older patients.**

REFERENCES

1. Gracia F, Koch J, Aziz N: Downbeat nystagmus as a side effect of lithium carbonate: Case report. J Clin Psychiatry 46:292–293, 1985.
2. Williams DP, Troost BT, Rogers J: Lithium-induced downbeat nystagmus. Arch Neurol 45:1022–1023, 1988.
3. Halmagyi GM, Lessell I, Curthoys IS, Lessell S, Hoyt WF: Lithium-induced downbeat nystagmus. Am J Ophthalmol 107:664–670, 1989.
4. Corbett JJ, Jacobson DM, Thompson HS, Hart MN, Albert DW: Downbeating nystagmus and other ocular motor defects caused by lithium toxicity.
5. Leigh RJ, Zee DS: The Neurology of Eye Movements, ed 3. New York: Oxford University Press, 1999.
6. Wennmo K, Wennmo C: Drug-related dizziness. Acta Otolaryngol 455(Suppl):11–13, 1988.
7. Rascol O, Hain TC, Brefel C, Benazet M, Clanet M, Montastruc JL: Antivertigo medications and drug-induced vertigo. Drugs 50:777–791, 1995.

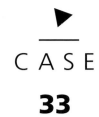

CASE

33

Syncope

HISTORY

A 15-year-old girl presented with a complaint of vertiginous attacks associated with fainting starting 6 months before evaluation. The patient described episodes occurring once or twice per month, characterized by the acute onset of leg weakness, vertigo, and disorientation. She occasionally noticed disequilibrium, loss of vision, and double vision. On several occasions, her mother thought that she had lost consciousness briefly. The family stated that during these episodes, the patient did not respond normally, and that when she spoke she sounded drunk. Following each episode, the patient had a sense of malaise and ataxia. These symptoms were followed some minutes later by headache and drowsiness. The symptoms were markedly reduced after sleep. Occasional tinnitus accompanied these episodes, but the patient had no complaint of hearing loss. She was not using medications. The family history was significant. Her mother had suffered from similar episodes when she was an adolescent, and as an adult she suffered from migraine headaches accompanied by a sense of dizziness.

Question 1: Based on the patient's history, what are the diagnostic considerations?

Answer 1: This patient's history is consistent with a vestibular system abnormality that involves central nervous system structures, considering the association of neurologic symptoms, especially syncope, that is, brief loss of consciousness. The conditions that should be considered include basilar artery migraine (see later text), vertebrobasilar insufficiency (see Case 12), Chiari malformation (see Case 40), posterior fossa neoplasm (see Case 2), and other causes of syncope such as loss of postural tone with brief loss of consciousness (see Table Case 33–1).

Table Case 33–1 Causes of Syncope

Loss of circulatory blood volume
Hyperventilation
Hypoglycemia
Cardiopulmonary disease such as cardiac arrhythmia
Orthostatic hypotension
Basilar artery migraine
Reflex (vasovagal) syncope
Raised intrathoracic pressure
Seizure disorder
Transient brainstem ischemia from structural lesions

Source: Adapted from Shen WK, Gersh BJ: Syncope: mechanisms, approach, and management. In: Low PA (ed). Clinical Autonomic Disorders: Evaluation and Management. Boston: Little, Brown and Company, 1993, pp 605–640.[4]

PHYSICAL EXAMINATION

The neurologic, otologic, and neurotologic examinations were normal. There was no orthostatic hypotension.

LABORATORY TESTING

An MRI scan of the brain and a magnetic resonance angiogram were normal.

A complete blood count, electrolytes, metabolic screen, electroencephalogram (EEG), and Holter monitor recording were normal.

Question 2: What are the clinical characteristics of basilar artery migraine?

Answer 2: Basilar artery migraine, a condition described by Bickerstaff,[1] is associated with symptoms referable to the region supplied by the basilar artery. The diagnosis of basilar artery migraine is somewhat controversial in that many of the symptoms of migraine of any type can be ascribed to territory supplied by the basilar artery; in this sense, all migraine is basilar artery migraine. Nonetheless, basilar artery migraine is a well-defined, distinct diagnostic entity that should be considered in patients with recurrent neurologic symptoms referable to the vertebrobasilar system followed by headache in a patient with a strong family history of migraines.[2]

The clinical manifestations of basilar artery migraine include (*1*) visual symptoms such as tunnel vision and hallucinations; (*2*) ataxia, vertigo, and sometimes tinnitus; and (*3*) parathesias of the face and limbs. Other symptoms include loss of consciousness, nystagmus, double vision, internuclear ophthalmoplegia, and cranial neuropathy.[2]

DIAGNOSIS/DIFFERENTIAL DIAGNOSIS

Because other causes for loss of consciousness were ruled out, the patient was given the diagnosis of basilar artery migraine.

TREATMENT/MANAGEMENT

The patient was treated with dietary restriction of possible migraine-triggering foods and instructed to keep a diary so that precipitant factors could be identified.[3] Additionally, she was treated with propranolol. The frequency of the attacks decreased to one every 2 or 3 months.

SUMMARY

A 15-year-old girl presented with episodes of abrupt onset of leg weakness followed by vertigo, disequilibrium, and poor balance. Her level of consciousness was reduced with some of the episodes. These symptoms were followed by headaches and were relieved by sleep. The patient had a family history of migraine headaches. Laboratory studies appropriate for the evaluation of syncope were all normal. She was given the diagnosis of basilar artery migraine. Treatment consisted of dietary restrictions and propranolol. The frequency of her episodes was reduced.

TEACHING POINTS

1. **Syncope, that is, brief loss of consciousness, may be associated with symptoms suggestive of a vestibular disorder.** However, syncope caused by impaired central nervous system function cannot be the result of a peripheral vestibular abnormality alone.
2. **Basilar artery migraine, vertebrobasilar insufficiency, Chiari malformation, and posterior fossa neoplasm are the causes of syncope most likely to have vestibular symptoms as part of their presentation.**
3. **Basilar artery migraine is a distinct diagnostic entity that can be associated with syncope.**

REFERENCES

1. Bickerstaff E: Basilar artery migraine. Lancet 1:15–17, 1961.
2. Hockaday JM (ed): Migraine in Childhood. London: Butterworths, 1988.
3. American Council for Headache Education, Constantine LM, Scott S: Migraine: The Complete Guide. New York: Dell, 1994.
4. Shen WK, Gersh BJ: Syncope: mechanisms, approach, and management. In: Low PA (ed). Clinical Autonomic Disorders: Evaluation and Management. Boston: Little, Brown and Company, 1993, pp 605–640.

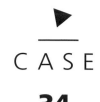

Drop Attacks

HISTORY

A 36-year-old female librarian presented with a complaint of episodic loss of balance. These attacks had occurred approximately once each month during the 2 years before evaluation. They were stereotyped and characterized by an abrupt loss of balance, causing the patient to feel that she was being pulled to the ground. There was no associated vertigo or nausea. The patient was unaware of any precipitating factors. No episodes occurred while the patient was driving. However, on several occasions, she fell and suffered bruises.

The patient was evaluated by her primary care physician, who was unable to reach a diagnosis. That evaluation included a negative MRI scan of the brain and negative blood studies including hematologic, metabolic, and rheumatologic parameters.

Question 1: What are the possible explanations for this patient's attacks, and what further historical information would be helpful?

Answer 1: The patient's attacks of loss of balance could indicate brief episodes of loss of consciousness. Thus, detailed questioning of the patient and her family regarding evidence of loss of consciousness is essential. If the patient is suffering from episodic loss of consciousness, her attacks should be labeled *syncope*, whose differential diagnosis is discussed in Case 33.

If the patient does not lose consciousness during the episodes, the attacks should be labeled *drop attacks*, which have been defined as a falling spell occurring without warning or postical symptoms, with immediate righting, and without loss of awareness or consciousness.[1,2]

Because the patient's attacks occur monthly, any association with menses should be ascertained. Additional important information includes the past med-

Table Case 34–1
Causes of Drop
Attacks

Tumarkin's otolithic crisis
Migraine
Epilepsy
Misinterpreted syncope

---

ical history, especially of any otologic or neurologic abnormality, past or present medication use, and family history.

ADDITIONAL HISTORY

The patient and her family were adamant that the patient did not lose consciousness during these episodes. Despite the abrupt onset and seemingly immediate fall of the patient to the floor, she remembered each episode and was alert, oriented, and conversant immediately afterward. There was no apparent postictal lethargy or confusion. The patient noted no association between her episodes and menses. Her family history was significant. Her mother and sister suffered from typical migraine headaches. Also, the patient's past history was significant for "sick headaches" as a teenager, usually associated with menses. These headaches had stopped approximately 15 years before evaluation, when the patient was in her early 20s. She was not currently using any medications.

Question 2: What are the causes of drop attacks?

Answer 2: Drop attacks can be a manifestation of several disease states (Table Case 34–1), and their origin is often difficult to determine with certainty. In patients with endolymphatic hydrops (see Cases 9, 16, 21, 25), drop attacks sometimes occur and have been labeled *Tumarkin's otolithic crisis.*[3,4] Presumably, this crisis results from abrupt alterations in otolithic function with concomitant changes in the vestibulospinal system and loss of postural tone without an alteration in level of consciousness. Drop attacks may also be a component of migraine (see Cases 8, 21, 24). Abrupt loss of postural tone could represent a migraine aura akin to so-called basilar artery migraine, although this is quite unusual. According to Meissner et al.,[1] of 108 patients with drop attacks, 17 had migraines with no other obvious cause. Drop attacks also can be seen in patients with partial and generalized epilepsy. In addition to these possibilities, one should always be concerned that a patient thought to have drop attacks is actually suffering from syncopal episodes associated with very brief loss of consciousness. Thus, the conditions discussed in Case 33 should also be considered, especially vertebrobasilar insufficiency, postural hypotension, and simple "faints."

PHYSICAL EXAMINATION

The general, neurologic, otologic, and neurotologic examinations were normal.

Question 3: Based on the history and physical examination, what laboratory tests should be ordered?

Answer 3: Based on the above discussion, laboratory tests should include vestibular laboratory tests and an audiogram to search for subclinical hearing loss that may suggest endolymphatic hydrops. Electrocochleography (see Chapter 5) should also be considered to detect the presence of endolymphatic hydrops. The patient should also undergo electroencephalography and Holter monitoring.

LABORATORY TESTING

Videonystagmography was normal.
    Rotational testing was normal.
    Posturography was normal.
    An audiogram and electrocochleography were normal.
    Electroencephalography and Holter monitoring were both normal.

DIAGNOSIS/DIFFERENTIAL DIAGNOSIS

Question 4: Based on the history, physical examination, and laboratory studies, what is this patient's most likely diagnosis?

Answer 4: The patient's diagnosis is uncertain. An unusual variant of migraine or an unusual presentation of endolymphatic hydrops are the most likely diagnostes.

TREATMENT/MANAGEMENT

Question 5: Based on the differential diagnosis, what treatment, if any, should be instituted?

Answer 5: This patient should be treated for either endolymphatic hydrops or migraine. Treatment for migraine with a migraine prophylactic agent poses little risk to this patient, who has no other medical problems. Treatment for endolymphatic hydrops with a diuretic and salt restriction also has little risk.

FOLLOW-UP

The patient was advised to restrict her consumption of foods known to provoke migraine (see Case 13) and was treated with a combination of hydrochlorothiazide and triamterene and salt restriction for possible endolymphatic hydrops. She continued to have further episodes of loss of postural control for an additional 2 months. Diuretic therapy was discontinued, and the patient was started on a calcium channel blocking agent. She immediately noticed a reduction in the frequency of her attacks. The patient continued to use this medication for 6 months, during which the attacks tapered off completely. She then discontinued all medications and has been symptom-free.

    Based on the patient's response to therapy, she received the presumptive and uncertain diagnosis of drop attacks in association with migraine.

SUMMARY

A 36-year-old woman presented with episodes of abrupt loss of postural tone without loss of consciousness. Episodes occurred approximately once each month but were not associated with menses. An extensive evaluation did not uncover any objectifiable abnormalities. The patient was treated presumptively for endolymphatic hydrops without success. She was then treated with a calcium channel blocking agent. Her episodes resolved. Following discontinuation of medication, the patient remained symptom-free.

TEACHING POINTS

1. **A drop attack is a falling spell occurring without warning or postictal symptoms, with immediate righting, and without loss of awareness or consciousness.** It is essential that patients with presumed drop attacks be questioned carefully about even brief episodes of loss of consciousness because this would suggest syncope, which has a different and more ominous differential diagnosis.
2. **Drop attacks can be a manifestation of several disease states (see Table Case 34–1), and their cause is often difficult to determine with certainty.**
3. **Tumarkin's otolithic crisis consists of drop attacks in some patients with endolymphatic hydrops (Meniere's disease).** Presumably, Tumarkin's otolithic crises result from abrupt alterations in otolithic function. If a patient is believed to have Tumarkin's otolithic crisis, treatment for endolymphatic hydrops with a diuretic and salt restriction is the most appropriate initial therapy.

REFERENCES

1. Meissner I, Wiebers DO, Swanson JW, O'Fallon WM: The natural history of drop attacks. Neurology 36:1029 1034, 1986.
2. Kubala MJ, Millikan CH: Diagnosis, pathogenesis, and treatment of "drop attacks." Arch Neurol 11:107–113, 1964.
3. Black FO, Effron MZ, Burns DS: Diagnosis and management of drop attacks of vestibular origin: Tumarkin's otolithic crisis. Otolaryngol Head Neck Surg 90:256 262, 1982.
4. Baloh RW, Jacobson K, Winder T: Drop attacks with Meniere's syndrome: Ann Neurol 28:384–387, 1990.

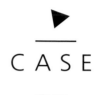

Ramsay Hunt Syndrome

HISTORY

A 55-year-old male physician presented with ear pain, hearing loss, vertigo, and progressive facial paralysis. The symptoms began 3 days before evaluation with the acute onset of severe left ear pain. Two days before evaluation, he had noticed distortion of hearing in the left ear, tinnitus, and disequilibrium when he moved quickly. By that evening, he had severe vertigo, nausea and vomiting, and a definite loss of hearing in the left ear. He also noticed that he could not fully close his left eye, his smile was asymmetric, his voice had become slightly hoarse, and his swallowing felt "funny." Worried about a possible stroke, he went to the emergency room for evaluation. The patient's past medical history and family history were negative.

Question 1: What is the differential diagnosis for this patient's combination of symptoms?

Answer 1: The combination of hearing loss, vertigo, facial paralysis, and bulbar symptoms suggests brainstem dysfunction, possibly as a result of cerebrovascular disease (See Case 30) or encephalitis. Another possibility is a cranial polyneuropathy.

PHYSICAL EXAMINATION

General examination was normal. Cranial nerve examination revealed full extraocular movements. Saccadic and pursuit movements were normal. No nystagmus present with visual fixation. Facial sensation to light touch and pinprick was normal. On testing of corneal reflexes, the left eye did not close when the left cornea was touched but the right eye closed when either cornea was touched.

There was weakness of the left side of the face; the patient was unable to raise his eyebrow or fully close his left eye; he had only a slight amount of movement of his left levator labii. Facial function was graded as House-Brackmann grade 4.[1] The gag reflex was intact. However, visualization of the larynx revealed a left vocal cord paresis, suggesting a lesion of the left vagus nerve. The patient had normal strength during shoulder shrug and was able to lift his arms over his head. However, his left sternocleidomastoid muscle appeared to be weak.

The patient had normal strength and muscle tone in the extremities. Romberg's test demonstrated increased sway without falls. Gait was within normal limits, although the patient tended to veer slightly to the left when he made sharp turns.

On otologic examination, the left pinna, external auditory canal, and eardrum revealed multiple vesicles in the concha and external ear canal and a few on the eardrum. The left eardrum appeared to be slightly reddened, but there was no evidence of acute otitis media. Examination of the oral cavity revealed a number of small vesicles on the left buccal mucosa. Tuning-fork examination revealed a positive Rinne test bilaterally and a midline Weber's test with 512 and 1024 Hz tuning forks.

Neurotologic examination revealed a right-beating jerk nystagmus using infrared glasses. The head thrust was abnormal toward the left. The patient could not stand on a foam pad with his eyes closed. Stepping testing showed that he deviated 90 degrees to the left.

Question 2: Based on the results of the physical examination, what is this patient's most likely diagnosis?

Answer 2: The presence of vesicles on the auricle and in the mouth is highly suggestive of an acute viral process, most likely herpes zoster. J. Ramsay Hunt[2] described a syndrome consisting of facial paralysis, inner ear disturbances, and painful herpetiform blisters of the auricle in 1907. The cause of the syndrome has been confirmed to be herpetic infection involving the seventh and eighth cranial nerves.[3,4] Thus, this patient's most likely diagnosis is Ramsay Hunt syndrome, also known as *herpes zoster oticus*. Facial paralysis is seen in about 60% of patients, and eighth nerve dysfunction, consisting of either sensorineural hearing loss or vertigo, appears in about 40% of patients with herpes zoster oticus. Histopathologic studies have confirmed the direct involvement of the seventh nerve by an inflammatory process marked by hemorrhage, extravasation of blood, inflammatory cell infiltration, and ultimately nerve fiber degeneration. It is not known if this effect is the result of an autoimmune phenomenon or of the viral infection itself. The histopathologic correlate of the eighth nerve disturbance has not been elucidated. Some patients, like this one, have a more widely distributed cranial neuropathy that can affect the tenth and eleventh cranial nerves.

LABORATORY TESTING

Videonystagmography: Ocular motor testing revealed a right-beating spontaneous vestibular nystagmus. Caloric testing revealed a reduced vestibular response on the left with absent bithermal responses. The patient refused ice-water testing.

Rotational testing revealed a mild right directional preponderance.

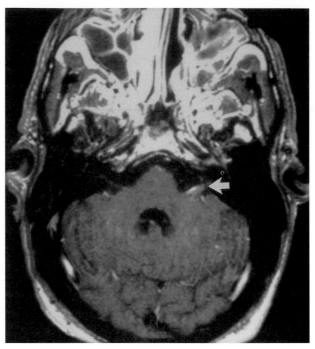

Figure Case 35–1 Axial magnetic resonance image of the head showing enhancement of the seventh and eighth cranial nerves within the internal auditory canal suggestive of an inflammatory neuritis. White arrow = vestibular cochlear nerve bundle within the internal auditory canal. (*Source*: With permission from Hirsch BE et al: Localizing retrocochlear hearing loss. Am J Otol 17(4):537–546, 1996.[10])

Posturography indicated excessive sway on conditions 5 and 6, that is, a vestibular pattern.

An audiogram showed a high-frequency sensorineural hearing loss in the left ear; the word recognition score was 80% in the left ear. The right ear was normal. A brainstem auditory-evoked potential revealed normal amplitudes and latencies in the right ear. However, the left ear showed a slight delay between waves 1 and 3 and a slight delay of wave 5. Otoacoustic emissions were normal bilaterally.

An MRI scan of the head showed enhancement of the seventh and eighth cranial nerves within the internal auditory canal suggestive of an inflammatory neuritis (Fig. Case 35–1). No mass lesions or other abnormalities were noted.

Question 3: How does the laboratory tests help to localize the site of viral involvement?

Answer 3: The abnormal audiogram and loss of caloric function in the left ear suggest involvement of both the vestibular and cochlear subdivisions of the inner ear or eighth cranial nerve on the left. The otoacoustic emissions were normal, suggesting that the hearing loss is a result of neural rather than sensory dysfunction. The brainstem auditory evoked potential suggests a lesion between the spiral ganglion and the brainstem. As in this case, inflammatory cranial neuritis, which may be of viral origin, can be demonstrated on MRI.[5]

Question 4: Can viruses other than herpes zoster or infectious agents cause neuritis leading to hearing loss or vestibular system disturbances?

Answer 4: Several other viruses can cause hearing loss or vestibular disturbance, including rubella, rabies, mumps, cytomegalic viruses, and human immunodeficiency virus (HIV). In addition to the viral causes of neuritis, several bacterial infections can also produce inner ear disturbances, including tetanus, typhoid fever, leptospirosis, syphilis, diphtheria, and Lyme disease.

Question 5: Can Lyme disease cause both facial nerve paralysis and inner ear disturbances?

Answer 5: Lyme disease, a systemic spirochetal (*Borrelia burgdorferi*) infection that follows the bite of an infected tick (*Ixodes dammini*), should be considered as a possible cause of any inflammatory polyneuritis.[6] Lyme disease is well known to cause facial paralysis, but it may also cause decreased hearing, tinnitus, and vertigo.[7]

During the first stage of Lyme disease, erythema chronicum migrans, characterized by a small expanding papula that forms an annular lesion with a central clear zone and an erythematous outer border, is reported in 60% to 80% of patients. During stage 2 Lyme disease, about 15% to 20% of patients develop neurologic complications. Although facial paralysis is one of the most common neurologic signs, both hearing loss and vertigo are common. Krejcova et al.[7] reported that 44% of their patients had hearing abnormalities and 81% had vestibular abnormalities.

DIAGNOSIS/DIFFERENTIAL DIAGNOSIS

This patient was given the diagnosis of Ramsay Hunt syndrome, that is, herpes zoster oticus.

TREATMENT/MANAGEMENT

This patient was treated with a combination of acyclovir, 4 g daily in divided doses, and prednisone, 1 mg/kg per day for 10 days.[8,9] Phenergan, 25 to 50 mg intramuscularly, was needed for 2 days to control nausea and vomiting. Ophthalmic ointments were prescribed because of exposure of the left cornea as a result of the facial paralysis. The skin lesions of the auricle were treated with mupirocin ointment. There was no apparent secondary infection of the skin by staphylococcal or streptococcal bacteria, so no systemic antibiotic therapy was needed.

The patient was followed closely over the ensuing 2 weeks. No further progression of the cranial nerve deficits or significant side effects from the medications occurred. The ear pain and vesicles on the ear resolved within 2 weeks. Facial movement returned to nearly normal within 3 months. The tenth and eleventh cranial nerve abnormalities recovered completely. The patient reported the continued presence of mild disequilibrium, hearing impairment, and unilateral left-sided tinnitus at 6-month follow-up.

SUMMARY

A 55-year-old man presented with ear pain, hearing loss, vertigo, and progressive facial paralysis. Physical examination suggested the diagnosis of a polyneuritis with involvement of cranial nerves 7, 8, 10, and 11. A vesicular eruption of the pinna along with facial paralysis and audiovestibular symptoms suggested Ramsay Hunt syndrome. Treatment consisted of acyclovir, steroids, skin care, eye care, and vestibular-suppressant medications. The patient recovered nearly completely, with only residual mild dizziness, hearing impairment, and tinnitus.

TEACHING POINTS

1. **Ramsay Hunt syndrome consists of facial paralysis, inner ear disturbances, and painful herpetiform blisters of the auricle.** The cause of the syndrome has been confirmed to be herpetic infection involving the seventh and eighth cranial nerves. Occasionally, viral involvement of other cranial nerves also occurs.
2. **Viruses other than herpes zoster can cause hearing loss and vestibular system disturbances. These viruses include rubella, rabies, mumps, cytomegalic viruses, and HIV.**
3. **Inflammatory cranial neuritis may be demonstrated on MRI.**
4. **The treatment of Ramsay Hunt syndrome includes acyclovir, 4 g daily in divided doses, and prednisone, 1 mg/kg per day for 10 days.** Vestibular suppressants may be required for nausea and vomiting. Ophthalmic ointments may be needed if exposure of the cornea occurs as a result of the facial paralysis. The skin lesions of the auricle can be treated with medicated ointments. Secondary infection of the skin by staphylococcal or streptococcal bacteria can occur in severe cases and should be treated appropriately.
5. **Bacterial infection also may produce inner ear disturbances.** Examples include tetanus, typhoid fever, leptospirosis, syphilis, diphtheria, and Lyme disease. In particular, Lyme disease causes both facial nerve paralysis and inner ear disturbances. Lyme disease is caused by a systemic spirochetal (*B. burgdorferi*) infection that follows the bite of an infected tick (*I. dammini*) and should be considered as a possible cause of any inflammatory polyneuritis.

REFERENCES

1. House JW, Brackmann DE: Facial nerve grading system. Otolaryngol Head Neck Surg 93:146–147, 1985.
2. Hunt JR: Herpetic inflammations of the geniculate ganglion: A new syndrome and its aural complications. Arch Otol 36:371–381, 1907.
3. Weller TH: Varicella and herpes zoster: Changing concepts of the natural history, control, and importance of a not-so-benign virus. N Engl J Med 309:1434–1440, 1983.
4. Wackym PA: Molecular temporal bone pathology: II. Ramsay Hunt syndrome (herpes zoster oticus). Laryngoscope 107(9):1165–1175, 1997.
5. Korzec K, Sobol SM, Kubal W, Mester SJ, Winzelberg G, May M: Gadolinium-enhanced magnetic resonance imaging of the facial nerve in herpes zoster oticus and Bell's palsy: Clinical implication. Am J Otol 12:163–168, 1991.
6. Moscatello AL, Worden DL, Nadelman RB, Wormser G, Lucente F: Otolaryngologic aspects of Lyme disease. Laryngoscope 101:592–595, 1991.
7. Krejcova H, Bojar M, Jerabek J, Thomas J, Jirous J: Otoneurological symptomatology in Lyme disease. Adv Otorhinolaryngol 42:210–212, 1988.
8. Dickins JRE, Smith JT, Graham SS: Herpes zoster oticus: Treatment with intravenous acyclovir. Laryngoscope 98:776–779, 1988.
9. Murakami S, Hato N, Horiuchi J, Honda N, Gyo K, Yanagihara N: Treatment of Ramsay Hunt syndrome with acyclovir-prednisone: Significance of early diagnosis and treatment. Ann Neurol 41(3):353–357, 1997.
10. Hirsch BE, Durrant JD, Yetiser S, Kamerer DB, Martin WH: Localizing retrocochlear hearing loss. Am J Otol 17(4):537–546, 1996.

CASE
36

Convergence Spasm

HISTORY

A 35-year-old woman presented with dizziness that began following head trauma 6 months prior to evaluation. The patient slipped on ice and fell on her right arm and shoulder, after which her head struck the ground. She did not lose consciousness but did develop a small subdural hematoma. The patient described her dizziness as a sense of lightheadedness and disequilibrium without vertigo. She did not notice symptoms when turning in bed or looking up. The patient noted neck discomfort without localized pain, and there was no association between the neck discomfort and her dizziness. There was no complaint of hearing loss or tinnitus. The patient's past medical history was significant for migraine and a single panic attack several weeks prior to evaluation. Within the last 6 months, the patient was treated unsuccessfully with meclizine, which she discontinued. She was using ibuprofen on an as-needed basis.

Question 1: Based upon the patient's history, what are the possible diagnoses?

Answer 1: This patient's dizziness complaints are nonspecific. The temporal relationship with head trauma suggests the possibility of a labyrinthine concussion. A brainstem concussion seems unlikely since the head trauma appears mild and did not cause loss of consciousness. The patient's history does not suggest benign paroxysmal positional vertigo (see Cases 7, 22, 25, 31, 39) despite its frequent onset following head trauma. Also, the patient's history does not suggest cervicogenic dizziness (Case 53). Posttraumatic endolymphatic hydrops (Case 9, 16, 21, 25) also does not seem likely given the absence of hearing loss and tinnitus.

265

PHYSICAL EXAMINATION

Neurologic examination revealed apparent bilateral sixth nerve palsies. Specifically, when the patient gazed to the right or left, she was unable to adduct the right or the left eye. However, when she attempted lateral gaze, her pupils were noted to constrict. The remainder of the neurologic examination was normal. Otologic examination was normal. Neurotologic examination revealed unusual eye movements during a search for spontaneous nystagmus using infrared video goggles. Specifically, the patient was noted to have intermittent convergence with associated pupillary constriction. During these episodes the patient complained of an odd sensation of eyestrain. The head thrust test, positional test, and stability on a foam pad all were normal.

Question 2: What is the significance of the patient's abnormal physical examination?

Answer 2: The pupillary constriction during gaze testing suggests that the patient's apparent bilateral sixth nerve palsies are a result of the superimposition of convergence and lateral gaze. That is, the patient's physical examination suggests convergence spasm, an abnormality in which there is excessive and inappropriate convergence.[1–6] The spontaneous convergence seen with infrared video goggles also suggests convergence spasm. The patient had no evidence for a vestibular system abnormality.

Question 3: How might convergence spasm lead to complaints of dizziness?

Answer 3: A patient with convergence spasm will experience abnormal vision intermittently. Visual difficulties may result from abnormal focusing, excessive accommodation, or ocular misalignment, that is, strabismus, during convergence spasms. Such visual difficulties can be interpreted by the patient as dizziness.

LABORATORY TESTING

Videonystagmography: Ocular motor, positional, and caloric tests were normal.
    Rotational testing was normal.
    Posturography revealed increased sway in all sway conditions in a nonspecific pattern.
    MRI scan of the brain was normal.

Question 4: What are the causes of convergence spasm? What is the likely cause of convergence spasm in this patient?

Answer 4: Convergence spasm has been seen with numerous disorders, which are listed in Table Case 36–1. This patient has no evidence of any of the disorders listed other than functional convergence spasm. The term *functional* refers to the absence of a medically defined etiology.

DIAGNOSIS/DIFFERENTIAL DIAGNOSIS

This patient was given the diagnosis of convergence spasm of uncertain etiology.

Table Case 36–1
Causes of Convergence
Spasm

Thalamic hemorrhage
Pineal tumor
Encephalitis
Wernicke-Korsakoff syndrome
Vertebrobasilar insufficiency
Chiari malformation
Multiple sclerosis
Metabolic encephalopathy
Phenytoin intoxication
Functional convergence spasm

TREATMENT

Question 5: What treatment strategies are appropriate for a patient with convergence spasm of uncertain etiology?

Answer 5: Referral of such patients to an ophthalmologist or neuro-ophthalmologist is appropriate. For patients with one of the well-defined etiologies in Table Case 36–1, specific treatment of the underlying condition should be instituted. For patients with functional convergence spasm, cycloplegic eye drops, correction of refractive error or the addition of minus lenses, and occlusion of the medial third of the visual field of each eye have been advocated (see Schwartze et al.[7]).

Question 6: What is convergence insufficiency? Can convergence insufficiency present with dizziness?

Answer 6: Convergence insufficiency is a somewhat controversial disorder characterized by decreased positive fusional vergence at near.[8–11] Convergence insufficiency can be associated with dizziness presumably because of blurry vision and possibly even double vision when looking at nearby objects. These visual abnormalities can be interpreted as dizziness by some patients.

FOLLOW-UP

The patient was referred to a neuro-ophthalmologist, who confirmed the diagnosis of convergence spasm. The patient did not respond to cycloplegic medication. At a follow-up evaluation 3 months later, the patient had a normal examination and was nearly symptom-free.

SUMMARY

A 35-year-old woman presented with dizziness that began following head trauma 6 months prior to evaluation. There was no loss of consciousness, but a small subdural hematoma was identified. Dizziness symptoms included lightheadedness and disequilibrium. Vertigo was absent. Physical examination was normal except for apparent bilateral sixth nerve palsies. Pupillary constriction during attempted lateral gaze and spontaneous convergence behind infrared video goggles suggested convergence spasm as the etiology for the patient's dizziness. Cycloplegic eye drops were not helpful.

TEACHING POINTS

1. **Patients with convergence spasm, that is, frequent inappropriate or excessive convergence, may experience abnormal vision intermittently.** Visual difficulties may result from abnormal focusing, excessive accommodation, or ocular misalignment, that is, strabismus, during convergence spasms. Such visual difficulties can be interpreted by the patient as dizziness.
2. **Convergence spasm is associated with numerous disorders, which are listed in Table Case 36–1.** The term *functional* refers to the absence of a medically defined etiology.
3. **For patients with a well-defined etiology for convergence spasm, specific treatment of the underlying condition should be instituted.** For patients with functional convergence spasm, cycloplegic eye drops, correction of refractive error or the addition of minus lenses, and occlusion of the medial third of the visual field of each eye have been tried with limited success.
4. **Convergence insufficiency is a somewhat controversial disorder characterized by decreased positive fusional vergence at near.** It can be associated with dizziness presumably because of visual abnormalities such as blurry vision and possibly even double vision when looking at nearby objects.

REFERENCES

1. Cogan DG, Freese CG: Spasm of the near reflex. Arch Ophthalmol 54:752–759, 1955.
2. Griffin JF, Wray SH, Anderson DP: Misdiagnosis of spasm of the near reflex. Neurology 26:1018–1020, 1976.
3. Nirankari VS, Hameroff SB: Spasm of the near reflex. Ann Ophthalmol 12:1050–1051, 1980.
4. Sarkies NJC, Sanders MD: Convergence spasm. Trans Ophthalmol 104:782–786, 1985.
5. Rabinowitz Dagi LR, Chrousos GA, Cogan DC: Spasm of the near reflex associated with organic disease. Am J Ophthalmol 103:582–585, 1987.
6. Goldstein JH, Schneekloth BB: Spasm of the near reflex: A spectrum of anomalies. Surv Ophthalmol 40:269–278, 1996.
7. Schwartze GM, McHenry LC Jr, Proctor RC: Convergence spasm-treatment by amytal interview: a case report. J Clin Neuroophthalmol 3:123–125, 1983.
8. Daum KM: Characteristics of convergence insufficiency. Am J Optom Physiol Optics 65(6):426–438, 1988.
9. Cohen M, Groswasser Z, Barchadski R, Appel A: Convergence insufficiency in brain-injured patients. Brain Injury 3(2):187–191, 1989.
10. Lepore FE: Disorders of ocular motility following head trauma. Arch Neurol 52:924–926, 1995.
11. Birnbaum MH, Soden R, Cohen AH: Efficacy of vision therapy for convergence insufficiency in an adult male population. J Am Optom Assoc 70:225–232, 1999.

▶
───

C A S E

37

Congenital Inner Ear Malformations

HISTORY

A 16-year-old girl reported an acute onset of hearing loss, tinnitus, and disequilibrium. These symptoms began following a high school football game 7 days earlier. The patient, a majorette in the high school band, was seated in the grandstand in front of the bass drum. The game was very exciting, and the drummer had enthusiastically beaten his drum. The patient had felt pain in her ears several times and then a full feeling in her right ear. Following the game, she noted bilateral loss of hearing, nonlocalized tinnitus, and unsteadiness. She claimed that she could not hear at all and that the world around her seemed to bounce or jiggle when she moved her head quickly.

There was a past history of a left-sided hearing loss of unknown etiology that was first noticed at age 5.

The following day, the patient was seen by an otolaryngologist, who examined her ears and performed an audiogram that confirmed a profound loss of hearing in both ears. The otolaryngologist prescribed oral prednisone and referred the patient for further evaluation.

Question 1: What are the possible causes of this patient's new loss of hearing and of her vestibular symptoms?

Answer 1: The patient may have suffered from acoustic trauma or a temporary threshold shift (see later text) from the pounding of a bass drum close to her ears during the football game. *Acoustic trauma* generally refers to a single high-intensity acoustic event such as a firecracker or gun discharging near an unprotected ear. Acoustic trauma can damage hair cells within the cochlea, causing an immediate and permanent sensorineural hearing loss that involves the midfrequency hearing range between 3 and 6 kHz and is typically centered at 4 kHz. Mild temporary vestibular symptoms are not unusual in cases of acoustic trauma. In this patient's case, it is possible that a single note, aggressively played from the bass drum close to the patient's unprotected ear, caused acoustic trauma.

A *temporary threshold shift* is a temporary increase in auditory thresholds of 10 to 20 dB usually involving the middle to high frequencies (3 to 6 kHz). It often occurs after sustained exposure to high-intensity noise. Associated symptoms include high-pitched tinnitus and a sense of fullness in the ear. Vestibular symptoms are not generally noted during temporary threshold shifts. The symptoms of a temporary threshold shift are usually fully reversible over 12 to 24 hours and are thought to be the result of an acute excessive consumption of essential metabolic factors within the inner ear. A permanent shift in hearing thresholds primarily affecting the high-frequency range can occur following repeated temporary threshold shifts and is referred to as *noise-induced hearing loss*. The incidence of both temporary threshold shifts and noise-induced hearing loss has increased recently in teenagers, primarily because of noise exposure at rock concerts and from the use of personal musical devices at high loudness levels.

Because this patient's hearing loss did not resolve and because she has vestibular symptoms, she is probably suffering from the results of acoustic trauma caused by the proximity to a loud bass drum rather than from a temporary threshold shift.

Question 2: What are the possible causes of this patient's preexisting unilateral hearing loss?

Answer 2: The differential diagnosis for hearing loss discovered during childhood is summarized in Table Case 37–1. Most disorders that cause an inherited or congenital hearing loss present with bilateral profound sensorineural hearing loss at birth.[1] Although the incidence of vestibular abnormalities in congenitally deaf individuals is unknown, symptoms of vestibular dysfunction are rarely reported. A few reports of vestibular laboratory tests performed in conjunction with cochlear implantation suggest that many profoundly deaf individuals have decreased or absent vestibular function. The lack of vestibular symptoms despite abnormal vestibular function may be a result of substitution of other sensory modalities for the abnormal vestibular function. Also, patients with bilateral vestibular loss rarely have vertigo (see Cases 4 and 27).

Inherited hearing loss that develops beyond infancy may be associated with other nonotologic abnormalities such as kidney disease (e.g., Alport's syndrome), ocular disease (e.g., Usher's syndrome), pigmentary disorders (e.g., Waardenburg's syndrome), bony abnormalities (e.g., osteogenesis imperfecta), and mucopolysaccharide storage disease (e.g., Hurler's syndrome and Hunter's syndrome).

Inherited noncongenital hearing loss may or may not be associated with vestibular abnormalities. There are many patterns of hearing loss and vestibular function; they vary in the relative affliction of hearing versus balance and in severity, age of onset, and rate of progression. For example, Usher's syndrome Type I, an inherited autosomal recessive disorder characterized by severe to profound hearing loss and retinitis pigmentosa, is associated with absent vestibular responses. Mixed X-linked progressive deafness with stapes fixation, a condition in

Table Case 37–1 Summary
of the Differential Diagnosis
of Sensorineural Hearing
Loss in Children

Inherited
  Congenital
  Noncongenital
Acquired
  Prenatal
    Infectious
    Inner ear malformations
  Perinatal
    Infectious
    Hyperbilirubinemia
    Prematurity, birth trauma, anoxia
    Persistent fetal circulation
  Postnatal
    Infectious
    Head trauma
    Acoustic trauma
    Noise-induced
    Perilymphatic fistula
    Endolymphatic hydrops

which males show progressive moderate to severe mixed hearing loss, is also associated with abnormal vestibular function. Female carriers of this disorder have only mild hearing loss and normal vestibular function.

Acquired prenatal hearing loss, whether infectious or a result of inner malformations (dysplasias or dysgenesis), may cause vestibular dysfunction. Many patients with inner ear malformations have other abnormalities that comprise a syndrome, such as Klippel-Feil syndrome, Pendred's syndrome, trisomy syndrome, and DiGeorge's syndrome.

A spectrum of inner ear malformations can occur, ranging from total agenesis to various combinations of bony and membranous abnormalities of the cochlea and semicircular canals.[2,3] Examples include Mondini dysplasia, the enlarged vestibular aqueduct syndrome, and cochlear-saccular dysgenesis (i.e., Sheibe dysplasia). Individuals with inner ear dysplasias may present with sudden or progressive hearing loss in childhood or young adulthood. The hearing loss may be unilateral or bilateral. Vestibular symptoms are frequently noted but generally are mild, although acute vertigo may occasionally be the most prominent symptom of an inner ear malformation. A bump on the head, a strong sneeze, or straining during a bowel movement may worsen the hearing or vestibular symptoms associated with inner ear malformations.

Inner ear dysplasias can also be associated with an abnormal communication between the middle ear space and the cerebrospinal fluid space, that is, a perilymphatic fistula (see Case 52). Children with this condition are at risk of recurrent meningitis.[4]

The perinatal causes of hearing loss are listed in Table Case 37–1. These abnormalities can usually be ruled out by reviewing the child's history of perinatal hospitalization or complications at birth. The postnatal causes of childhood hearing loss include infections, such as bacterial or viral meningitis. Mumps labyrinthitis is the most common cause of unilateral hearing loss. Head trauma, acoustic trauma, and noise-induced hearing loss are common causes of hearing loss, especially affecting teenagers, and should be sought in the patient interview.[5] Perilymphatic fistula can cause both hearing loss and vestibular disturbances.[6] The presence of inner ear malformations or head trauma may contribute to the formation of a perilymphatic fistula (see Case 52).

Endolymphatic hydrops can occur in childhood and produces a symptom complex of recurrent vertigo, fluctuating hearing loss, tinnitus, and aural fullness similar to that seen in adults.[7]

ADDITIONAL HISTORY

Further history revealed no known familial hearing loss or history of consanguinity. The patient was a full-term infant, and there were no reported maternal complications of pregnancy or delivery. The parents reported two episodes of high fever of unknown cause during childhood. There was no history of head trauma or noise exposure.

Question 3: What is the most likely cause of this patient's prior hearing loss? How does this relate to the likely cause of the patient's new hearing loss?

Answer 3: The negative maternal and perinatal history does not reveal the cause of the prior left-sided profound hearing loss first noticed at age 5. It is possible that the hearing loss may have been related to a viral labyrinthitis during one of the episodes of high fever. It may also have been caused by an occult inner ear malformation.[8] This idea is supported by the sudden loss of hearing in the contralateral ear precipitated by acoustic trauma, which is suggestive of a bilateral inner ear malformation.

PHYSICAL EXAMINATION

Neurologic examination was normal. Otoscopic examination was normal. The patient could not hear a whispered voice or finger rub in either ear. Neurotologic examination revealed no spontaneous nystagmus with infrared goggles. The head thrust test was normal. No nystagmus or vertigo was noted during pressure changes in the external auditory canal induced by a pneumatic otoscope. The patient could not stand on a compliant foam pad with her eyes open or closed. The stepping test revealed a significant 90 degree deviation to the right.

Question 4: How should the possibility of an inner ear malformation be evaluated with laboratory tests?

Answer 4: Audiometric and vestibular testing can help to define the extent of audiovestibular abnormalities including severity and laterality. A high-resolution CT scan of the temporal bones is most frequently used to diagnose an inner ear anatomic malformation. Because most inner ear malformations include some degree of bony labyrinthine abnormalities, they are easily detected and characterized by CT imaging, which provides bony detail of the inner ear superior

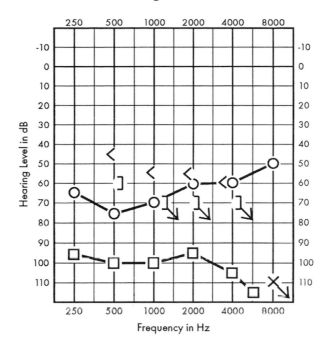

Word Recognition Score		Air	unmasked	Right	Left

Word Recognition Score
Right : 66%
Left : 0%

			Right	Left
Air	unmasked		O———O	✗———✗
	masked		△———△	□———□
Bone	unmasked		◄---<	>--- >
	masked		E---[	}---]

Figure Case 37–1 Audiogram.

to that of MRI. However, recent advances in MRI have led to visualization of the labyrinthine fluid spaces in sufficient detail to characterize many inner ear malformations.

LABORATORY TESTING

Videonystagmography: Ocular motor and positional tests were normal. Caloric testing indicated an absent response to bithermal stimulation and minimal responses to ice-water irrigation, that is, a severe bilateral vestibular reduction.

Rotational testing revealed severely reduced gain and increased phase lead.

Posturography indicated excessive sway on conditions 4, 5, and 6, that is, a surface-dependent pattern.

An audiogram (Fig. Case 37–1) showed a profound sensorineural hearing loss in the left ear. The right ear showed a flat severe sensorineural hearing loss. Word recognition was 0% in the left ear and 66% in the right ear.

CT imaging of the temporal bones showed the presence of a bilateral inner ear malformation consistent with the enlarged vestibular aqueduct syndrome (Fig. Case 37–2).

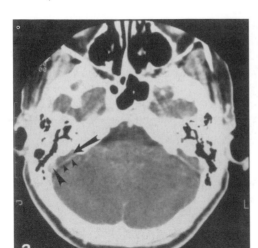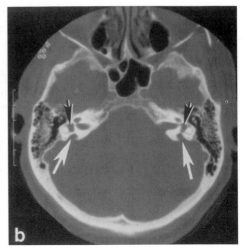

Figure Case 37–2 Axial computed tomographic images showing bilateral dilated vestibular aqueducts. (a) Soft-tissue algorithm shows the dilated endolymphatic sac (arrow), seen here better on the left side. The sac is a fluid-density structure adjacent to the contrast-enhanced sigmoid sinus (large arrowhead). Enhancing dura defines the medial border of the sac (small arrowheads). (b) Bone algorithm demonstrates the osseous anatomy of the inner ear. The osseous vestibular aqueduct is markedly enlarged (white arrows). The labyrinthine vestibules (highlighted arrows) are slightly dysplastic. (*Source*: With permission from Hirsch BE et al: Magnetic resonance imaging of the large vestibular aqueduct. Arch Otolaryngol Head Neck Surg 118:1124–1127, 1992.[10])

DIAGNOSIS/DIFFERENTIAL DIAGNOSIS

This patient was given the diagnosis of enlarged vestibular aqueduct syndrome.

Question 5: What is the enlarged vestibular aqueduct syndrome?

Answer 5: The enlarged vestibular aqueduct syndrome is a congenital malformation of the temporal bone in which the vestibular aqueducts are abnormally enlarged.[9] The syndrome predisposes children to develop progressive sensorineural hearing loss and vestibular dysfunction at a relatively early age.[2–4] An abnormally large vestibular aqueduct can occur as an isolated finding or it can accompany more widespread congenital malformations of the cochlea and semicircular canals. The vestibular aqueduct syndrome is four times more common than Mondini dysplasia.

Question 6: What is the mechanism whereby acoustic trauma or barotrauma (a gradual but large, rather than an abrupt but modest, change in external auditory canal pressure) causes or exacerbates hearing loss and vestibular dysfunction in patients with inner ear malformations?

Answer 6: Although the exact mechanism of hearing loss and vestibular dysfunction as a result of acoustic trauma or barotrauma in patients with inner ear malformations is unknown, two theories are most commonly proffered: (*1*) hearing and vestibular dysfunction may result from an abnormal susceptibility to rupture of the membranous labyrinth or (*2*) hearing and vestibular dysfunction may result from a perilymphatic fistula. In addition to avoiding acoustic trauma, that is, exposure to excessively loud sounds and barotrauma, patients and their parents should be told to avoid activities such as weight lifting, contact sports, and scuba diving, which increase intrathoracic and cerebrospinal fluid pressure, thereby increasing the likelihood of either rupture of inner ear membranes or the development of a perilymphatic fistula.

TREATMENT/MANAGEMENT

The possibility of exploring the right ear for a perilymphatic fistula was discussed with the patient and her family. It was decided that the patient would complete a 2-week course of oral prednisone at a dose of 1 mg/kg per day and remain at bed rest with minimal activity for 2 weeks in case the recent worsening of symptoms was a result of a pressure-induced membrane rupture. The patient's symptoms stabilized. One month later, she resumed normal activities and was counseled regarding avoidance of contact sports, straining, and lifting heavy objects. She was fitted with a hearing aid in the right ear and asked to enroll in a lip-reading class to help improve her communication skills. At 6-week follow-up, the patient reported no further vertigo or disequilibrium and some subjective improvement in hearing. Follow-up audiometric testing showed that word recognition scores had increased to 85%, although pure tone thresholds were unchanged.

SUMMARY

A 16-year-old girl presented with disequilibrium and a loss of hearing and tinnitus in an only-hearing ear following acoustic trauma. A congenital bilateral inner ear malformation was subsequently discovered by CT scanning. Treatment included consideration of middle ear exploration for repair of a possible perilymphatic fistula, a short course of steroids, and 2 weeks of bed rest. Surgery was not performed. The patient's vestibular symptoms resolved, and partial hearing returned. She was fitted with a hearing aid and counseled to avoid strenuous activities and contact sports. The patient also was enrolled in a lip-reading class in order to improve her communication skills and to prepare her for the possibility of future bilateral profound hearing loss.

TEACHING POINTS

1. **Acoustic trauma is a single high-intensity acoustic event discharging near an unprotected ear.** It can damage hair cells within the cochlea, thereby causing an immediate and permanent sensorineural hearing loss that is typically centered at 4 kHz. Mild, temporary vestibular symptoms are not unusual in cases of acoustic trauma.

2. **A temporary threshold shift is a temporary increase in auditory thresholds of 10 to 20 dB, primarily involving the middle to high frequencies.** It often occurs following sustained exposure to high-intensity noise. Associated symptoms include high-pitched tinnitus and a sense of fullness in the ear. Vestibular symptoms are not generally

noted. The symptoms of a temporary threshold shift are usually fully reversible over 12 to 24 hours and are thought to be caused by an acute excessive consumption of essential metabolic factors within the inner ear. A permanent shift in hearing thresholds primarily affecting the high-frequency range can occur following repeated temporary threshold shifts and is referred to as *noise-induced hearing loss*.

3. **Hearing loss discovered during childhood has many causes.** The differential diagnosis is summarized in Table 37–1.

4. **Inner ear dysplasia may present with sudden or progressive hearing loss in childhood or young adulthood.** The hearing loss can be unilateral or bilateral. Vestibular symptoms are frequently noted but generally are mild, although acute vertigo may occasionally be the most prominent symptom of an inner ear malformation. A bump on the head, a strong sneeze, or straining during a bowel movement may worsen the hearing or vestibular symptoms associated with inner ear malformations. Inner ear dysplasias can also be associated with a perilymphatic fistula.

5. **Inner ear malformations often include some degree of bony labyrinthine abnormalities.** They are easily detected and characterized by CT imaging. MRI scan lacks the ability to visualize the bony detail necessary to characterize inner ear malformations.

6. **The enlarged vestibular aqueduct syndrome is a congenital malformation of the temporal bone in which the vestibular aqueducts are abnormally enlarged.** The syndrome predisposes children to develop progressive sensorineural hearing loss and vestibular dysfunction at a relatively early age. An abnormally large vestibular aqueduct can occur as an isolated finding or can accompany more widespread congenital malformations of the cochlea and semicircular canals.

7. **The mechanism of acoustic trauma-induced or barotrauma-induced otologic dysfunction in patients with congenital inner ear malformations is unknown.** In addition to avoiding acoustic trauma and exposure to barotrauma, patients with congenital inner ear malformations and their parents should be counseled concerning avoidance of activities such as weight lifting, contact sports, and scuba diving, which increase intrathoracic and cerebrospinal fluid pressure, thereby increasing the likelihood of either rupture of inner ear membranes or the development of a perilymphatic fistula.

8. **Treatment for an acute worsening of hearing loss and acute vestibular symptoms associated with congenital inner ear malformations should include consideration of middle ear exploration, a short course of corticosteroids, and a period of reduced activity and bed rest.** Surgery directed at the endolymphatic sac should not be performed.

REFERENCES

1. Meyerhoff WL, Cass S, Schwaber MK, Sculerati N, Slattery WH: Progressive sensorineural hearing loss in children. Otolaryngol Head Neck Surg 110:569–579, 1994.
2. Schuknecht HF: Mondini dysplasia: A clinical and pathological study. Ann Otol Rhinol Laryngol 89(Suppl 65):3–23, 1980.

3. Jackler RK, De La Cruz A: The large vestibular aqueduct syndrome. Laryngoscope 99:1238–1243, 1989.
4. Parisier SC, Birken EA: Recurrent meningitis secondary to idiopathic oval window CSF leak. Laryngoscope 86:1503–1515, 1976.
5. Brookhouse PE, Worthington DW, Kelly WJ: Noise-induced hearing loss in children. Laryngoscope 102:645–655, 1992.
6. Supance JS, Bluestone CD: Perilymph fistulas in infants and children. Otolaryngol Head Neck Surg 91:663–671, 1983.
7. Meyerhoff WL, Paperella MM, Shea D: Meniere's disease in children. Laryngoscope 88:1504–1511, 1978.
8. Jackler RK, Dillon WP: Computed tomography and magnetic resonance imaging of the inner ear. Otolaryngol Head Neck Surg 99:494–504, 1988.
9. Levenson MJ, Parisier SC, Jacobs M, Edelstein DR: The large vestibular aqueduct syndrome in children. Arch Otolaryngol Head Neck Surg 115:54–58, 1989.
10. Hirsch BE, Weissman JL, Curtin HD, Kamerer DB: Magnetic resonance imaging of large vestibular aqueduct. Arch Otolaryngol Head Neck Surg 118:1124–1127, 1992.

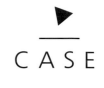

CASE

38

Ocular Tilt Reaction

HISTORY

A 68-year-old man presented with a chief complaint of abnormal vision and continuous vertigo. His vision seemed slanted, and he felt as if he were not upright. The patient was evaluated 1 day after the onset of symptoms. There was no complaint of hearing loss or tinnitus. There were no obvious exacerbating or remitting factors. His past medical history was significant for hypertension and diabetes. The patient's medication included a calcium channel blocker and an oral hypoglycemic agent. The family history was noncontributory.

PHYSICAL EXAMINATION

On general examination, it was noted that the patient's head was tilted to the left. Cranial nerve examination revealed a skew deviation with a right hypertropia, a vertical ocular misalignment unaffected by gaze. The remainder of the cranial nerve examination was normal. There were no abnormalities of strength or sensation and no limb dysmetria. The patient could not stand or walk without assistance. Otologic examination was normal. Neurotologic examination revealed no spontaneous nystagmus.

Question 1: Based on the patient's history and physical examination, what is the likely diagnosis?

Answer 1: The patient's history and physical examination suggest a vestibular system abnormality because of the vertigo and the inability to stand. The patient's abnormal vision and skew deviation suggest a central nervous system lesion. Con-

278

sidering the risk factors of hypertension and diabetes, the patient has probably suffered from a brainstem infarction.

Question 2: What is the significance of this patient's skew deviation?

Answer 2: Skew deviation is thought to be a manifestation of abnormalities in the otolith-ocular pathways that create a left–right otolith-ocular imbalance.[1] This idea is somewhat controversial, however, since a vertical misalignment of the eyes is never appropriate for frontal-eyed animals because such a misalignment always leads to a misalignment of the visual axes. However, there may be a vestigial pathway in the otolith-ocular system that causes a vertical misalignment, because lateral-eyed animals require such a vertical disconjugacy when the head is tilted.

Question 3: What is the significance of the patient's head tilt? What is the ocular tilt reaction? In what disorders is the ocular tilt reaction commonly seen?

Answer 3: This patient's head tilt and skew deviation suggest a condition known as the *ocular tilt reaction,*[2] presumably as a result of damage to otolith ocular connections in the brainstem. The ocular tilt reaction is the combination of head tilt, skew deviation, and ocular torsion, all in the same direction, presumably as a result of imbalance in tonic otolith-ocular drive. Figure Case 38–1 illustrates skew deviation and ocular torsion in a patient (not the individual in this case study) with the ocular tilt reaction. The ocular tilt reaction can be seen with acute pe-

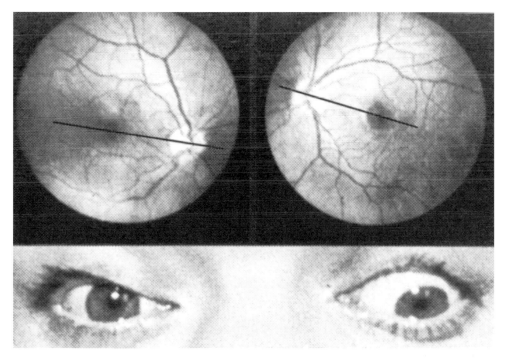

Figure Case 38–1 Photograph of the ocular fundi and eyes of a patient with an ocular tilt reaction. Note the torsion of the fundi and the left hypertropia indicating a leftward ocular tilt reaction. (*Source*: With permission from Halmagyi GM et al: Tonic controversive ocular tilt reaction due to unilateral mesodiencephalic lesion. Neurology 40:1503–1509, 1990.[3])

ripheral vestibular abnormalities that involve the otolith organs or their connections to the vestibular nuclei, and with lesions of brainstem otolith-ocular pathways.[3,4] Thus, brainstem infarctions, brainstem hemorrhages, and mass lesions are common causes of this condition. The ocular tilt reaction often goes unrecognized because (1) severely ill bedridden patients may have an unnoticed head tilt, especially while supine; (2) ocular torsion can be diagnosed objectively only with fundus photography; and (3) the most obvious sign, skew deviation, is a subtle eye movement abnormality that requires a high index of suspicion and an experienced examination for diagnosis.

LABORATORY TESTING

An MRI scan of the brain demonstrated a lesion in the brainstem that was thought to be a small infarction.

DIAGNOSIS/DIFFERENTIAL DIAGNOSIS

This patient was given the diagnosis of ocular tilt reaction secondary to a brainstem infarction.

TREATMENT/MANAGEMENT

Treatment consisted of supportive care and control of the patient's hypertension and diabetes.

Question 4: What is the otolith-ocular reflex? What are manifestations of otolith-ocular reflex abnormalities?

Answer 4: The *otolith-ocular reflex* is that portion of the VOR wherein linear acceleration or changes of the head with respect to gravity lead to eye movements.

The otolith-ocular reflex is best known through the phenomenon of *ocular counterrolling*, wherein a roll of the head, that is, a movement of the ear to the shoulder, is associated with a torsion of the eye about its visual axis in the opposite direction. Presumably, the otolith organs of the inner ear, specifically the utricle and saccule, sense a change in orientation with respect to gravity and drive the eyes torsionally to counteract this tilt. With static tilts of the head, the amount of ocular counterrolling is far less than that required to counteract entirely the effect of head tilt on the orientation of the retina.[5,6] For example, a 45 degree head tilt is associated with approximately only a 9 degree ocular torsion (counterroll),[7] resulting in a large tilt of the retina with respect to upright.

Other forms of the otolith-ocular reflex include eye movements generated by linear acceleration of the head such as that experienced in trains and motor vehicles. Linear motion along the interaural axis, that is, left and right, causes horizontal eye movement, whereas linear motion along the rostral-caudal body axis, that is, up and down, causes vertical eye movement. Because many movements of the head, for example those that occur during walking, are a mixture of linear and rotational motion, the otolith-ocular reflex must combine with the semicircular canal–ocular reflex to maintain stable vision. Currently, there are no routine laboratory tests to assess the otolith-ocular reflex.

SUMMARY

A 68-year-old man with hypertension and diabetes suffered from the acute onset of slanted vision and vertigo. The patient was found to have an ocular tilt reaction consisting of head tilt and skew deviation. MRI revealed a small area of infarction in the brainstem. The patient was thought to have damage to the central otolith-ocular pathways. Treatment consisted of supportive care and control of the patient's hypertension and diabetes.

TEACHING POINTS

1. **The otolith-ocular reflex is that portion of the VOR wherein linear acceleration or changes of head position with respect to gravity lead to eye movements.** Currently, there are no routine laboratory tests to assess the otolith-ocular reflex.
2. **The ocular tilt reaction is a triad of head tilt, skew deviation, and ocular torsion in the same direction**—for example, a leftward head tilt, a right hypertropia, and ocular torsion with the upper poles of eyes deviated to the left. The ocular tilt reaction can be seen with acute peripheral vestibular abnormalities and with lesions of brainstem otolith-ocular pathways.
3. **The ocular tilt reaction often goes unrecognized because severely ill bedridden patients may have an unnoticed head tilt, especially while supine, and skew deviation and ocular torsion are subtle eye movement abnormalities that requires a high index of suspicion for diagnosis.**

REFERENCES

1. Leigh RJ, Zee DS: The Neurology of Eye Movements, ed 3. New York: Oxford University Press, 1999.
2. Westheimer G, Blair S: The ocular tilt reaction—a brainstem oculomotor routine. Invest Ophthalmol 14:833–839, 1975.
3. Halmagyi GM, Brandt T, Dieterich M, Curthoys IS, Stark RJ, Hoyt WF: Tonic controversive ocular tilt reaction due to unilateral mesodiencephalic lesion. Neurology 40:1503–1509, 1990.
4. Mossman S, Halmagyi GM: Partial ocular tilt reaction due to unilateral cerebellar lesion. Neurology 49(2):491–493, 1997.
5. Collewijn H, Van der Steen J, Ferman L, Jansen TC: Human ocular counterroll: Assessment of static and dynamic properties from electromagnetic scleral coil recordings. Exp Brain Res 59:185–196, 1985.
6. Vogel H, Thumler R, Von Baumgarten RJ: Ocular counterrolling. Acta Otolaryngol (Stockh) 102:457–462, 1986.
7. Fluur E: A comparison between subjective and objective recording of ocular counterrolling as a result of tilting. Acta Otolaryngol 79:111–114, 1975.

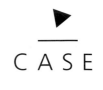

Horizontal Semicircular Canal Benign Paroxysmal Positional Vertigo

HISTORY

A 50-year-old man complained of 3 weeks of positional dizziness. He noted symptoms of brief vertigo that occurred only when rolling over in bed, either to the right or to the left. Otherwise, the patient, who worked as a design engineer, had no symptoms. His past medical history was significant for hypertension, which was treated with a diuretic. Ten years earlier, the patient had had 1 week of positional dizziness that resolved spontaneously. He had no significant family history.

Question 1: Based on the patient's history, what is the differential diagnosis?

Answer 1: This patient's history is highly suggestive of benign paroxysmal positional vertigo (see Cases 7, 22, 25, and 31). Although he may have another cause of episodic vertigo, which has a broad differential diagnosis, benign paroxysmal positional vertigo is most likely.

PHYSICAL EXAMINATION

The patient's general, neurologic, and otologic examinations were normal. On neurotologic examination, no nystagmus was seen with infrared glasses when the patient was sitting. Dix-Hallpike maneuvers were negative. However, when the patient was asked to move from the supine to the lateral position or to turn his head to the right or left while his torso was supine (roll maneuver), he became vertiginous for approximately 10 seconds and was noted to have horizontal nystagmus that lasted as long as the vertigo. The nystagmus was associated with nausea but no vomiting. The nystagmus was noted to be right-beating in the right-lateral and head-right positions and left-beating in the head-left and left-lateral positions. If the patient maintained a lateral or head-turned position, neither nystagmus nor vertigo persisted after they had decayed. The vertigo and nystagmus were much more intense with the right ear down.

LABORATORY TESTING

Videonystagmography: Ocular motor function was normal. There was no vestibular nystagmus when the patient was seated, and the caloric test was normal. On static positional testing, however, the patient was noted to have 10 to 15 seconds of nystagmus that was right-beating in the head-right and right-lateral positions and left-beating in the head-left and left-lateral positions. The amplitude of the nystagmus was much higher with the right ear down.

Rotational testing was normal.

Posturography was normal.

Question 2: What is the significance of the time course and direction of the patient's positional nystagmus?

Answer 2: The patient has a paroxymsal rather than a persistent horizontal nystagmus. This time course suggests free-floating debris in the horizontal semicircular canal rather than a mismatch of cupular and endolymphatic specific gravity (see Case 45). The direction of the nystagmus is geotropic, that is, right-beating with the right ear down and left-beating with the left ear down. This is consistent with excitation of the down ear or inhibition of the up ear during positional testing.

DIAGNOSIS/DIFFERENTIAL DIAGNOSIS

Question 3: Based on the patient's history, physical examination, and laboratory studies, what is the diagnosis?

Answer 3: This patient is suffering from horizontal semicircular canal benign paroxysmal positional vertigo (HCBPPV).[1-4] This entity is thought to result from free-floating debris in the horizontal semicircular canal endolymph in much the same way that typical (posterior semicircular canal) benign paroxysmal positional vertigo results from debris in the posterior semicircular canal endolymph. Interestingly, it is not uncommon to see HCBPPV occur transiently as a sequela of a particle-repositioning maneuver for posterior semicircular canal benign paroxysmal positional vertigo or spontaneously some time later after an episode of posterior semicircular canal benign paroxysmal positional vertigo resolves spontaneously.

Question 4: Because patients with HCBPPV experience vertigo and have geotropic nystagmus in both lateral positions, how can this condition be lateralized to one ear?

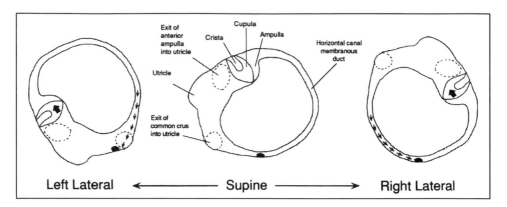

Figure Case 39–1 Schematic drawing showing the presumed pathophysiology of horizontal semicircular canal benign paroxysmal positional vertigo affecting the right ear. The right horizontal semicircular canal is illustrated in three panels: left lateral position, supine position, and right lateral position. Small arrows indicate movement of the debris within the endolymph. Large arrows indicate the direction of cupula deviation. Movement of the head from the supine position to the right lateral position causes movement of debris in an ampulopedal direction, which produces excitation of the right horizontal semicircular canal and, thus, right-beating horizontal nystagmus. Movement of the head from the supine position to the left lateral position produces movement of debris in an ampulofugal direction, which produces inhibition of the right horizontal semicircular canal ampulla and, thus, left-beating horizontal nystagmus. (*Source*: With permission from Baloh RW, Jacobson K, Honrubia V. Horizontal semicircular canal variant of benign paroxysmal vertigo. Neurology 43:2542–2549, 1993.[3])

Answer 4: Based on the presumed pathophysiology of this condition (Fig. Case 39–1), the affected ear is determined by the lateral position that provokes the more intense vertigo and nystagmus.

This patient was given the diagnosis of HCBPPV affecting the right ear.

TREATMENT/MANAGEMENT

Question 5: What is the treatment for patients with HCBPPV?

Answer 5: Analogous to the treatment for typical benign paroxysmal positional vertigo, which affects the posterior semicircular canal, treatment for HCBPPV also consists of a particle-repositioning maneuver.[5,6] The patient is turned in the appropriate manner to move the debris that is presumed to be floating in the endolymph of the horizontal semicircular canal into the vestibule. This particle repositioning is accomplished by rolling the patient 270 degrees from the supine position toward the unaffected ear, then to the prone position, then to the side-down position with the affected ear down, then back to the seated position (see Fig. Case 39–2). The maneuver should be performed slowly. Another treatment option is to have the patient lie on the side with the involved ear up for many hours.[7]

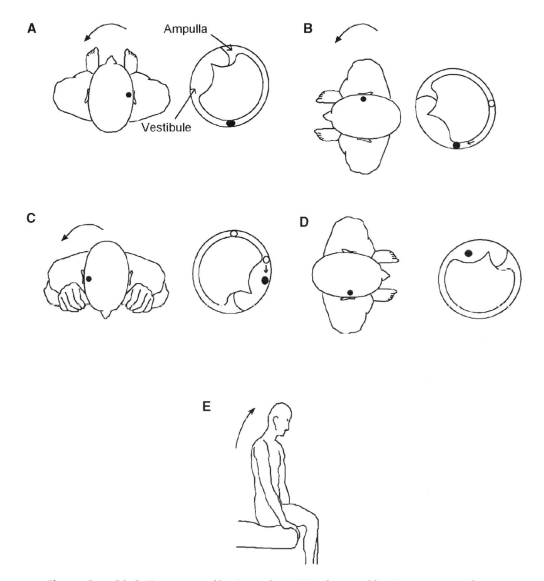

Figure Case 39–2 Treatment of horizontal semicircular canal benign paroxysmal positional vertigo affecting the right ear. Following establishment of the diagnosis, the patient is placed in the supine position (A). Note that the free-floating otolith debris reaches the most dependent position within the horizontal semicircular canal. Then, the patient is rotated toward the intact ear (in this case, the left ear) by 90 degrees to reach the left lateral position (B). Note the movement of the debris toward the vestibule. Then the patient is rotated another 90 degrees to reach the prone position (C). Note the presumed position of the debris in the vestibule. The patient is rotated a final 90 degrees to reach the right lateral position to complete the particle-repositioning procedure (D). The patient is then returned to the seated position (E). (*Source:* Adapted with permission from Nuti D et al: The management of horizontal-canal paroxysmal positional vertigo. Acta Otolaryngol (Stockh) 118:455–460, 1998.[7])

SUMMARY

A 50-year-old male design engineer presented with 3 weeks of positional vertigo. Physical examination disclosed a negative Dix-Hallpike maneuver, but paroxysmal vertigo and nystagmus were elicited during static positional testing. Laboratory tests were negative aside from paroxysmal nystagmus induced by assuming the head-right, head-left, right-lateral, and left-lateral positions. The patient received the diagnosis of HCBPPV. Treatment consisted of a special particle-repositioning maneuver comparable to that used for the treatment of typical posterior semicircular canal benign paroxysmal positional vertigo. After this maneuver, the patient was asymptomatic.

TEACHING POINTS

1. **HCBPPV is a variant of typical benign positional vertigo.** It is thought to result from debris in the endolymph of the horizontal semicircular canal, rather than in the posterior semicircular canal, as occurs in typical benign positional vertigo.

2. **The diagnosis of HCBPPV can be made by turning the patient's head to the right and to the left while the patient is supine.** The patient will become vertiginous for 10 to 30 seconds, and a paroxysmal horizontal nystagmus will be observed for as long as the vertigo persists. The nystagmus is right-beating in the head-right position and left-beating in the head-left position. Patients with HCBPPV have vertigo and nystagmus in both head—turned positions. However, when the affected ear is down, the vertigo and nystagmus that are provoked are more intense than those experienced with the unaffected ear down.

3. **Treatment for HCBPPV consists of a special particle-repositioning maneuver.** The patient is rolled 360 degrees from the supine position toward the unaffected ear, then to the prone position, and then to the side-down position with the affected ear down, then back to the supine position.

REFERENCES

1. McClure JA: Horizontal canal BPV. J Otolaryngol 14:30–35, 1985.
2. Pagnini P, Nuti D, Vannucchi P: Benign paroxysmal vertigo of the horizontal canal. ORL J Otorhinolaryngol Relat Spec 51:161–170, 1989.
3. Baloh RW, Jacobson K, Honrubia V: Horizontal semicircular canal variant of benign positional vertigo. Neurology 43:2542–2549, 1993.
4. De la Meilleure G, Dehaene I, Depondt M, Damman W, Crevits L, Vanhooren G: Benign paroxysmal positional vertigo of the horizontal canal. J Neurol Neurosurg Psychiatry 60:68–71, 1996.
5. Lempert T: Horizontal benign positional vertigo. Neurology 44:2213–2214, 1994.
6. Lempert T, Tiel-Wilck T: A positional maneuver for treatment of horizontal-canal benign positional vertigo. Laryngoscope 106:476–478, 1996.
7. Nuti D, Agus G, Barbieri MT, Passali D: The management of horizontal-canal paroxysmal positional vertigo. Acta Otolaryngol (Stockh) 118(4):455–460, 1998.

Chiari Malformation

HISTORY

A 19-year-old female college student complained of constant dizziness and disequilibrium for several years. The patient noted that she had gait instability, with veering to both the right and the left. There was no true vertigo. Rather, she experienced lightheadedness and disequilibrium, especially when tipping her head back, even while seated. The patient was not particularly bothered by rapid head movements and had no complaints of hearing loss or tinnitus. There was no significant past medical history. The family history was noncontributory.

Question 1: Based on the patient's history, what are the diagnostic considerations?

Answer 1: This patient's history is extremely nonspecific but does suggest a balance system disorder. The symptoms cannot be definitively localized to either the central or peripheral vestibular system. However, the absence of vertigo and the absence of symptoms with rapid head movements suggest a central rather than a peripheral vestibular system abnormality. The worsening of the patient's symptoms when tipping her head back suggests the possibility of a posterior fossa abnormality such as a posterior (vertebrobasilar) circulation abnormality (see Case 12) or a cervical abnormality (see Case 53).

PHYSICAL EXAMINATION

Neurologic examination revealed gaze-evoked nystagmus on left gaze, right gaze, and upward gaze. Oblique down and lateral gaze both to the right and to the left revealed an oblique-torsional (downbeating) nystagmus (Fig. Case 40–1). The pa-

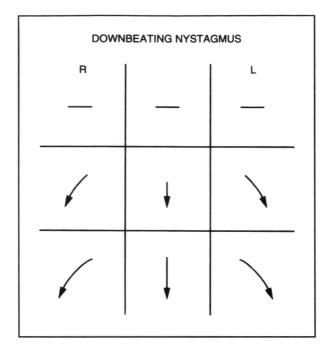

Figure Case 40–1 Downbeating nystagmus. Shown are the direction and magnitude of nystagmus in each of the nine cardinal positions of gaze. Note that the nystagmus is oblique-torsional on downgaze and lateral gaze and is abolished by upgaze. Although it is common for patients with downbeating nystagmus to have nystagmus in only downgaze and lateral gaze, some have nystagmus that persists even with upward gaze. (*Source*: With permission from Furman JM: Nystagmus and the vestibular system. In: Podos SM, Yanoff M (eds). Textbook of Ophthalmology. New York: Gower Medical, 1993, p 9.6.[6])

tient also had saccadic overshoot dysmetria when looking both to the right and to the left and abnormal ocular pursuit with "catch-up" saccades. The remainder of the patient's cranial nerve examination was normal. Strength and sensation were normal. The coordination test was normal. The patient had a widened base of gait. Romberg's test was negative. Otologic examination was normal. On neurotologic examination, she had no nystagmus in the primary position, but with infrared glasses she demonstrated a spontaneous right-beating nystagmus. The patient had difficulty standing on a compliant foam surface. Pastpointing was absent.

Question 2: Based on the physical examination, what is the most likely localization of this patient's lesion, and what are the likely diagnostic possibilities?

Answer 2: The patient's downbeating nystagmus is suggestive of a craniocervical junction abnormality. In combination with the gaze-evoked nystagmus, saccadic dysmetria, and abnormal ocular pursuit, the patient appears to have a lesion of the caudal midline cerebellum. Diagnostic considerations include a Chiari malformation, that is, caudally positioned cerebellar tonsils, a mass lesion, such as a foramen magnum meningioma, or demyelinating disease. Given the gradual worsening of symptoms and the patient's relatively benign history, less likely eti-

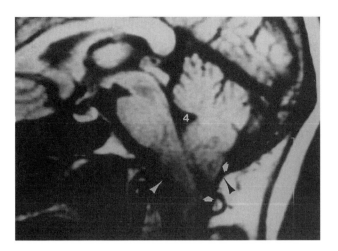

Figure Case 40–2 Sagittal magnetic resonance imaging scan demonstrating a Chiari malformation. The cerebellar tonsils extend into the vertebral canal, with no displacement of the fourth ventricle (4). The foramen magnum is seen between the white and black solid arrowheads. Arrows outline the cerebellar tonsil. (*Source*: With permission from Weber PC, Cass SP: Neurotologic manifestations of Chiari 1 malformation. Otolaryngol Head Neck Surg 109:853–860, 1993.[7])

ologies include an infectious process such as a viral or postviral syndrome, inflammatory disease, and olivocerebellar degeneration syndrome.

LABORATORY TESTING

An MRI scan of the brain revealed a Chiari malformation with the cerebellar tonsils approximately 5 mm below the foramen magnum and an obliterated ambient cistern (Fig. Case 40–2).

Question 3: What is the role, if any, of vestibular laboratory testing in patients with Chiari malformation? Should vestibular laboratory testing be ordered for this patient?

Answer 3: Although vestibular laboratory testing is not required to confirm the diagnosis of Chiari malformation, it may be helpful in planning management, for example, whether to request a neurosurgical consultation, and in following the patient's progress following posterior fossa decompression surgery if this procedure is performed. Vestibular laboratory testing provides a quantitative assessment of the extent of a patient's vestibular system abnormalities, including documentation of any vestibular nystagmus suspected on physical examination. Moreover, some patients with Chiari malformation manifest peripheral vestibular signs such as a caloric reduction. Such information may aid management.

Despite the fact that vestibular laboratory testing may have confirmed some of the abnormalities seen on physical examination, this patient's Chiari malformation is already thought to be symptomatic on the basis of the clinical evaluation, thereby justifying a referral to a neurosurgeon. Thus, vestibular laboratory testing was not obtained.

Question 4: What is the pathophysiologic basis for this patient's nystagmus?

Answer 4: This patient had three types of nystagmus: (1) gaze-evoked nystagmus, (2) downbeating nystagmus, and (3) spontaneous vestibular nystagmus. It is important to note that, by definition, gaze-evoked nystagmus is left-beating on left lateral gaze, right-beating on right lateral gaze, and upbeating on upward gaze. Gaze-evoked nystagmus is typically conjugate, that is, both eyes move equally. Nystagmus that beats down, even when seen only with downgaze, is considered downbeating nystagmus, not gaze-evoked nystagmus elicited by downgaze.

Gaze-evoked nystagmus is thought to be a result of poor gaze holding caused by an abnormal *neural integrator*,[1] that is, a central nervous system circuit that converts (integrates in the mathematical sense) an eye velocity command to an eye position signal. The mechanism of gaze-evoked nystagmus is as follows: The viscoelastic restoring forces of the globe tend to bring the eye toward the primary, that is, the straight-ahead position. These forces are strongest when the eye is deviated away from the primary position. In order to keep the eye on a target placed away from the primary position, a tonic level of neural activity is required to overcome these restoring forces. This required tonic level of activity during gaze away from the primary position declines more quickly than normal in patients with abnormalities of the neural integrator. With this decline of tonic activity, the eye gradually drifts back toward the primary position. This slow drift of the eyes during attempted gaze deviation is interrupted by quick (saccadic) eye movements that bring the eyes back toward the target, away from the primary position. This alternation of slow drift (as a result of a slowly declining tonic drive to the eye muscles) and rapid repositioning movements constitutes gaze-evoked nystagmus. Because the rapid repositioning movements are always in the direction of gaze, gaze-evoked nystagmus, by definition, always beats in the same direction as that of the gaze that evoked it.

There are multiple causes of gaze-evoked nystagmus. The most common causes are the effect of drugs such as anticonvulsants and structural abnormalities in the posterior fossa, especially those affecting the cerebellum. The precise location of the gaze-holding mechanism (i.e., the neural integrator) is unknown, but the nucleus prepositus hypoglossi, which is located in the medulla oblongata near the hypoglossal (twelfth cranial nerve) nucleus, is a likely candidate for horizintal gaze holding.[2] However, the integrity of the neural integrator probably also depends on the cerebellum because cerebellar lesions are frequently associated with gaze-evoked nystagmus.

Downbeating nystagmus is, by definition, a nystagmus wherein the quick component is down or obliquely down and lateral (Fig. Case 40–1). Often, with oblique downbeating nystagmus on down and lateral gaze, there is a torsional component, with the upper pole of the eye beating in the direction of lateral gaze. Downbeating nystagmus is thought to be caused by an imbalance of up versus down tonic drive to the eyes. This up–down imbalance may be a result of unequal central vestibular pathways so that there is a stronger tonic drive to move the eyes up rather than down,[3] resulting in a slow drift up and resetting quick movements down. An alternative hypothesis is that downbeating nystagmus is caused by a vertical ocular pursuit asymmetry so that the eyes drift up.[4] In any case, the slow drifts up are interrupted by quick resets down, leading to downbeating nystagmus. Downbeating nystagmus is most often seen with lesions of the craniocervical junction.

This patient's spontaneous vestibular nystagmus is likely to be caused by a central vestibular imbalance arising from an impairment of vestibular nuclear structures. As discussed in Chapter 1, spontaneous vestibular nystagmus usually results from a peripheral vestibular lesion. However, as in Case 29, medullary lesions involving the vestibular nuclei can also result in tonic vestibular imbalance and cause spontaneous vestibular nystagmus on a central basis. The fact that this patient's spontaneous primary position nystagmus was seen only with a loss of fixation suggests that her fixational abilities allowed her to suppress the vestibular nystagmus. This ability to suppress vestibular nystagmus is somewhat surprising because the patient demonstrated impairment of ocular pursuit, which is considered to be very important for visual–vestibular interaction. In some patients, however, there can be a discrepancy between pursuit and fixation suppression of the vestibulo-ocular reflex.[5]

DIAGNOSIS/DIFFERENTIAL DIAGNOSIS

This patient had a symptomatic Chiari malformation with associated ocular motor abnormalities and imbalance.

TREATMENT/MANAGEMENT

This patient was treated with a suboccipital craniectomy and decompression of her Chiari malformation. Following this treatment the patient was symptomatically much improved, with resolution of her spontaneous vestibular nystagmus. Abnormal ocular pursuit, gaze-evoked nystagmus, and downbeating nystagmus persisted.

SUMMARY

A 19-year-old woman with a complaint of several years of dizziness and disequilibrium had signs of a posterior fossa abnormality. An MRI scan disclosed a Chiari malformation. The patient was treated with a suboccipital craniectomy and decompression. Symptoms of dizziness and disequilibrium were markedly reduced. The spontaneous vestibular nystagmus disappeared, but gaze-evoked and downbeating nystagmus persisted.

TEACHING POINTS

1. **In downbeating nystagmus, the quick component is down or obliquely down on downgaze and torsional on down-lateral gaze.** Downbeating nystagmus is thought to be caused by an imbalance of up versus down tonic drive to the eyes.
2. **Downbeating nystagmus localizes the lesion to the craniocervical junction.** Causes include (1) Chiari malformation, (2) a mass lesion such as a foramen magnum meningioma, or (3) demyelinating disease. Less likely causes include (4) an infectious process such as a viral or

292 UNUSUAL DISEASE CASE STUDIES

postviral syndrome, (5) inflammatory disease, and (6) an olivocerebellar degeneration syndrome.

3. **Gaze-evoked nystagmus is a nystagmus that is left-beating on left lateral gaze, right-beating on right lateral gaze, and upbeating on upward gaze.** Gaze-evoked nystagmus is typically conjugate. Nystagmus that beats down, even when seen only with downgaze, is considered downbeating nystagmus, not gaze-evoked nystagmus. Gaze-evoked nystagmus is thought to result from impaired gaze holding arising from an abnormal neural integrator, a central nervous system circuit that converts (integrates in the mathematical sense) an eye velocity command into an eye position signal. The most common causes of gaze-evoked nystagmus are the effect of drugs such as anticonvulsants and structural abnormalities in the posterior fossa, especially those affecting the cerebellum.

REFERENCES

1. Leigh RJ, Zee DS (eds.): The Neurology of Eye Movements, ed 3. New York: Oxford University Press, 1999.
2. Cannon SC, Robinson DA: The final common integrator is in the prepositus and vestibular nuclei. In: Keller EL, Zee DS (eds): Adaptive Processes in Visual and Oculomotor Systems. Oxford: Pergamon Press, 1986, pp 307–312.
3. Baloh RW, Spooner JW: Downbeat nystagmus: A type of central vestibular nystagmus. Neurology 31:304–310, 1981.
4. Zee DS, Friendlich AL, Robinson DA: The mechanism of downbeat nystagmus. Arch Neurol 30:227–237, 1974.
5. Chambers B, Gresty M: The relationship between disordered pursuit and vestibulo-ocular reflex suppression. J Neurol Neurosurg Psychiatry 46:61–66, 1983.
6. Furman JM: Nystagmus and the vestibular system. In: Podos SM, Yanoff M (eds). Textbook of Ophthalmology. New York: Gower Medical, 1993, pp 9.1–9.7.
7. Weber PC, Cass SP: Neurotologic manifestations of Chiari 1 malformation. Otolaryngol Head Neck Surg 109:853–860, 1993.

CASE

41

Saccadic Fixation Instability

HISTORY

A 55-year-old man who worked as a shopkeeper complained of positional dizziness of 6 weeks' duration. He also complained of poor vision, especially when shifting his gaze from one point to another, constant disequilibrium, some tremulousness, palpitations, and a recent weight loss of several pounds. There was no complaint of hearing loss or tinnitus. The patient had no past medical history or family history of significance. He had recently been evaluated by his primary care physician, who could not establish a diagnosis. That evaluation included normal routine blood studies, a normal chest x-ray, and a normal electrocardiogram.

PHYSICAL EXAMINATION

The patient's general examination demonstrated a fine tremor of the head and limbs. He had a blood pressure of 150/100 and a heart rate of 95, with a regular rate and rhythm. The patient had no significant change in blood pressure or heart rate after standing for 3 and 5 minutes. His neurologic examination revealed full extraocular movements. He had no nystagmus. However, horizontal conjugate ocular flutter was noted. It occurred in bursts lasting for 1 to 2 seconds. These bursts of small left and right saccades typically occurred immediately following refixation of gaze. The patient had normal strength and sensation. There was mild limb dysmetria on heel-knee-shin and finger-to-nose testing. The patient's gait was wide-based, and he could not walk without assistance. Romberg's test could not be performed because the patient could not stand without assistance with the feet together. Otologic examination was normal. Dix-Hallpike maneuvers were negative.

294 UNUSUAL DISEASE CASE STUDIES

Question 1: What is ocular flutter? Are there other types of saccadic eye movement abnormalities? How does opsoclonus differ from ocular flutter?

Answer 1: Ocular flutter, unlike nystagmus, consists of a to-and-fro movement of the eyes wherein both components are rapid, that is, saccadic. Whereas nystagmus is defined as a to-and-fro movement of the eyes wherein at least one of the directions of movement is slow (less than about 40 degrees per second), in saccadic fixation instabilities, of which ocular flutter is one type, both leftward and rightward movements are rapid. Saccadic fixation instabilities include ocular flutter, opsoclonus, square-wave jerks, macro-square-wave jerks, and macro-saccadic oscillations[1–3] (Table Case 41–1).

Whereas ocular flutter is limited to horizontal eye movements, opsoclonus includes horizontal, vertical, and torsional saccades that may occur separately or in combination such that the eyes move in quite erratic patterns. As with ocular flutter, the intersaccadic interval in opsoclonus is brief or absent. Opsoclonus is considered a more severe form of saccadic fixation instability than ocular flutter. Some patients show different forms of saccadic fixation instabilities at different times in their illness. For example, ocular flutter can occur while a patient is recovering from opsoclonus.

Question 2: Based on the history and physical examination, what is the localization of this patient's problem?

Answer 2: Some of the patient's complaints are consistent with a vestibular abnormality. However, his tremulousness and weight loss, coupled with the finding of ocular flutter on physical examination, clearly suggest a central abnormality. The patient's incoordination and severe gait instability strongly suggest that his problem includes an abnormality in the cerebellum. The ocular flutter suggests an abnormality in the pons, because this is the region of the brain important for the generation of saccadic eye movements. The pons, however, receives powerful input from the cerebellum that may be used to trigger saccadic eye movements. In this way, a cerebellar abnormality can manifest itself as the abnormal occurrence of normally appearing saccadic eye movements. The patient's complaint of positional vertigo is unexplained.

Question 3: What are the diagnostic considerations for this patient?

Answer 3: The differential diagnosis for saccadic fixation instability is given in Table Case 41–2. The subacute onset of saccadic fixation instability can be caused by structural abnormalities of the pons or cerebellum, a viral brainstem encephalitis or cerebellitis, or a paraneoplastic syndrome. Some toxic agents and medications have been reported to cause saccadic fixation instability, but these would probably cause an acute onset of symptoms. Paraneoplastic-related saccadic fixation instability, typically in the form of opsoclonus, has been seen with carcinoma of the lung, especially oat cell carcinoma; carcinoma of the breast, especially ductal carcinoma; and uterine carcinoma. In children, saccadic fixation instabilities, typically in the form of opsoclonus, are seen with postviral encephalitis and with neuroblastoma.[4]

Question 4: What additional laboratory testing would help in establishing the cause of this patient's condition?

Answer 4: Quantitative laboratory testing could further elucidate whether or not the patient is suffering from a vestibular abnormality and document the ocular

Table Case 41-1 Types of Saccadic Fixation Instabilities

Category	Characteristics and Associated Ocular Motor Findings	Possible Pathophysiologic Substrate
Square-wave jerks	Small saccades (0.5–5 degrees) away from fixation and back with a 200-millisecond intersaccadic interval.	Can be normal, especially in the elderly. Common in cerebellar disease and progressive supranuclear palsy.
Macro-square-wave jerks	Saccadic intrusions (5–15 degrees) that take the eye away from fixation and return it within 70–150 milliseconds.	Multiple sclerosis and olivopontocerebellar atrophy.
Macrosaccadic oscillations	Oscillations around the fixation point that wax and wane. Intersaccadic interval of 200 milliseconds.	Lesions of dorsal vermis and fastigial nucleus.
Ocular flutter	Intermittent bursts of horizontal oscillations	Saccadic oscillation without an intersaccadic interval.
Opsoclonus	Combined horizontal, vertical, and torsional oscillations.	Saccadic oscillations without an intersaccadic interval.

Source: Adapted with permission from Leigh RJ, Zee DS: The Neurology of Eye Movements, ed 3. New York: Oxford University Press, 1999, p 450.[1]

Table Case 41–2 Causes of Saccadic Fixation Instability

Viral encephalitis
Neuroblastoma
Paraneoplasia
Trauma (in association with hypoxia and sepsis)
Meningitis
Intracranial tumors
Hydrocephalus
Thalamic hemorrhage
Multiple sclerosis
Hyperosmolar coma
Viral hepatitis
Sarcoid
Acquired immune deficiency syndrome
Side effects of drugs: lithium, amitriptyline, phenytoin and diazepam, phenelzine and imipramine, cocaine
Toxins: chlordecone, thallium, strychnine, toluene, organophosphates
As a component of the syndrome of myoclonic encephalopathy of infants (dancing eyes and dancing feet)
As a transient phenomenon of healthy neonates

Source: Adapted with permission from Leigh RJ, Zee DS: The Neurology of Eye Movements, ed 3. New York: Oxford University Press, 1999, p. 454.[1]

flutter. MRI of the brain is critical to rule out structural disorders. Because this patient may be suffering from a paraneoplastic syndrome, laboratory testing, including CT or MRI of the chest, should include a search for a remote carcinoma, especially of the lung. A lumbar puncture may uncover a viral meningoencephalitis. Blood studies should include anti-Ri, anti-Yo and, anti-Hu antibody titers.

LABORATORY TESTING

Videonystagmography: Ocular motor testing revealed the presence of ocular flutter. Also, the patient had difficulty tracking a slowly moving target. There was a left-reduced vestibular response on caloric testing.

Rotational testing revealed a left-directional preponderance.

An MRI scan of the brain was normal.

A search for a remote carcinoma, including antibody studies, a complete blood count and differential, urinalysis, and chest CT was negative. Cerebrospinal fluid examination was normal.

DIAGNOSIS/DIFFERENTIAL DIAGNOSIS

Question 5: Based on the additional information from laboratory testing, what is this patient's likely diagnosis?

Answer 5: Laboratory testing suggested both an ocular motor abnormality, namely ocular flutter, and a vestibular system abnormality. Imaging studies revealed no structural abnormality. The two most likely diagnoses of this patient's condition are the remote effects of a non–central nervous system neoplasm, that is, a paraneoplastic disorder, or a viral brainstem-cerebellar encephalitis. A toxic exposure is unlikely considering the lack of an appropriate history.

Question 6: What is the underlying pathophysiologic mechanism for saccadic fixation instability, and how does it differ from the mechanism for the generation of nystagmus?

Answer 6: Saccadic fixation instabilities are presumably caused by an abnormality of the saccadic generation circuitry. The paramedian pontine reticular formation is particularly important for the generation of horizontal saccades. The saccadic eye movement generation circuitry contains several types of cells, including the *burst* cells that fire during a saccade and the *pause* cells that are active between saccades but shut off during saccades. The pause cells are thought to inhibit saccades. Presumably, inappropriate saccades occur when pause cells in the pons stop inappropriately, allowing a rapid, that is, saccadic, eye movement to occur.[5] Because this triggering mechanism is premotor and does not involve the neural mechanism for generating conjugate eye movements, saccades caused by inappropriate pause cell behavior have normal velocity and are conjugate, even though they occur spontaneously at unwanted times. Also, the obligatory refractory period between two voluntary saccades (about 200 milliseconds) is violated by abnormal pause cell behavior. Whether saccadic fixation instabilities are a result of abnormal function of the pause cells themselves or of the triggers to the pause cells is uncertain.

The patient was given the diagnosis of ocular flutter of undetermined etiology. A viral infection of the central nervous system or a paraneoplastic syndrome were both considered possibilities, despite negative laboratory studies. Additionally, the patient had a vestibular imbalance of uncertain etiology.

TREATMENT/MANAGEMENT

In the hope of reducing the central nervous system inflammatory response, the patient was treated with prednisone, 60 mg daily for 2 weeks, followed by a gradually tapering dose. He had significant symptomatic recovery, with reduction of tremulousness and resolution of the ocular flutter. He was enrolled in a vestibular rehabilitation program for gait and balance training, with gradual resolution of his imbalance. One year after presentation, the patient was asymptomatic. Despite this positive response to steroid therapy, the patient should be followed closely since subsequent manifestation of a tumor remote from the nervous system is possible.[6]

SUMMARY

A 55-year-old man presented with a 6-week history of dizziness, disequilibrium, and tremulousness. Physical examination revealed ocular flutter in addition to mild limb dysmetria and ataxic gait. Vestibular laboratory studies disclosed a vestibular asymmetry in addition to the saccadic instability. A definitive diagnosis could not be reached, but a viral syndrome or a remote effect of carcinoma was suspected. The patient was treated with prednisone. Symptoms resolved, and the patient's balance improved during the subsequent 3 to 6 months. At 1-year follow-up, the patient was asymptomatic.

TEACHING POINTS

1. **Saccadic fixation instabilities, unlike nystagmus, consist of a to-and-fro eye movement wherein both components are rapid, that is, saccadic.** With nystagmus, at least one of the directions of movement is slow, that is, less than about 40 degrees per second. Saccadic fixation instabilities include ocular flutter, opsoclonus, square-wave jerks, macro-square-wave jerks, and macrosaccadic oscillations (Table Case 41–1).

2. **Opsoclonus, which includes horizontal, vertical, and torsional saccades, is the most severe form of saccadic fixation instability.** Ocular flutter, a purely horizontal form of saccadic fixation instability, is less severe and may occur while a patient is recovering from opsoclonus.

3. **Causes of ocular flutter and opsoclonus include structural abnormalities of the pons or cerebellum, brainstem encephalitis or cerebellitis, a paraneoplastic syndrome, and several toxic agents and medications.** In children, saccadic fixation instabilities, typically in the form of opsoclonus, can be seen with viral or postviral encephalitis and with neuroblastoma.

4. **The pathophysiology of saccadic fixation instability is an abnormality of the saccadic generation circuitry.**

REFERENCES

1. Leigh RJ, Zee DS: The Neurology of Eye Movements, ed 3. New York: Oxford University Press, 1999.
2. Sharpe JA, Fletcher WA: Saccadic intrusions and oscillations. Can J Neurol Sci 11:426–433, 1984.
3. Abel LA, Traccis S, Dell'Osso L, Daroff R, Troost B: Square wave oscillation. Neuroophthalmology 4:21–25, 1984.
4. Digre KB: Opsoclonus in adults. Arch Neurol 43:1165–1175, 1986.
5. Zee DS, Robinson DA: A hypothetical explanation of saccadic oscillations. Ann Neurol 5:405–414, 1979.
6. Furman JM, Eidelman BH, Fromm GH: Spontaneous remission of paraneoplastic saccadic fixation instability. Neurology 38:499–501, 1988.

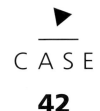

C A S E

42

Congenital Nystagmus

HISTORY

A 49-year-old man presented with a chief complaint of dizziness for 5 years. The patient had daily symptoms that were characterized by a sense of light-headedness, difficulty focusing his vision, a sense of movement just after turning his head, and poor balance while walking. He stated that his symptoms had been particularly noticeable since a head injury sustained 1 year ago while working as a corrections officer. The patient had no complaints of vertigo, positional sensitivity, hearing loss, or tinnitus. His past history was significant for 10 years of high blood pressure, for which he was under the care of a physician. The family history was noncontributory.

Question 1: Based on the patient's history, what are the diagnostic considerations? What further historical information should be obtained?

Answer 1: This patient's complaints suggest a vestibular system abnormality. There are features that suggest both peripheral (e.g., illusory motion) and central nervous system (e.g., chronic imbalance) involvement. The patient's long course of symptoms suggests either a chronic stable condition or a slowly progressive abnormality. The role of the head trauma sustained 1 year earlier is uncertain. Additional information on the patient's head trauma would be useful, as well as information about any prior evaluations for dizziness because his problem is long-standing.

ADDITIONAL HISTORY

The patient related that the head trauma he suffered 1 year before evaluation was minor. Evidently, he was pushed to the ground and struck his head against a wall, but he did not lose consciousness and was able to stand and to return to work immediately. He did note, however, a worsened problem with balance following that episode. He was evaluated by his primary care physician, who was uncertain about the cause of the patient's disequilibrium but noted unusual eye movements. His physician ordered a CT scan of the head, which was normal, and prescribed meclizine, which was of no benefit to the patient.

PHYSICAL EXAMINATION

The patient had full extraocular movements but had a primary position nystagmus that did not have clearly defined fast and slow components. The nystagmus appeared to be irregular, with both fast and slow components to the right and to the left. With infrared glasses, the nystagmus did not change. On horizontal gaze deviation, the patient had a typical gaze-evoked nystagmus, which was also seen on upward gaze but not on downward gaze. In fact, on downgaze, the nystagmus diminished somewhat. The patient was unable to follow a target smoothly. The remainder of the cranial nerve examination was normal. The patient's motor, sensory, and coordination examinations were normal. Romberg's test was negative. Gait was slightly wide-based and slow. Otologic examination was normal. The head thrust test could not be interpreted because of nystagmus with the eyes open in the light. The patient could stand on a foam pad without falling even with his eyes closed.

Question 2: Based on the history and physical examination, what is this patient's likely diagnosis and what further information would be helpful?

Answer 2: This patient's examination revealed unusual eye movements. It would be helpful to know how long these movements have existed. Moreover, since this condition may represent congenital nystagmus, it would be helpful to assess the influence of convergence. An oculographic recording of the patient's nystagmus might help determine its origin. A vestibular laboratory evaluation might help uncover the basis for the patient's complaints of dizziness.

ADDITIONAL HISTORY AND ADDITIONAL PHYSICAL EXAMINATION INFORMATION

The patient was unaware of his nystagmus but said that as a child he was evaluated by an ophthalmologist for "jumpy eyes." With convergence, his nystagmus decreased in amplitude.

LABORATORY TESTING

Videonystagmography: Ocular motor testing revealed nystagmus in the primary position during visual fixation that had an unusual pattern. There were no clearly defined quick and slow components, but a repeating complex pattern was observed. The nystagmus was unchanged with the eyes open in darkness. With horizontal gaze deviation, the patient developed gaze-evoked nystagmus. He was unable to track a slowly moving target smoothly. Optokinetic nystagmus was severely impaired, without clearly defined nystagmus. During positional testing, the nystagmus persisted without change. Caloric testing revealed bilaterally reduced responses with about 5 degrees per second peak velocity of nystagmus during each irrigation of a binaural bithermal caloric testing sequence.

Rotational testing revealed reduced responses with extremely abnormal dynamics, that is, a large phase lead and a short time constant of only about 5 seconds.

DIAGNOSIS/DIFFERENTIAL DIAGNOSIS

Question 3: What is this patient's diagnosis, and what is the significance of the laboratory tests? What role did the patient's head trauma play in the generation of his symptoms?

Answer 3: The patient's laboratory study results are consistent with congenital nystagmus, the characteristics of which are listed in Table Case 42–1. This patient had many of the typical features, although there was no null region; that is, there was no direction of gaze wherein the nystagmus was minimal. Vestibular studies suggested bilateral vestibular loss. However, the vestibulo-ocular studies also demonstrated abnormal VOR dynamics. Because congenital nystagmus is usually associated with abnormalities of the VOR even in the absence of dizziness,[1–3] it is impossible to say whether or not the reduced VOR was a feature of the patient's congenital nystagmus, a sign of vestibular abnormality, or in any way related to the head trauma. Thus, it is impossible to say whether or not the patient suffered from a labyrinthine or brainstem concussion related to the head trauma suffered 1 year before evaluation. The history alone, however, suggests some exacerbation of the patient's underlying disability from the head trauma, but his abnormal eye movements complicate interpretation of both the physical examination and the laboratory test abnormalities. Possibly, the patient did suffer a peripheral vestibular injury and his ability to compensate was impaired by a central nervous system abnormality, one of whose manifestations was congenital nystagmus.

Table Case 42–1 Characteristics of Congenital Nystagmus

Present since infancy
Irregular waveforms
Conjugate
Almost always horizontal
Accentuated by fixation, attention, and anxiety
Decreased by convergence and active eyelid closure
Often a null region
No complaint of oscillopsia
Occasionally inverted optokinetic nystagmus

Question 4: What is pendular nystagmus? What are its subtypes?

Answer 4: Jerk nystagmus, by definition, has clearly defined fast and slow components; pendular nystagmus, by definition, is a to-and-fro movement of the eyes without a clearly defined quick movement direction. By convention, the direction of jerk nystagmus is named for the direction of the quick movement, because this is what is most apparent clinically. There are numerous varieties of jerk nystagmus. Defining features include direction, influence of gaze, conjugacy, effect of visual fixation, and waveform.

Pendular nystagmus may be congenital or acquired. Congenital pendular nystagmus is known simply as *congenital nystagmus*, whereas acquired pendular nystagmus, which is very unusual, is called just that. Pendular nystagmus is more or less sinusoidal, but it can have an unusual pattern such as that of this patient, whose pendular nystagmus had a pseudoperiodic waveform.

The underlying pathophysiology of pendular nystagmus, congenital or acquired, is unknown. Patients with congenital (pendular) nystagmus have abnormalities of gaze-holding mechanisms that manifest as gaze-evoked nystagmus and abnormalities of ocular tracking. Patients with congenital nystagmus also have abnormal VOR dynamics.[1–3]

Acquired pendular nystagmus has been seen in patients with many disorders, including multiple sclerosis, and in those with brainstem infarctions. Although congenital nystagmus is almost always horizontal, acquired pendular nystagmus often has nonhorizontal components and may even be elliptical, presumably as a result of simultaneous horizontal and vertical pendular oscillations.[4] Although congenital nystagmus is often associated with excellent visual acuity, presumably because the pattern of eye movement allows brief periods of visual fixation, acquired pendular nystagmus is typically associated with oscillopsia and poor vision. Acquired pendular nystagmus is typically unaffected by visual fixation.

A variant of acquired pendular nystagmus, often purely vertical, is an oscillation of the eyes that can be seen in association with palatal myoclonus as a result of interruption of the so-called Mollaret's triangle, which includes the fiber pathways linking the inferior olive, the dentate nucleus, and the red nucleus.[5] Pendular nystagmus should not be confused with saccadic oscillations, which are discussed elsewhere (see Case 41).

This patient was given the diagnoses of congenital nystagmus and labyrinthine concussion.

TREATMENT/MANAGEMENT

There is no specific treatment for congenital nystagmus. Several medications have been tried, with limited success, as have optical remedies,[4,6] also with limited success. Based on the possibility that this patient had a vestibular system imbalance that could not be adequately assessed because of his congenital nystagmus, a course of vestibular rehabilitation was instituted. This had little effect on the patient's condition or complaints. A vestibular-suppressant medication was prescribed. This, too, was not beneficial. The patient continued working but planned to take early retirement.

SUMMARY

A 49-year-old man complained of long-standing disequilibrium that worsened following minor head trauma. Examination revealed pendular nystagmus that was diminished by convergence. A diagnosis of congenital nystagmus was made. Vestibular laboratory testing also suggested abnormal VOR dynamics and a reduced magnitude of responses. The vestibular laboratory test abnormalities may have been the result of congenital nystagmus rather than peripheral vestibular dysfunction. The patient's worsening balance following minor head trauma may have been a result of labyrinthine concussion, but this could neither be confirmed nor ruled out. Treatment with both balance therapy and vestibular-suppressant medication was unsuccessful.

TEACHING POINTS

1. **Pendular nystagmus, a to-and-fro movement of the eyes without a clearly defined quick movement direction, differs from jerk nystagmus, which has clearly defined fast and slow components.** Pendular nystagmus may be congenital or acquired. Congenital pendular nystagmus is known simply as *congenital nystagmus*. Pendular nystagmus usually has an unusual, somewhat repetitive pattern.

2. **Congenital nystagmus differs from acquired pendular nystagmus. Congenital pendular nystagmus is almost always horizontal.** Acquired pendular nystagmus often has both horizontal and nonhorizontal components. Also, although congenital nystagmus is often associated with excellent visual acuity, presumably because the pattern of eye movement allows brief periods of visual fixation, acquired pendular nystagmus is typically associated with oscillopsia and poor vision.

3. **The pathophysiology of pendular nystagmus, whether congenital or acquired, is unknown.** Abnormalities associated with congenital (pendular) nystagmus include poor gaze holding, poor ocular tracking, and a diminished VOR.

REFERENCES

1. Carl JR, Optiacan LM, Chu FC, Zee DS: Head shaking and vestibulo-ocular reflex in congenital nystagmus. Invest Ophthalmol Vis Sci 26:1043–1050, 1985.
2. Demer JL, Zee DS: Vestibulo-ocular and optokinetic deficits in albinos with congenital nystagmus. Invest Ophthalmol Vis Sci 25:739–745, 1984.
3. Gresty MA, Barratt HJ, Page NG, Ell JJ: Assessment of vestibulo-ocular reflexes in congenital nystagmus. Ann Neurol 17:129–136, 1985.
4. Leigh JR, Zee DS (eds): The Neurology of Eye Movements, ed 3. New York: Oxford University Press, 1999.
5. Nakada T, Kwee I: Oculopalatal myoclonus. Brain 109:431–441, 1986.
6. Yee C, Baloh R, Honrubia V: Effect of Baclofen on congenital nystagmus. In: Lennerstrand G, Zee D, Keller E (eds). Functional Basis of Ocular Motility Disorders. Oxford: Pergamon Press, 1982, pp 151–158.

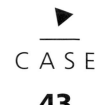

Otosclerotic Inner Ear Syndrome

HISTORY

A 47-year-old female social worker complained of dizziness for 6 months. The dizziness had been quite variable, consisting of one major episode of vertigo 3 months earlier associated with nausea and vomiting that lasted for hours and several minor episodes of vertigo lasting for seconds. Between episodes, the patient noticed daily dizziness that was worsened by rapid head movements. She also noticed some unsteadiness and veering of her gait to the left, especially in darkness.

The patient also complained of a bilateral hearing loss, first noticed at age 25, which had been slowly progressive in both ears. There was no fluctuation of hearing and no aural fullness. A bilateral low-pitched roaring sound, worse in the right ear, was present. There was no past medical history of otitis media, noise exposure, or trauma. The family history was positive for hearing loss in her mother and two maternal aunts.

PHYSICAL EXAMINATION

General and neurologic examinations were normal, except that the patient's casual walking was slow. Tandem walking was performed with slight difficulty. Romberg's test was negative. Otoscopy was normal. Tuning fork examination using a 512 Hz fork revealed lateralization to the right on Weber's test; the Rinne test was negative (bone conduction was greater than air conduction) bilaterally.

Question 1: What is the most likely cause of this patient's hearing loss?

Answer 1: The Rinne tuning fork examination suggests the presence of a bilateral conductive hearing loss. The result of Weber's test suggests either that the conductive hearing loss is slightly greater on the right or that a combined conductive and sensorineural hearing loss is present on the left. The finding of a conductive hearing loss, with no previous history of otitis media or trauma and a normal otoscopic examination, suggests a diagnosis of otosclerosis. The positive family history of hearing loss reinforces this diagnosis.

Question 2: What is otosclerosis?

Answer 2: Otosclerosis is a localized disease of bone remodeling involving the otic capsule. The abnormal remodeling begins with resorption of stable otic capsule bone in adults, followed by a reparative phase with bone deposition known as *sclerosis*. Conductive hearing loss develops when otosclerotic foci invade the stapedial ligament in the oval window and interfere with free motion of the stapes, causing conductive hearing loss. Sensorineural hearing loss may also be present.

Question 3: What pathologic changes are seen in the inner ear in otosclerosis?

Answer 3: Otosclerotic bone occurs when the original endochondral bone of the bony labyrinth is destroyed and replaced by highly cellular fibrous tissue. This fibrous tissue contains abundant lysosomes containing hydrolytic enzymes that are thought to be involved in bone resorption. After destruction of the endochondral bone, bony remodeling and production of immature otosclerotic bone occur. Repetition of the remodeling process results in areas of otosclerotic bone that often contain both inactive and active regions of bony remodeling. About 85% of otosclerotic foci are located in the oval window regions. This process of bony remodeling often results in fixation of the stapes footplate and progressive conductive hearing loss. As normal bone is replaced by otosclerotic bone, the original anatomic configuration of the bony labyrinth is usually preserved. Actual invasion of the labyrinthine spaces is rare and occurs only in the most active lesions.

Question 4: Is otosclerosis a common disorder?

Answer 4: Clinically diagnosed otosclerosis has an estimated incidence of 0.5% to 1% in the adult Caucasian population, making it the single most common cause of hearing impairment in this population. The incidence of subclinical otosclerosis, that is, otosclerosis found in the temporal bones of individuals without symptoms during life, ranges from 8% to 12%. In African Americans, otosclerosis is found in only 1% of temporal bones and has a clinical incidence of only 0.1%. The disease is rare to nonexistent in Asians and Native Americans. There is a female-to-male ratio of clinical otosclerosis of about 2:1.[1]

Question 5: What is the cause of otosclerosis?

Answer 5: Families with autosomal dominantly inherited otosclerosis have been described, but in most patients the etiology of the disease is unknown. Measles virus infection and autoimmunity may contribute to the disorder.

LABORATORY TESTING

Videonystagmography: Ocular motor function was normal. A low-amplitude left-beating spontaneous vestibular nystagmus was noted. There was no positional nystagmus. Caloric testing revealed a significant right reduced vestibular response.

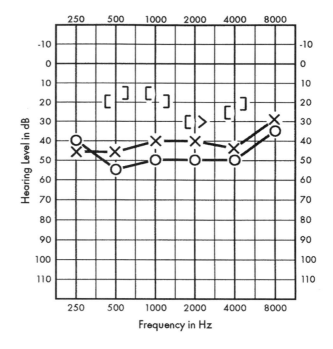

Figure Case 43–1 Audiogram.

Rotational testing revealed responses of normal amplitude and timing with a significant left directional preponderance.

Posturography was normal.

An audiogram was performed and showed a bilateral mixed conductive and sensorineural hearing loss (Fig. Case 43–1). The sensorineural component of the hearing loss was mild, ranging from 20 dB in the low frequencies to 30 dB in the high frequencies. The conductive component of the hearing loss produced a 40 to 50 dB hearing loss primarily affecting the lower frequencies in each ear. The conductive hearing loss was slightly greater in the right ear.

Question 6: This patient reported tinnitus, and the audiogram showed mild sensorineural hearing loss. Are these symptoms and findings commonly associated with otosclerosis, a disorder that primarily affects conduction of sound through the middle ear?

Answer 6: Although conductive hearing loss is the most common manifestation of otosclerosis, tinnitus is also very common and may be related to either fixation of the stapes or damage to the sensorineural elements of the cochlea. Sensorineural hearing loss is also frequently associated with otosclerosis. If sensorineural hearing loss is present, it is most commonly seen in combination with stapes fixation, which presumably causes a mixed conductive and sensorineural hearing loss. Occasionally, patients present with pure cochlear otosclerosis, that is, sensorineural hearing loss without a conductive component. Establishing that a sensorineural hearing loss is the result of otosclerosis is difficult. In advanced cases of cochlear otosclerosis, it is possible to detect the presence of abnormal otosclerotic bone surrounding the inner ear on high-resolution CT imaging of the temporal bone.

Question 7: Is dizziness commonly associated with otosclerosis? Are vestibular abnormalities common?

Answer 7: Vestibular symptoms are more common in individuals with otosclerosis than in the general population. The reported prevalence of dizziness in individuals with otosclerosis ranges from 7% to 40%.[2–4] Unilateral or bilateral reduced caloric function has been observed in up to 60% of otosclerotic patients complaining of vertigo.[4] It has also been suggested that the incidence of vestibular symptoms correlates with the presence of an associated sensorineural hearing loss.[4,5]

Question 8: What is the cause of dizziness associated with otosclerosis?

Answer 8: Dizziness in patients with otosclerosis may be caused either by the co-occurrence of a disorder other than otosclerosis, such as Meniere's disease, or by the pathologic process of otosclerosis itself, which can produce vestibular symptoms as a result of the otosclerotic inner ear syndrome discussed below. Surprisingly, the otosclerotic inner ear syndrome appears to occur less frequently than combined otosclerosis and Meniere's disease.[3]

The combination of Meniere's disease and otosclerosis has been reported by a number of authors[6,7] and has also been confirmed by temporal bone histopathology.[8] The clinical diagnosis of combined Meniere's disease and otosclerosis is based on the findings of a low-frequency sensorineural hearing loss, fluctuation of hearing, aural fullness, and vertigo, that is, a symptom complex typical of endolymphatic hydrops.[3,6,7]

The pathophysiology underlying the otosclerotic inner ear syndrome is uncertain. One proposed mechanism of vestibular injury caused by otosclerosis involves the encroachment of the cribriform area of the vestibule by otosclerotic bone[9] (Fig. Case 43–2). The cribriform area is pierced by vestibular nerve fibers from the internal auditory canal that innervate the vestibular end organs within the inner ear. Otosclerotic bone encroachment causes vestibular nerve degeneration, which has been observed in temporal bone specimens. Histopathologic studies have also demonstrated reduced cell counts in Scarpa's ganglion without evidence of otosclerotic encroachment of the cribriform areas, so other pathologic mechanisms are probably involved.[10] The otosclerotic inner ear syndrome seems to be more prevalent in individuals with cochlear otosclerosis, and thus the two conditions may have a common pathophysiology. The most popular theory of cochlear otosclerosis hypothesizes the release of toxic proteolytic enzymes into the inner ear by active areas of otosclerosis.[11,12] This pathologic mechanism may also affect the vestibular portion of the inner ear and result in symptoms of the otosclerotic inner ear syndrome.

Question 9: Are there any characteristic symptoms or signs of the otosclerotic inner ear syndrome?

Answer 9: No, historically the diagnosis of otosclerotic inner ear syndrome was created to describe vertigo in a patient with otosclerosis whose audiovestibular

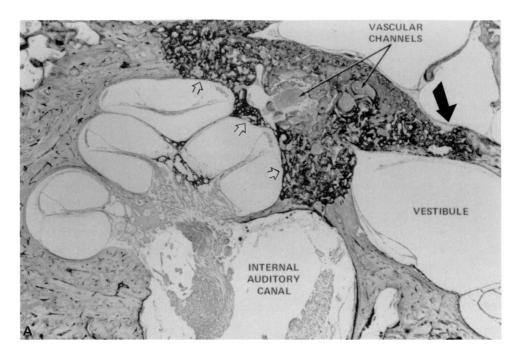

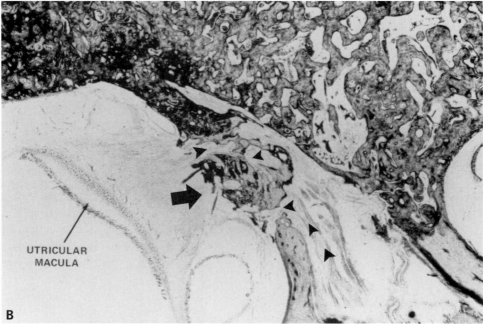

Figure Case 43–2 Histopathology of otosclerosis. (A) Low-power view of temporal
bone showing a focus of otosclerotic bone bordering the cochlea and vestibule and
infiltrating the stapes footplate. Note the presence of abnormal vascular channels
within the otosclerotic bone. Open arrowheads = portion of cochlea bordered by otosclerosis; solid arrow = stapes footplate. (*Source*: Reprinted by permission of the publisher from Schuknecht HF: Pathology of the Ear. Cambridge, MA: Harvard University Press. Copyright 1974 by the President and Fellows of Harvard College.) (B)
High-power view of temporal bone showing otosclerotic encroachment of the lamina cribosa (the region that transmits the vestibular nerve from the internal auditory
canal to the labyrinth). Thick arrow = lamina cribosa; arrowheads = vestibular nerve
fibers. (This histology section was given by Dr. H.F. Schuknecht to the Eye and Ear
Institute of Pittsburgh. The temporal bone specimen from which this section was
made belongs to The Massachusetts Eye and Ear Infirmary, Boston.)

symptoms do not suggest Meniere's disease or any other known vestibular syndrome. Symptoms of otosclerotic inner ear syndrome can include episodic vertigo lasting for 20 minutes to 6 hours, vague feelings of floating or lightheadedness, and nonspecific imbalance or disequilibrium.

Question 10: Why is it important to distinguish between vestibular system dysfunction based solely on otosclerotic inner ear syndrome versus vestibular system dysfunction based on combined Meniere's disease and otosclerosis?

Answer 10: Surgical treatment of the conductive hearing loss associated with otosclerosis is highly successful.[13] Although there is no contraindication to surgery for otosclerosis in an ear with the otosclerotic inner ear syndrome, surgery, for whatever reason, in an ear affected by active Meniere's disease is associated with an increased incidence of profound hearing loss.

DIAGNOSIS/DIFFERENTIAL DIAGNOSIS

The patient was given the diagnosis of otosclerosis and otosclerotic inner ear syndrome.

TREATMENT/MANAGEMENT

The patient elected to undergo surgical correction of the conductive hearing loss in the right ear. A stapedectomy was performed under local anesthesia and resulted in substantial improvement in hearing and reduction of tinnitus. The vestibular symptoms remained unchanged. The patient requested surgical correction of hearing in her left ear, but this was deferred for at least 6 months.

The presence of a sensorineural component of the hearing loss is suggestive of mild cochlear otosclerosis. Sodium fluoride supplementation has been proposed as a treatment of cochlear otosclerosis. Sodium fluoride is thought to reduce the amount of proteolytic enzymes released into the inner ear by an active focus of otosclerosis, thus reducing the progression of sensorineural hearing loss. However, the lack of controlled clinical trials, the potential complications (gastritis, skeletal fluorosis), and the cost of large doses of sodium fluoride have limited its widespread use.

The vestibular symptoms in this patient consisted of both episodic vertigo and daily dizziness and unsteadiness associated with quick head movements. Vestibular rehabilitation was recommended to improve the chronic movement-induced disequilibrium, and a vestibular suppressant (promethazine, 25 mg orally twice a day) was provided on an as-needed basis for the episodic spells.

SUMMARY

A 47-year-old woman presented with 6 months of dizziness. A long-standing bilateral hearing loss was also a problem. The family history was significant for hearing loss. The patient's hearing loss was found to be primarily conductive, and a diagnosis of otosclerosis was reached. Additionally, she had a sensorineural hearing loss and vestibular laboratory test abnormalities that suggested the otosclerotic inner ear syndrome. The patient underwent surgery for otosclerosis, which improved her hearing. Vestibular rehabilitation also was ordered.

TEACHING POINTS

1. **Otosclerosis is a disorder of the bony labyrinth that most commonly causes a progressive stiffening and fixation of the stapes footplate by the formation of abnormal otosclerotic bone.**

2. **Otosclerosis is a common disorder with a subclinical incidence of about 10% and a clinical incidence of up to 1% in the Caucasian population.** The incidence of otosclerosis varies by ethnic background and is greatest in Caucasians, uncommon in African Americans, and rare in Asians and Native Americans. There is a female-to-male ratio of clinical otosclerosis of about 2:1. Families with autosomal dominantly inherited otosclerosis have been described.

3. **Otosclerosis causes a conductive hearing loss. The finding of a conductive hearing loss with no previous history of otitis media or trauma and a normal otoscopic examination suggests a diagnosis of otosclerosis.** The presence of a conductive hearing loss can be inferred clinically through the use of the Rinne and Weber tuning fork tests.

4. **Tinnitus and sensorineural hearing loss may be associated with otosclerosis.** Cochlear otosclerosis (i.e., sensorineural hearing loss without a conductive component) can also occur but is difficult to diagnose. In suspected cases of cochlear otosclerosis, CT imaging of the temporal bones can confirm the diagnosis.

5. **Vestibular symptoms are more common in individuals with otosclerosis than in the general population.** The reported prevalence of dizziness in individuals with otosclerosis ranges from 7% to 40%. Dizziness in patients with otosclerosis may be caused by either the co-occurrence of a disorder other than otosclerosis, such as Meniere's disease, or by the pathologic process of otosclerosis itself, which can produce vestibular symptoms as a result of the otosclerotic inner ear syndrome.

6. *Otosclerotic inner ear syndrome* **is a term used to describe patients with vertigo and otosclerosis whose audiovestibular symptoms do not suggest Meniere's disease or any other known vestibular syndrome.** Symptoms of the otosclerotic inner ear syndrome can include episodic vertigo, vague feelings of floating or lightheadedness, and nonspecific imbalance or disequilibrium.

7. **Stapedectomy, the surgical treatment for conductive hearing loss associated with otosclerosis, is highly successful.** However, it is important to distinguish the otosclerotic inner ear syndrome from combined Meniere's disease and otosclerosis because surgery in an ear affected by active Meniere's disease is associated with an increased incidence of profound hearing loss, whereas there is no contraindication to surgery in patients with the otosclerotic inner ear syndrome alone.

8. **Treatment for the otosclerotic inner ear syndrome is nonspecific.** Occasionally, patients report improvement of their vestibular symptoms

following stapedectomy. Treatment may include vestibular-suppressant medications as needed and vestibular rehabilitation. Sodium fluoride supplementation has been advocated as a treatment for progressive sensorineural hearing loss associated with cochlear otosclerosis. The efficacy of sodium fluoride in the otosclerotic inner ear syndrome has not been established.

REFERENCES

1. Mackenzie M, Wolfenden N: Otosclerosis. J Laryngol Otol 69:437–456, 1955.
2. Paparella MM, Chasen WD: Otosclerosis and vertigo. J Laryngol Otol 80:511–517, 1966.
3. McCabe BF: Otosclerosis and vertigo. Trans Pacific Coast Oto-Ophthalmol Soc Ann Meeting 47:37–42, 1966.
4. Cody DT, Baker HL: Otosclerosis: Vestibular symptoms and sensorineural hearing loss. Ann Otol 87:778–796, 1978.
5. Morales-Garcia C: Cochleo-vestibular involvement in otosclerosis. Acta Otolaryngol 73:484–492, 1972.
6. Paparella MM, Mancini F, Liston SL: Otosclerosis and Meniere's syndrome: Diagnosis and treatment. Laryngoscope 94:1414–1417, 1984.
7. Shea JJ, Ge X, Orchik DJ: Endolymphatic hydrops associated with otosclerosis. Am J Otol 15:348–357, 1994.
8. Black FO, Sando I, Hildyard VH, Hemenway WG: Bilateral multiple otosclerotic foci and endolymphatic hydrops. Ann Otol Rhinol Laryngol 78:1062–1073, 1969.
9. Sando I, Miller D, Hemenway WG, Black FO: Vestibular pathology in otosclerosis. Temporal bone histopathological report. Laryngoscope 84(4):593–605, 1974.
10. Richter E, Schuknecht HF: Loss of vestibular neurons in clinical otosclerosis. Arch Otorhinolaryngol 234:1–9, 1982.
11. Lawrence M: Possible influence of cochlear otosclerosis on inner ear fluids. Ann Otol Rhinol Laryngol 75:553–558, 1966.
12. Causse JR, Uriel J, Berges J, Shambaugh GE Jr, Bretlau P, Causse JB: The enzymatic mechanism of the otospongiotic disease and NaF action on the enzymatic balance. Am J Otol 3:297, 1982.
13. Hillel AD: History of stapedectomy. Am J Otolaryngol 4:131–140, 1983.
14. Schuknecht HF: Pathology of the Ear. Cambridge: Harvard University Press, 1974.

CASE

44

Progressive Supranuclear Palsy

HISTORY

A 58-year-old woman who did not work outside the home complained of frequent falling. The patient's symptoms had begun several years previously, were gradually worsening, and did not fluctuate on a day-to-day basis. There was particular difficulty going down steps and stepping from the sidewalk to the street. The patient's spouse stated that she had some slowing of mentation and slurred speech. The patient had no complaint of vertigo or of hearing loss or tinnitus. There was no past medical history of significance and no family history of neurologic or otologic disease. The patient's primary care physician had performed a CT scan, which was normal, and had given the patient a diagnosis of Parkinson's disease. The patient had not responded to dopaminergic or anticholinergic agents.

Question 1: Based on the patient's history, what is the differential diagnosis?

Answer 1: This patient's history is most consistent with a progressive neurodegenerative syndrome, such as progressive supranuclear palsy, Parkinson's disease, striatonigral degeneration, or dementia with associated cerebellar signs. The differential diagnosis also includes multiple cerebral infarctions, hypothyroidism, central nervous system vasculitis, and a central nervous system neoplastic condition such as central nervous system lymphoma.

PHYSICAL EXAMINATION

The general examination revealed a disheveled woman who appeared to be depressed. Neurologic examination revealed limitation of vertical gaze, especially

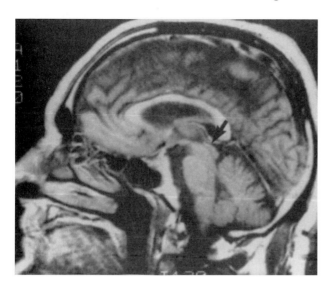

Figure Case 44–1 Sagittal MRI of a patient with progressive supranuclear palsy. Note the flattened quadrigeminal plate indicated by the arrow. (*Source*: With permission from Scully RE et al: Weekly clinicopathological exercises. N Engl J Med 329:1560, 1993.[6])

downward gaze during voluntary eye movements. There was severe slowing of vertical saccades and minimal slowing of horizontal saccades. Square-wave jerks were noted. There was saccadic pursuit and abnormal convergence. Doll's eyes (oculocephalic reflexes) revealed a full range of extraocular motion vertically and horizontally. The patient had a masked facies with a decreased blink rate. There was a hyperactive gag reflex. Motor system examination revealed increased tone with increased deep tendon reflexes that were symmetric. The plantar response was equivocal bilaterally. Sensation was normal. Coordination revealed slowing of alternating movements and slowing on finger-to-nose testing without dysrhythmia. Romberg's test was negative. Evaluation of the patient's gait revealed a widened base, short stride length, and retropulsion. The otologic examination was normal.

Question 2: Based upon the additional information from the physical examination, what is this patient's likely diagnosis? What laboratory testing is appropriate?

Answer 2: This patient's physical examination is consistent with progressive supranuclear palsy. Because of the poor prognosis for progressive supranuclear palsy and its poor response to treatment, an MRI scan should be performed before giving this diagnosis. Also, hematologic and thyroid blood studies should be performed and the erythrocyte sedimentation rate should be obtained.

LABORATORY TESTING

An MRI scan of the brain suggested midbrain atrophy (Fig. Case 44–1).
A complete blood count was normal.

DIAGNOSIS/DIFFERENTIAL DIAGNOSIS

This patient was given a diagnosis of progressive supranuclear palsy.

Table Case 44–1
Manifestations of
Progressive Supranuclear
Palsy

Decreased cognitive ability
Abnormal ocular motor function
  Square-wave jerks
  Limitation of vertical eye movement
  Slow or absent vertical saccades
  Hypometric horizontal saccades
  Saccadic pursuit
  Abnormal convergence
  Normal oculocephalic reflexes
  Bell's phenomenon typically absent
Masked facies
Dysarthria
Dysphagia
Rigidity
Abnormal gait
Midbrain atrophy on CT

Question 3: What are the manifestations of progressive supranuclear palsy?

Answer 3: The manifestations of progressive supranuclear palsy are given in Table Case 44–1.

Question 4: What is the pathophysiology of progressive supranuclear palsy?

Answer 4: Progressive supranuclear palsy is characterized by cell loss in many locations including the midbrain (substantia nigra, red nucleus, superior colliculus), the corpus striatum (especially the globus pallidus), and the dentate nucleus of the cerebellum.[1,2]

As discussed in Chapter 1, the midbrain is important for vertical and torsional eye movements in much the same way that the pons is important for horizontal eye movements. A premotor center in the midbrain important for vertical saccades is the rostral interstitial nucleus of the medial longitudinal fasciculus.[3] It is comparable to the paramedian pontine reticular formation, which is important for horizontal saccades. Other structures that are important for the vertical and torsional VOR include the posterior commissure; the interstitial nucleus of Cajal; the third and fourth cranial nerve nuclei; and the medial longitudinal fasciculus, which carries signals from the medulla and the pons to the midbrain.[3,4] The midbrain is also important for vergence eye movements. Thus, midbrain lesions can cause limitation of vertical eye movements, vertical nystagmus, skew deviation (a vertical ocular misalignment), abnormal vergence, and an abnormal vertical and/or torsional VOR.

Question 6: What disease states are associated with midbrain dysfunction?

Answer 6: Disorders that affect the midbrain include degenerative disorders, such as progressive supranuclear palsy; mass lesions, such as pinealoma; infarction, such as the "top of the basilar syndrome"[5]; midbrain hemorrhage; hydrocephalus; and encephalitis.

TREATMENT/MANAGEMENT

The patient was treated with a course of bromocryptine. This provided minimal symptomatic relief for several months, after which time the patient began a progressive and relentless decline.

SUMMARY

A 58-year-old woman presented with a chief complaint of frequent falling, slowed cognition, blurred vision, and personality change. Examination revealed marked limitation of downgaze, square-wave jerks, and retropulsion of gait. The MRI scan suggested midbrain atrophy. The patient was given the diagnosis of progressive supranuclear palsy. She had been unresponsive to dopaminergic and anticholinergic agents. A course of bromocryptine provided minimal benefit.

TEACHING POINTS

1. **The gradual onset and worsening of imbalance in the absence of vertigo suggests a progressive neurologic disorder.**
2. **Progressive supranuclear palsy is a disorder characterized by the gradual onset of cognitive decline and poor balance.** Progressive supranuclear palsy is caused by cell loss in many locations, including the midbrain (substantia nigra, red nucleus, superior colliculus), the basal ganglia (especially the globus pallidus), and the dentate nucleus of the cerebellum.
3. **The midbrain is important for vertical, torsional, and vergence eye movements.** Thus, midbrain lesions can cause limitation of vertical eye movements, vertical nystagmus, skew deviation, an abnormal vertical and/or torsional VOR, and abnormal vergence.
4. **The midbrain is also important for vergence eye movements.**
5. **Disorders that affect the midbrain include degenerative disorders, such as progressive supranuclear palsy; mass lesions, such as pinealoma; infarction, such as the top of the basilar syndrome; midbrain hemorrhage; hydrocephalus; and encephalitis.**

REFERENCES

1. Steele JC, Richardson JC, Olszewski J: Progressive supranuclear palsy. Arch Neurol 10:333–359, 1964.
2. Behrman S, Carroll JD, Janota I, Matthews WB: Progressive supranuclear palsy. Brain 92:663–678, 1969.
3. Buttner-Ennever JA (ed): Neuroanatomy of the Oculomotor System. Amsterdam: Elsevier, 1988.
4. Leigh RJ, Zee DS: The Neurology of Eye Movements, ed 3. New York: Oxford University Press, 1999.
5. Caplan L: Top of the basilar syndrome. Neurology 30:72–79, 1980.
6. Scully RE, Mark E, McNeely W, McNeely B: Weekly clinicopathological exercises. N Engl J Med 329:1560, 1993.

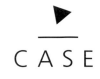

Solvent Exposure

HISTORY

A 30-year-old male welder presented with a chief complaint of dizziness after a mishap at work 3 months before evaluation. The patient was welding inside a large tank that previously had been used for storing industrial solvents. He was not wearing any breathing protection. He remembers vaporizing some "goo." Then he felt giddy and was observed by fellow workers giggling and rolling in the snow outside the storage tank. The patient was taken to a local emergency room, where no abnormalities were found. He experienced persistent dizziness and disequilibrium characterized by a sense of lightheadedness and worsened by head movement. The patient's symptoms were also worsened by standing for prolonged periods and by walking on uneven surfaces. He also complained of intolerance to exposure to any solvents or household cleaning agents. The patient had no complaint of hearing loss, tinnitus, or fullness or stuffiness of the ears. There was no positional sensitivity. He had no prior history of dizziness or any other significant prior medical history. The family history was noncontributory. The patient had undergone an extensive evaluation before presentation because of the legal implications of the accident. The brain imaging scan, blood studies, and audiometric test were normal.

Question 1: Based on the patient's history, what is the likely diagnosis?

Answer 1: This patient is likely to have suffered from industrial chemical or solvent exposure.[1] The chance occurrence of any unrelated illness or exacerbation of a preexisting condition is unlikely. He also seems to have acquired an intolerance to solvents.[2]

316

PHYSICAL EXAMINATION

The general and otologic examinations were normal. Neurologic examination showed that the patient had full extraocular movements with saccadic pursuit. There was bilateral horizontal gaze-evoked nystagmus. The patient had a wide-based gait and an unsteady tandem gait. Romberg's test was normal. The remainder of the neurologic examination was normal. With infrared glasses there was no nystagmus while seated, but on positional testing he had a direction-changing positional nystagmus with left-beating nystagmus in the head-left and left-lateral positions and right-beating nystagmus in the head-right and right-lateral positions. There was no paroxysmal positional nystagmus on Dix-Hallpike maneuvers. He could not maintain balance on a foam pad with his eyes closed. Stepping in place revealed wide-based and ataxic stepping but no rotational deviation.

LABORATORY TESTING

Videonystagmography: Ocular motor and positional testing confirmed the abnormalities seen during physical examination that included saccadic pursuit, bilateral horizontal gaze-evoked nystagmus, and a direction-changing positional nystagmus. Additionally, the patient could suppress his positional nystagmus with vision. There was a 35% left reduced vestibular response on caloric testing.

Rotational testing revealed a mild right directional preponderance.

Posturography indicated excessive sway on all conditions in a nonspecific pattern.

Question 2: Based on the history, physical examination, and laboratory studies, what structures are likely to be involved in this patient's problem?

Answer 2: Some of this patient's abnormalities, such as gaze-evoked nystagmus and saccadic pursuit, suggest brainstem and cerebellar involvement, whereas peripheral vestibular involvement (on the left) is suggested by a mildly reduced response on caloric testing unilaterally. His posturography is nonlocalizing and thus does not support or rule out a peripheral vestibular disorder. The patient's directional preponderance on rotational testing suggests an ongoing vestibulo-ocular asymmetry due either to impaired compensation for his peripheral vestibular disorder (see Case 3) or to a central vestibular abnormality.

Question 3: What is the pathophysiology of direction-changing positional nystagmus, and what is its localizing value?

Answer 3: Direction-changing positional nystagmus was once thought to be indicative of a central nervous system disorder, but more recent studies have suggested that direction-changing positional nystagmus can be caused by either a peripheral or a central vestibular disorder.[3] A well-recognized peripheral vestibular cause of direction-changing positional nystagmus is acute ethanol intoxication. However, direction-changing positional nystagmus that is not acute and not a result of ethanol cannot be localized. Direction-changing positional nystagmus of peripheral vestibular origin, either alcoholic or otherwise, is probably based on an inequality between the specific gravity of the cupula of the horizontal semicircular canal and the specific gravity of the surrounding endolymph.[4] Such an inequality of specific gravity could result from either a heavy cupula, a light cupula, or debris adherent to the cupula.

The most common cause of direction-changing positional nystagmus is an inequality of the specific gravity of the horizontal semicircular canal cupula and the surrounding endolymph caused by ethanol intoxication.[5] So-called positional alcohol nystagmus (PAN) occurs both early (about 30 minutes to 3 hours) and late (about 4 to 13 hours) following the ingestion of ethanol. The presumed mechanism relates to a difference in diffusion rates into and out of the horizontal semicircular canal cupulae and the surrounding semicircular canal endolymph. Thus, in the early stage of PAN (PAN I), the horizontal semicircular canal cupulae are light and "float" when the head is in the lateral, that is, the ear-down, position. The direction-changing positional nystagmus of PAN I is geotropic, that is, left-beating in the left lateral position and right-beating in the right lateral position. In the later stage of ethanol intoxication the cupulae "sink," thereby causing an ageotropic direction-changing positional nystagmus, PAN II. A less frequent but well-understood peripheral vestibular cause of direction-changing positional nystagmus is that of horizontal semicircular canal cupulolithiasis.[6] This condition is thought to be caused by debris, possibly degenerated otoconia, adherent to the horizontal semicircular canal cupula of either the right or the left ear. Patients with this condition have a persistent ageotropic positional nystagmus and, like patients with PAN, have a nystagmus that persists for as long as a head-lateral position is maintained.

Well-documented cases of direction-changing positional nystagmus resulting from central nervous system lesions have been described,[7] but the underlying pathophysiology for this association is unknown. Thus, this patient's direction-changing positional nystagmus may be based upon either central or peripheral vestibular involvement.

Question 4: What are some of the industrial solvents known to cause vestibular system impairment, and what is the pathophysiologic basis for this impairment?

Answer 4: Very little is known about industrial solvent exposure, including exactly which chemicals are responsible and the underlying pathophysiology. However, xylene, styrene, trichlorethylene, and methylchloroform are industrial agents thought to be toxic to the vestibular system. The most consistent vestibular abnormalities following exposure to these agents in animals are a persistent, that is, a nonparoxysmal, positional nystagmus[8] and impaired visual–vestibular interaction.[9–11] Other reported abnormalities include an increased VOR.[12]

The pathophysiology of the vestibular dysfunction seen in industrial solvent exposure probably relates to central vestibular pathways, including the cerebellum. The direction-changing positional nystagmus seen with solvent exposure is not thought to be caused by a cupula-endolymph specific gravity mismatch (see above), because the positional nystagmus can be blocked by the GABA agonist baclofen.[8]

Chronic exposure to volatile hydrocarbons can cause chronic toxic encephalopathy, which can be associated with abnormal visual–vestibular interaction and abnormal smooth pursuit.[13]

DIAGNOSIS/DIFFERENTIAL DIAGNOSIS

This patient was given the diagnosis of industrial solvent toxicity causing a combination of peripheral and central vestibular disorders.

TREATMENT/MANAGEMENT

This patient was treated with a course of vestibular rehabilitation therapy. He was advised to avoid exposure to all industrial solvents, including paint fumes and household cleaning products. The patient was also advised to avoid situations that required balance for safety. His symptoms improved somewhat, but he was unable to return to work as a welder.

SUMMARY

A 30-year-old male welder was accidentally exposed to a vaporized mixture of industrial solvents and became acutely dizzy. He gradually recovered but was left with a chronic imbalance. The patient was found to have objective evidence of a vestibular system disorder, including direction-changing positional nystagmus, which is a nonlocalizing abnormality. Other abnormalities, such as unilateral caloric reduction and an abnormal ocular motor test, suggested impairment of peripheral and central vestibular structures, respectively. The patient was treated with a course of vestibular rehabilitation therapy and his symptoms decreased somewhat, but he could not return to work.

TEACHING POINTS

1. **Industrial solvents can cause vestibular system impairment. Xylene, styrene, trichlorethylene, and methylchloroform are industrial agents thought to be toxic to the vestibular system.** The most consistent vestibular abnormality following exposure to these agents is a persistent positional nystagmus.
2. **The pathophysiology of industrial solvent–induced vestibular dysfunction is unknown but probably involves central vestibular pathways including the cerebellum.**
3. **Treatment for industrial solvent–induced vestibular dysfunction is nonspecific.** Affected individuals should be advised to avoid subsequent exposure to all industrial solvents, including paint fumes and household cleaning products, and to avoid situations that require balance for safety. Vestibular rehabilitation may help promote improved balance and adaptation to vestibular deficits.

REFERENCES

1. Hodgson MJ, Furman J, Ryan C, Durrant J, Kern E: Encephalopathy and vestibulopathy following short-term hydrocarbon exposure. J Occup Med 31:51–54, 1989.
2. Gyntelberg F, Vesterhauge S, Fog P, Isager H, Zillstorff K: Acquired intolerance to organic solvents and results of vestibular testing. Am J Ind Med 9:363–370, 1986.
3. Brandt T: Background, technique, interpretation, and usefulness of positional and positioning testing. In: Jacobson GP, Newman CW, Kartush JM (eds). Handbook of Balance Function Testing. St Louis: Mosby Year Book, 1993, pp 123–155.
4. Money K, Johnson W, Corlett R: Role of semicircular canals in positional alcohol nystagmus. Am J Physiol 208:1065–1070, 1965.
5. Baloh RW, Honrubia V: Clinical Neurophysiology of the Vestibular System, ed 3. New York: Oxford University Press, 2001.

6. Baloh RW, Yue Q, Jacobson KM, Honrubia V: Persistent direction-changing positional nystagmus: Another variant of benign positional nystagmus? Neurology 45:1297–1301, 1995.
7. Lin J, Elidan, J Baloh RW, Honruba V: Direction-changing positional nystagmus: Incidence and meaning. Am J Otolaryngol 7:306–310, 1986.
8. Odkvist LM, Larsby B, Fredrickson MF, Liedgren SR, Tham R: Vestibular and oculomotor disturbances caused by industrial solvents. J Otolaryngol 9:53–59, 1980.
9. Niklasson M, Tham R, Larsby B, Eriksson B: Effects of toluene, styrene, trichloroethylene, and trichloromethane on the vestibulo- and opto-oculo motor system in rats. Neurotoxicol Teratol 15:327–334, 1993.
10. Hyden D, Larsby B, Andersson H, Odkvist LM, Liedgren SR, Tham R: Impairment of visuo-vestibular interaction in humans. ORL J Otorhinolaryngol Relat Spec 45:262–269, 1983.
11. Odkvist LM, Larsby B, Tham R, Ahlfeldt H, Andersson B, Eriksson B, Liedgren SR: Vestibulo-oculomotor disturbances in humans exposed to styrene. Acta Otolaryngol 94:487–493, 1982.
12. Biscaldi GP, Mingardi M, Pollini G, Moglia A, Bossi MC: Acute toluene poisoning. Electroneuro-physiological and vestibular investigations. Toxicol Eur Res 3:271–273, 1981.
13. Odkvist LM, Moller C, Thuomas K-A: Otoneurologic disturbances caused by solvent pollution. Otolaryngol Head Neck Surg 106:687, 1992.

CASE

46

Wernicke's Encephalopathy

HISTORY

A 54-year-old woman who did not work outside the home presented with a chief complaint of 2 weeks of forgetfulness, "wandering eyes," and very poor balance. The patient's past history was significant for left hemiglossectomy and left radical neck dissection 6 months before presentation. The patient had no complaints of vertigo or hearing loss and no tinnitus. There was no prior history of balance disorder. The family history was negative.

Question 1: Based on the patient's history, what are the diagnostic considerations? What additional historical details should be obtained?

Answer 1: The patient's history is consistent with a wide differential diagnosis that includes a vestibular system abnormality because of imbalance. However, abnormal eye movements and impaired cognition suggest a central nervous system disorder. A single condition that includes all three of this patient's signs and symptoms—eye movement abnormalities, mental status change, and ataxia—is Wernicke's encephalopathy. Many other conditions can account for one or two of these signs and symptoms, and these should be considered. Because Wernicke's encephalopathy is a result of vitamin B_1 deficiency, further information from the patient regarding nutrition is extremely important. Also, further details should be obtained regarding the patient's recent mental status.

ADDITIONAL HISTORY

This patient had become depressed following recent surgery for head and neck cancer and had limited her caloric intake severely. In the month before evaluation, her sole caloric intake consisted of ethanol. During the past 2 weeks, the patient had become increasingly forgetful and confused and was brought in for evaluation by her family when she became disoriented.

PHYSICAL EXAMINATION

The patient was an emaciated woman with a supine blood pressure of 100/60. Neurologic examination revealed that she was not oriented to person, place, or time. She was unable to remember any objects at 1 minute during memory testing. Cranial nerve examination revealed upbeating nystagmus in the primary position that was diminished with upgaze and increased with downgaze, the reverse of that expected from Alexander's law (see Case 1). The patient could not move her eyes horizontally when asked to do so. There was facial asymmetry and an inability to protrude the tongue, both presumably caused by the radial neck dissection and hemiglossectomy. Coordination testing revealed a severe dysmetria of the upper and lower extremities. The deep tendon reflexes were normal. Sensation could not be assessed reliably. Romberg's test could not be performed because the patient could not stand with her eyes open without assistance. Her gait was severely ataxic. Otoscopic examination was normal.

Question 2: What is the etiology and the pathophysiologic basis of upbeating nystagmus?

Answer 2: The etiology of upbeating nystagmus is highly varied and given in Table Case 46–1. Note that abnormalities in numerous locations in the nervous system can be associated with upbeating nystagmus and that many disorders associated with upbeating nystagmus have an uncertain or distributed localization.

The pathophysiology of upbeating nystagmus is uncertain. Several mechanisms have been hypothesized including an imbalance in vertical vestibulo-ocular pathways, abnormal gaze-holding, and asymmetric vertical pursuit signals.[1]

Table Case 46-1 Etiologies of Upbeating Nystagmus

Cerebellar degeneration and atrophy
Multiple sclerosis
Infarction of medulla, cerebellum, or superior cerebellar peduncle
Tumors of medulla, cerebellum, or midbrain
Wernicke's encephalopathy
Brainstem encephalitis
Bechet's syndrome
Meningitis
Congenital visual abnormalities
Thalamic arteriovenous malformation
Organophosphate poisoning
Tobacco

Source: Adapted with permission from Leigh RJ, Zee DS: The Neurology of Eye Movements, ed 3. Oxford University Press, New York, 1999, p. 420.[1]

This patient's upbeating nystagmus diminished with up gaze and increased with downgaze. This reversal of Alexander's law suggests that abnormal gaze-holding is unlikely in this case.

LABORATORY TESTING

Videonystagmography: Ocular motor testing revealed upbeating nystagmus that was not changed when the patient was placed in darkness. Caloric testing revealed bilaterally reduced responses; there was a minimal response to ice water irrigations bilaterally.

Rotational testing revealed reduced responses with markedly increased phase lead.

An MRI scan of the brain was normal. Cerebrospinal fluid evaluation was normal.

DIAGNOSIS/DIFFERENTIAL DIAGNOSIS

Question 3: Based on the patient's history, physical examination, and laboratory tests, what is the likely diagnosis?

Answer 3: This patient is probably suffering from Wernicke's encephalopathy. Table Case 46–2 lists the clinical features of this condition, which is a result of hypovitaminosis B_1. The characteristic clinical features of this condition include eye movement abnormalities, mental status change, and gait ataxia. An additional commonly seen feature of this condition is vestibular paresis, either unilaterally or bilaterally, as assessed by caloric testing.[2] This patient had each of these four features. Presumably, the patient's head and neck surgery and her depression contributed to her poor nutritional habits and vitamin B_1 deficiency.

Question 4: In what clinical settings is Wernicke's encephalopathy seen?

Answer 4: Table Case 46–3 indicates the conditions that predispose to Wernicke's encephalopathy. Alcoholism is the most common of these conditions.

Question 5: This patient demonstrated markedly increased phase lead on rotational testing. What is the basis of this abnormality?

Answer 5: This patient's abnormal phase lead on rotational testing suggests an abnormality in the so-called velocity storage system.[3] *Velocity storage* refers to a

Table Case 46–2 Clinical Features of Wernicke's Encephalopathy

Ocular motor abnormalities such as nystagmus and gaze palsy
Ataxia
Global confusional state
Vestibular paresis
Hypotension
Hypothermia

Table Case 46–3
Conditions Associated
with Wernicke's
Encephalopathy

Alcoholism
Prolonged intravenous feeding
Intravenous hyperalimentation
Hyperemesis gravidarum
Anorexia nervosa
Prolonged fasting
Refeeding after starvation
Gastric plication

central nervous system circuit that maintains vestibular information beyond the cessation of activity of the eighth nerve afferents induced by vestibular stimulation. Thus, following a brief acceleratory stimulus, eighth nerve afferent activity will return to baseline in 5 to 7 seconds, whereas vestibular-induced eye movements may persist for about three to four times longer, that is, 15 to 30 seconds. A possible purpose of the velocity storage system is to improve the function of the VOR, especially for slow head movements. The velocity storage system is also critical for the generation of optokinetic nystagmus and thus probably plays a role during exposure to prolonged moving visual stimuli such as during walking.[4]

The central nervous system structures important for the velocity storage mechanism include the vestibular nucleus and the cerebellar uvula and nodulus.[5] Thus, abnormalities in these structures or their interconnections can impair velocity storage. However, despite their central nervous system localization, abnormalities of velocity storage are also seen with damage to the peripheral vestibular system.[6]

Abnormalities of the velocity storage system appear as increased phase lead during sinusoidal rotation and as a shortened VOR time constant, that is, an increased rate of decay of postrotatory nystagmus following abrupt changes in head velocity. There are no clinical correlates that are specific for abnormalities of the velocity storage system. Many different disorders can cause abnormalities in the velocity storage mechanism. Abnormal VOR dynamics indicative of abnormal velocity storage are a sensitive but nonspecific indicator of vestibular system damage.

Question 6: What is the basis of this patient's caloric reduction and abnormal VOR dynamics?

Answer 6: Wernicke's encephalopathy leads to reduced vestibular sensitivity, presumably because of damage to the vestibular nuclei in the medulla.[2]

This patient was given a diagnosis of Wernicke's encephalopathy.

TREATMENT/MANAGEMENT

This patient was treated with intravenous thiamine. Her nystagmus resolved, and she became less confused but had a persistent memory deficit. The gait ataxia persisted, though to a somewhat lesser degree. The patient's vestibular sensitivity improved so that bithermal responses were reduced but not absent. Her VOR dynamics remained abnormal, as evidenced by an increased phase lead of eye movements induced by sinusoidal rotation.

SUMMARY

A 54-year-old woman presented with forgetfulness and abnormal eye movements several months following hemiglossectomy for head and neck cancer. The patient was found to have poor memory, upbeating nystagmus, and gait ataxia. Laboratory testing revealed bilaterally reduced vestibular responses. The brain scan was normal. The patient was given the diagnosis of Wernicke's encephalopathy. Treatment consisted of intravenous thiamine. The patient improved somewhat but was left with a persistent deficit in memory and balance.

TEACHING POINTS

1. **Wernicke's encephalopathy, which is caused by vitamin B1 deficiency, is characterized by the combination of abnormal eye movements, mental status change, and ataxia.** The most common condition in which Wernicke's encephalopathy is seen is alcoholism.
2. **Eye movement abnormalities in Wernicke's encephalopathy include various types of nystagmus and gaze palsies.**
3. **Vestibular paresis, either unilaterally or bilaterally, is common in Wernicke's encephalopathy, probably as a result of damage to the vestibular nuclei in the medulla.**
4. **Abnormal vestibulo-ocular reflex dynamics, for example, increased phase lead on rotational testing, suggests dysfunction of the so-called velocity storage system.** The velocity storage system maintains central nervous system activity after activity in the eighth nerve decays.

REFERENCES

1. Leigh RJ, Zee DS: The Neurology of Eye Movements, ed 3. New York: Oxford University Press, 1999.
2. Ghez C: Vestibular paresis: A clinical feature of Wernicke's disease. J Neurol Neurosurg Psychiatry 32:132–139, 1969.
3. Furman JM, Becker JT: Vestibular responses in Wernicke's encephalopathy. Ann Neurol 26:669–674, 1989.
4. Cohen B, Matsuo V, Raphan T: Quantitative analysis of the velocity characteristics of optokinetic nystagmus and optokinetic after-nystagmus. J Physiol 270:321–344, 1977.
5. Waespe W, Cohen B, Raphan T: Dynamic modification of the vestibulo-ocular reflex by the nodulus and uvula. Science 288:199–202, 1985.
6. Zee D, Yee R, Robinson D: Optokinetic responses in labyrinthine-defective human beings. Brain Res 113:423–428, 1976.

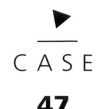

CASE
47

Vestibular Epilepsy

HISTORY

A 52-year-old female schoolteacher presented with a chief complaint of episodic dizziness. The first episode occurred 2 years before evaluation. The patient recalled having four other episodes prior to the last month, when she had about one episode each week. Each episode included a feeling of vertigo and blurred vision lasting for at most 1 minute, followed by a feeling of lethargy. There was no positional sensitivity, associated hearing loss, or tinnitus. The patient's past medical history was significant for migraine headaches. These headaches began when she was a teenager and remitted after menopause, which had occurred approximately 2 years before presentation. She also had a remote history of a generalized seizure disorder treated with phenobarbital, which she had not taken for as long as she could remember. She could not recall when she had last had a seizure. There was no family history of neurologic or otologic disease.

Question 1: Based on the patient's history, what is the differential diagnosis?

Answer 1: This patient's report of episodic vertigo suggests a peripheral vestibular abnormality, but the etiology is uncertain. Other diagnostic considerations are vertebrobasilar insufficiency, panic disorder, cardiac arrhythmia, hypoglycemia, and migraine-associated dizziness. The history of a seizure disorder is interesting and possibly of clinical significance because vertigo can be a rare manifestation of a seizure.

PHYSICAL EXAMINATION

The general, neurologic, otologic, and neurotologic examinations were entirely normal.

LABORATORY TESTING

Videonystagmography: Ocular motor, positional, and caloric tests were normal.
Rotational test was normal.
Posturography testing was normal.
An MRI scan of the brain was normal.
Blood studies including a glucose tolerance test were normal. A Holter monitor record was normal, although the patient did not have an episode while wearing the monitor.

Question 2: Based on the additional information from the patient's physical examination and laboratory studies, what is the differential diagnosis and what further tests should be ordered?

Answer 2: The physical examination and laboratory tests do not provide information to establish a definitive diagnosis, although they help to rule out a large number of diseases. A peripheral vestibulopathy such as a vestibular form of Meniere's disease or migraine-associated dizziness are still diagnostic possibilities. A seizure disorder, which could account for the patient's episodic vertigo, should be considered further. An electroencephalogram (EEG) should be ordered.

ADDITIONAL LABORATORY TESTING

The EEG was normal.

Question 3: Should the patient be treated?

Answer 3: The patient probably has a peripheral vestibulopathy of uncertain etiology. Treatment with a vestibular suppressant will probably prove ineffective because of the brief duration of the patient's episodes unless she uses a medication daily. Close follow-up should be instituted, especially regarding symptoms during episodes. The patient's family should be instructed to observe several episodes and determine the patient's level of consciousness during and after the episodes.

ADDITIONAL HISTORY

The patient returned in 2 weeks with her daughter and husband, who had both witnessed an episode of dizziness. During this episode, the patient had a depressed awareness of her surroundings but could converse and answer simple questions. Afterward, she could not recall the nature of the conversation during her episode, despite the fact that she had participated in it.

Question 4: What does this additional history suggest, and what, if any, additional laboratory tests should be ordered?

Answer 4: The additional history suggests that the patient may have an active seizure disorder, considering the disorientation during the episodes. Vertebrobasilar insufficiency, panic disorder, and a cardiac arrhythmia are still possibilities. Panic disorder is unlikely because the patient had no anxiety symptoms before, during, or after the episodes, and cardiac arrhythmia is unlikely given the normal Holter monitor record, although not during an episode.

The patient should be scheduled for prolonged EEG monitoring with simultaneous video monitoring and a simultaneous electrocardiogram (EKG).

FURTHER LABORATORY TESTING

During prolonged EEG monitoring, a vertiginous episode occurred, during which time the patient evidenced nystagmus that could be seen on the video monitor and on the frontal EEG leads. She had modest tachycardia during the episode. Her EEG during this episode showed rhythmic fast activity in the left posterior temporal region. An EKG obtained during the EEG monitoring was normal.

DIAGNOSIS/DIFFERENTIAL DIAGNOSIS

The patient was given the diagnosis of vestibular epilepsy, also known as *tornado epilepsy.*

Question 5: What is the pathophysiologic basis for vertigo during a seizure?

Answer 5: Vertigo during seizures is presumably a result of activation of cortical areas that are associated with the perception of motion.[1–3] These areas are difficult to specify with certainty. However, the posterior aspect of the superior temporal gyrus and the parietotemporal junction, that is, the angular gyrus, are probably the regions most consistently associated with vestibular perceptions.[4] Vertiginous sensations can occur as the aura before a seizure.[5]

Question 6: What is the pathophysiologic basis for epileptic nystagmus?

Answer 6: In adults, epileptic nystagmus is probably less common than vertigo during a seizure. However, there are many well-described cases of epileptic nystagmus,[6] some of these including electro-oculographic recordings. Nystagmus during seizures is of uncertain cause but may be the result of activation of pursuit tracking pathways that drive the eyes toward the side of the cerebral focus, with quick components in the opposite direction.[7,8]

TREATMENT/MANAGEMENT

This patient was treated with carbamazepine, which markedly reduced the frequency of her vertiginous episodes to only a few per year. She was restricted from driving and advised to avoid activities in which a vertiginous episode or seizure could be injurious.

SUMMARY

A 52-year-old woman presented with episodic vertigo without associated hearing loss or tinnitus. The patient had a past history of migraine headaches and a remote history of a generalized seizure disorder without seizures for at least 20 years. Her physical examination, MRI, and vestibular laboratory tests were normal. Additional history suggested a seizure disorder. EEG revealed a focal abnormality during a vertiginous episode that occurred while the patient was undergoing prolonged video EEG. She was given the diagnosis of vertiginous epilepsy and treated successfully with carbamazepine.

TEACHING POINTS

1. **Vestibular epilepsy, also known as *tornado epilepsy*, is a disorder in which vertigo occurs during seizures, presumably as a result of activation of cortical areas that are associated with the perception of motion.**
2. **A diagnosis of vestibular epilepsy should be considered in any patient with a history of a seizure disorder who presents with vertigo of uncertain etiology.** A careful inquiry regarding changes in level of consciousness during or following vertiginous episodes is essential. Prolonged video EEG monitoring may be required to capture an ictal episode.
3. **Nystagmus may or may not be associated with vestibular epilepsy.** When present during a seizure, nystagmus may indicate activation of ocular pursuit pathways.

REFERENCES

1. Kogeorgos J, Scott DF, Swash M: Epileptic dizziness. Br Med J 282:687–689, 1981.
2. Kluge M, Beyenburg S, Fernandez G, Elger CE: Epileptic vertigo: Evidence for vestibular representation in human frontal cortex. Neurology 55(12):1906–1908, 2000.
3. Lobel E, Kleine J, Le Bihan D, Leroy-Willig A, Berthoz A: Functional MRI of galvanic vestibular stimulation. J Neurophysiol 80:2699–2709, 1998.
4. Smith BH: Vestibular disturbances in epilepsy. Neurology 10:465–469, 1960.
5. Nielsen JM: Tornado epilepsy simulating Meniere's syndrome. Neurology 9:794–796, 1959.
6. Stolz SE, Chatrian G-E, Spence A: Epileptic nystagmus. Epilepsia 32:910–918, 1991.
7. Furman JM, Crumrine PK, Reinmuth OM: Epileptic nystagmus. Ann Neurol 27:686–688, 1990.
8. Tusa RJ, Kaplan PW, Hain TC, Naidu S: Ipsiversive eye deviation and epileptic nystagmus. Neurology 40:662–665, 1990.

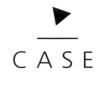

Prion Disease

HISTORY

A 50-year-old male sales representative presented with a chief complaint of dizziness of 2 months' duration. The patient noted that his symptoms were constant, characterized by a sense of lightheadedness and disequilibrium associated with poor balance. Additional symptoms included some difficulty with vision and poor concentration. The patient's symptoms had been slowly progressive following a subacute onset. He had no complaint of hearing loss or tinnitus. There was no family history of neurologic or otologic disease. The patient had no significant past medical history and used no medications.

Question 1: Based on the patient's history, what are the diagnostic considerations?

Answer 1: This patient has a very nonspecific history consistent with both vestibular and nonvestibular causes of dizziness. His condition appears to be progressive, and the complaints of poor vision and difficulty with concentration, although consistent with a vestibular system abnormality, are more likely to be symptoms of a central nervous system abnormality. Physical examination and appropriate laboratory testing are required to further define this patient's problem.

PHYSICAL EXAMINATION

The patient had a normal general examination except that he was disheveled. He was cooperative and oriented to person and place but was unsure of the date. He was unable to recall any of three objects at 3 minutes. There was some slowing of speech with mild dysarthria but no aphasia. Eye movement examination revealed poor upgaze and poor convergence, with gaze-evoked nystagmus. There were no other cranial nerve abnormalities. Coordination testing revealed mild dysmetria of both the upper and lower extremities. Strength and sensation were normal. The patient had a wide-based gait and could not tandem walk. He had great difficulty standing with his feet together, even with his eyes open, and could not stand with his eyes closed without assistance. Otologic examination was normal.

Question 2: Based on the history and physical examination, what are the diagnostic considerations and what laboratory tests, if any, would be appropriate?

Answer 2: This patient's history and physical examination are consistent with a central nervous system abnormality apparently affecting the cerebellum and possibly the midbrain, given the poor upgaze and poor convergence. There is little to suggest a vestibular system abnormality. Laboratory testing should certainly include brain imaging and routine blood studies. A lumbar puncture should be considered.

LABORATORY TESTING

An MRI scan of the brain was normal. Cerebrospinal fluid examination was normal.

Blood tests, including a complete blood count, electrolytes, metabolic parameters, thyroid function tests, and rheumatologic parameters were negative.

ADDITIONAL HISTORY

No firm diagnosis was established, and the patient was treated with a course of steroids without benefit. The patient's balance and cognitive function progressively declined. Several weeks after the initial evaluation, he was noted to have intermittent myoclonic jerks. He underwent EEG, which revealed diffuse slowing with some sharp waves.

Question 3: With the laboratory results and additional history, what are the diagnostic considerations?

Answer 3: The differential diagnosis includes spinocerebellar degeneration (see Case 19) with an associated cognitive deficit, paraneoplastic cerebellar degeneration (see Case 41), Alzheimer's disease, an unusual central nervous system neoplasm such as lymphoma, acquired immune deficiency syndrome (AIDS), progressive multifocal leukoencephalopathy, and the ataxic form of Creutzfeldt-Jakob disease. The last disorder is the most likely because of the constellation of symptoms and signs, especially the myoclonic jerks and the rate of progression.

The patient had a relentless course and died 3 months after evaluation. Neuropathologic evaluation was consistent with a spongiform encephalopathy.

Question 4: What are the clinical features of Creutzfeldt-Jakob disease? What are the features of the ataxic form of Creutzfeldt-Jakob disease? What is the pathophysiology of this condition?

Answer 4: The typical clinical characteristics of Creutzfeldt-Jakob disease include subacute onset of difficulty with memory and concentration. Patients may suffer from disequilibrium, double vision, incoordination, dysarthria, and tremor. Most patients go on to develop myoclonus, including startle-myoclonus, and can also develop corticospinal tract and extrapyramidal symptoms. Patients with the ataxic form of Creutzfeldt-Jakob disease typically present with abnormalities of gait and limb incoordination. Dysarthria and nystagmus occur early in the course. With time, patients with the ataxic form develop the other symptoms of Creutzfeldt-Jakob disease noted above. Patients deteriorate over a period of weeks to months, with a relentless decline in neurologic function.[1,2]

Creutzfeldt-Jakob disease, including the ataxic form, is thought to be caused by prions.[3,4] *Prion* is a loose acronym for a small proteinaceous infectious particle that resists inactivation by procedures that modify nucleic acids. The agent that causes Creutzfeldt-Jakob disease is thought to be related to the agent or agents that cause other dementing illnesses such as kuru and the Gerstmann-Straussler syndrome.[3,4]

Neuropathologically, there is loss of granule cells, with relative sparing of the Purkinje cells in the cerebellum.[2,5] Spongy degeneration, neuronal loss, gliosis, and amyloid plaques also affect vestibular nuclei,[6] the inferior olive, and the dentate nucleus.[7]

DIAGNOSIS/DIFFERENTIAL DIAGNOSIS

This patient's diagnosis was the ataxic form of Creutzfeldt-Jakob disease. Unfortunately, there is no effective treatment for this disease.

SUMMARY

A 50-year-old man presented with a 2-month history of progressively worsening dizziness, disequilibrium, and poor concentration. The patient had no significant past medical history and was using no medications. Incoordination suggested cerebellar system abnormalities. Eye movement abnormalities suggested a cerebellar and possibly a midbrain abnormality. The MRI scan was normal. A course of steroids was not helpful. The patient's clinical condition worsened; he developed dementia and myoclonus. The EEG was diffusely abnormal. The patient died 3 months after evaluation, at which time a neuropathologic evaluation indicated spongiform encephalopathy. The patient's clinical course suggested that he had the ataxic form of Creutzfeldt-Jakob disease.

TEACHING POINTS

1. **Creutzfeldt-Jakob disease is an unusual neurologic disorder that presents with the subacute onset of difficulty with memory and concentration, disequilibrium, double vision, incoordination, dysarthria, and tremor.** Most patients go on to develop myoclonus, including startle-myoclonus, and can also develop corticospinal tract and extrapyramidal symptoms.

2. **An ataxic form of Creutzfeldt-Jakob disease affects a subgroup of patients with this disorder, who present with poor balance, ataxia, and limb incoordination. Dysarthria and nystagmus also may occur early in the course of the disease.** With time, patients develop the other typical symptoms of Creutzfeldt-Jakob disease. They deteriorate over a period of weeks to months, with a relentless decline in neurologic function.

3. **The cause of Creutzfeldt-Jakob disease, including its ataxic form, is thought to be caused by an unconventional virus.** Such agents, called *prions,* also have been called *slow viruses,* which cause *slow infections.*

4. **The balance abnormalities seen in Creutzfeldt-Jakob disease can be explained by the loss of granule cells in the cerebellum and spongy degeneration, neuronal loss, gliosis, and amyloid plaques in the inferior olive and dentate nucleus.**

REFERENCES

1. Gomori AJ, Partnow MJ, Horoupian DS: The ataxic form of Creutzfeldt-Jakob disease. Arch Neurol 29:318–323, 1973.
2. Brownell B, Oppenheimer DR: An ataxic form of subacute presenile polioencephalopathy (Creutzfeldt-Jakob disease). J Neurol Neurosurg Psychiatry 28:350–361, 1965.
3. Prusiner SB: Prions and neurodegenerative diseases. N Engl J Med 317:1571–1581, 1987.
4. Yee RD, Farlow MR, Suzuki DA, Betelak KF, Ghetti B: Abnormal eye movements in Gerstmann-Straussler-Scheinker disease. Arch Ophthalmol 110:68–74, 1992.
5. Lafarga M, Berciano MT, Suarez I, Viadero CF, Andres MA, Berciano J: Cytology and organization of reactive astroglia in human cerebellar cortex with severe loss of granule cells: A study of the ataxic form of Creutzfeldt-Jakob disease. Neuroscience 40:337–352, 1991.
6. Manolidis LS, Balojannis SJ: Ultrastructural alterations of the vestibular nuclei in Jacob-Creutzfeld disease. Acta Otolaryngol 95:508–521, 1983.
7. Jellinger K, Heiss WD, Deisenhammer E: The ataxis (cerebellar) form of Creutzfeldt-Jakob disease. J Neurol 207:289, 1974.

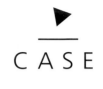

Orthostatic Tremor

HISTORY

A 70-year-old man presented with the complaint of unsteadiness while standing. The patient's symptoms had been present for the past 7 years and were
gradually worsening. He complained that after standing for 2 to 3 minutes, he
felt very unsteady and fatigued and needed to lean against something for support. He did not complain of dizziness. He was asymptomatic when sitting or
walking. There was no positional dizziness. His past medical history was significant for bilateral hearing loss and arthritis. His past surgical history included resection of a colon cancer and prostate surgery. Medications included a cholesterol-lowering agent. He did not consume alcohol. He had no complaints of double
vision, numbness, weakness, confusion, or difficulty with speech.

Question 1: What are the diagnostic considerations for this patient?

Answer 1: The patient's history does not suggest a vestibular disorder because
of the absence of dizziness and gait instability. Rather, the patient's symptoms
suggest a central nervous system abnormality affecting the postural control system. The complaint of difficulty standing but not walking is quite unusual for
both vestibular disorders and central nervous system abnormalities that affect
motor control such as Parkinson's disease.

PHYSICAL EXAMINATION

Neurologic examination revealed a palpable tremor in the lower extremities while
the patient was standing. This tremor was noted only after the patient had been

334

Table Case 49–1. Typical Symptoms and Signs of
Orthostatic Tremor

Onset of unsteadiness within 1 minute of standing
Progressive unsteadiness while standing still
Complaint of fear of falling
Complaint of stiffness
Stress increases the tremor
Tremor increases with prolonged standing
May be unable to walk slowly
Normal neurologic examination except tremor of legs while standing

standing for 1 to 2 minutes. No upper extremity tremor was seen at rest, with action, or with attention. The remainder of the neurologic examination was normal, with the exception of mildly impaired tandem gait. Otologic examination was normal. Neurotologic examination was normal.

Question 2: Based on the additional information from the physical examination, what are the possible diagnoses?

Answer 2: The patient's physical examination revealed an *orthostatic tremor*.[1-3] There were no signs suggesting a vestibular system abnormality. The typical symptoms and signs of orthostatic tremor are listed in Table Case 49–1. Note that a key feature of the diagnosis is unsteadiness while standing rather than unsteadiness while walking. The tremor may worsen in the Romberg position. Also, patients with orthostatic tremor may have a wide-based stance and yet are able to stand with the eyes closed without falling.

Orthostatic tremor is a clinical diagnosis. Most patients present with a high-frequency tremor primarily in the lower extremities of approximately 14 to 16 Hz.[4] The tremor may be a result of a synchronous co-contraction of the agonist and antagonists muscles of the legs or a result of alternately firing antagonists and antagonists. Typically, orthostatic tremor is difficult to see visually but it can be palpated, especially in the calves.

LABORATORY TESTING

Videonystagmography: Ocular motor function was normal. There was no positional nystagmus, and caloric responses were normal.

Rotational responses were normal.

The amount of sway during posturography was normal. However, the patient's record during posturography revealed extremely high shear (horizontal) forces.

An MRI scan of the brain revealed deep white matter changes consistent with the patient's age.

Question 3: What further diagnostic information is available from the results of laboratory testing?

Answer 3: Laboratory testing confirmed in the absence of a demonstrable vestibular abnormality. Also, posturography disclosed an unusual finding in the shear (horizontal) forces. High-frequency shear forces have been seen with orthostatic tremor, and this further supports the diagnosis. The patient's MRI scan, consistent with his age, revealed nonspecific abnormalities. Although disequilibrium of aging (see Case 10) is associated with deep white matter lesions, this patient's history and physical examination did not suggest a diagnosis of disequilibrium of aging, although an added effect of age must be considered.

DIAGNOSIS/DIFFERENTIAL DIAGNOSIS

The patient was given a diagnosis of orthostatic tremor.

Question 4: What treatments should be considered for a patient with orthostatic tremor?

Answer 4: Various medications have been used to treat orthostatic tremor. The most common ones include clonazepam, primidone, phenobarbital, valproic acid, clorazepate, gabapentin, propranolol, and carbidopa-levodopa. Gabapentin is currently the medication of choice for the treatment of orthostatic tremor.[5,6] In our experience, clonazepam is another medication that has been used successfully, although it appears that gabapentin is better for persons with orthostatic tremor. Vestibular rehabilitation may be a useful adjunct to pharmacotherapy in these patients.

TREATMENT

The patient was treated with gabapentin, 100 mg three times a day, and was referred for vestibular rehabilitation.

FOLLOW-UP

Three months following initiation of treatment with gabapentin and vestibular rehabilitation, the patient reported that his symptoms were decreased, though still present.

SUMMARY

A 70-year-old man presented with the complaint of unsteadiness while standing He was asymptomatic when sitting or walking. There was no dizziness. Neurologic examination revealed a palpable tremor in the lower extremities while the patient was standing. During posturography, the patient was noted to have extremely high shear (horizontal) forces. He was given a diagnosis of orthostatic tremor. The patient was treated with gabapentin, 100 mg three times a day, and was referred for vestibular rehabilitation. Three months following initiation of treatment with gabapentin and vestibular rehabilitation, the patient reported that his symptoms were decreased, though still present.

TEACHING POINTS

1. **Orthostatic tremor is a very unusual disorder characterized by unsteadiness while standing but not while walking.** The tremor may worsen in the Romberg position. Patients may have a wide-based stance and are able to stand with the eyes closed without falling. Typically, orthostatic tremor is difficult to see visually but it can be palpated, especially in the calves.
2. **Treatment options for orthostatic tremor include pharmacotherapy, for example, with gabapentin.** Vestibular rehabilitation may be a useful adjunct to pharmacotherapy in patients with orthostatic tremor.

REFERENCES

1. Heilman KM: Orthostatic tremor. Arch Neurol 41:880–881, 1984.
2. Britton TC, Thompson PD, van der Kamp W, Rothwell JC, Day BL, Findley LJ, Marsden CD: Primary orthostatic tremor: Further observation in six cases. J Neurol 239:209–217, 1992.
3. Veilleux M, Sharbrough FW, Kelly JJ, Westmoreland BF, Daube JR: Shaky-legs syndrome. J Clin Neurophysiol 4(3):304–305, 1987.
4. Thompson PD: Orthostatic tremor. J Neurol Neurosurg Psychiatry 66:278, 1999.
5. Evidente VG, Adler CH, Caviness JN, Gwinn KA: Effective treatment of orthostatic tremor with gabapentin. Movement Dis 13(5):829–831, 1998.
6. Onofrj M, Thomas A, Paci CF, D'Andreamatteo G: Gabapentin in orthostatic tremor: Results of a double-blind crossover with placebo in four patients. Neurology 51:880–882, 1998.

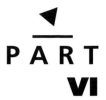

PART
VI

Clinically Controversial Case Studies

Acoustic Neuroma— Management

What is controversial about the management of dizziness associated with acoustic neuroma? For many patients with an acoustic neuroma, treatment options include stereotactic irradiation (gamma knife), conventional micro-surgery, and watchful waiting. Dizziness following stereotactic irradiation has been reported, but the cause and the optimal treatment remain uncertain.

HISTORY

A 68-year-old woman presented with the complaints of dizziness and unsteadi-ness for several months. The patient reported that these symptoms were getting worse and began shortly after she underwent stereotactic irradiation for treatment of a small acoustic neuroma. The neuroma was discovered during evaluation of left-sided hearing loss and tinnitus. The patient had noticed minimal dizziness at the time the neuroma was diagnosed. Her symptoms were exacerbated by fatigue and exertion. The patient reported veering to the left when walking, especially in dimly lit environments. She also complained of a pressure sensation around the left eye and blurred vision. Certain visual environments such as store aisles and sidewalks bothered her. The patient had been prescribed meclizine, but it pro-vided no relief.

Question 1: What are the treatment options for small acoustic neuromas?

Answer 1: The most common treatment of acoustic neuroma is microsurgical ex-cision of the tumor. Other treatment options include observation,[1,2] planned subtotal removal, and stereotactic irradiation. Selection of the appropriate treat-ment option depends on many factors and must be individualized.[3] The most im-

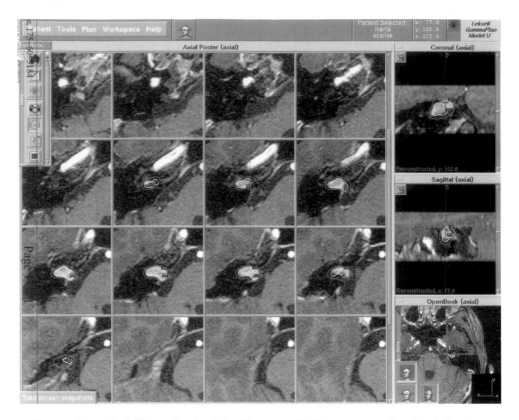

Figure Case 50–1 Example of a Leksell gamma knife treatment plan for delivering stereotactic radiation to an acoustic neuroma. The concentric lines that outline the tumor are 50% and 30% isodose curves that represent the distribution of radiation.

portant factors to consider include the size and location of the tumor, the age and health of the patient, and the severity of symptoms.

Question 2: What is stereotactic irradiation?

Answer 2: Stereotactic irradiation involves the use of precisely directed doses of radiation to treat tumors within the head while minimizing damage to surrounding structures. The radiation dose is designed to injure or kill the tumor cells or their supporting blood vessels. An acoustic neuroma does not disappear following irradiation, but it stops increasing in size. An example of an irradiation treatment plan is shown in Figure Case 50–1.

PHYSICAL EXAMINATION

Neurologic examination was normal, with the exception of mild gait instability. The patient could not tandem walk. Otologic examination revealed that on Weber's test, she lateralized to the right, and the Rinne test was positive bilaterally. Audibility of a finger rub was reduced on the left side. Neurotologic examination revealed no spontaneous nystagmus using infrared glasses. The head thrust was normal in both directions. A low-amplitude right-beating post-head-shake nystagmus was noted. The patient was unable to maintain her balance while standing on a compliant foam pad with the eyes closed. The stepping test revealed 30 degrees of rotation toward the left. Pastpointing was absent.

Question 3: What is the significance of the patient's physical examination abnormalities?

Answer 3: The patient's physical examination confirms a hearing loss on the left. Additionally, the normal head thrust suggests a preserved or partially preserved VOR bilaterally. Despite this evidence of preserved vestibular function, the patient's post-head-shake nystagmus suggests an ongoing vestibular asymmetry. The patient's inability to stand on a compliant foam pad with the eyes closed, inability to tandem walk, and mildly abnormal stepping test suggest a problem in the vestibulospinal system. Taken together, these findings suggest uncompensated vestibular dysfunction.

LABORATORY TESTING

Videonystagmography: Ocular motor testing was normal, and there was no spontaneous or positional nystagmus. Caloric testing showed no response to warm and cold irrigations bilaterally. Ice-water responses were present bilaterally.

Rotational testing revealed a decreased magnitude of responses (low gain) with a mild right directional preponderance.

Posturography testing revealed falls on conditions 5 and 6, indicating a vestibular loss pattern.

Audiometric testing revealed a mild high-frequency sensorineural hearing loss in the right ear. The left ear showed a profound sensorineural hearing loss, with a pure tone average of 72 dB and 0% word recognition.

An MRI scan of the brain revealed a neoplasm that filled the left internal auditory canal and extended into the cerebellopontine angle less than 1 cm (Fig. Case 50–2). The neoplasm was consistent with an acoustic neuroma. Comparison with the pretreatment study showed no tumor growth. The brain appeared normal.

Question 4: What is the significance of the vestibular laboratory test results?

Answer 4: The vestibular laboratory test results revealed a bilaterally reduced VOR, vestibulo-ocular asymmetry, and vestibulospinal dysfunction. The caloric reduction on the left is not surprising, as unilateral caloric weakness is commonly associated with acoustic neuroma. However, the caloric reduction on the unaffected right side is unexpected and may be due to a preexisting unrelated peripheral vestibular loss or may possibly be the result of central cerebellar inhibition. The reduced gains on rotational chair testing corroborate the results of caloric testing and suggest that overall vestibular sensitivity is reduced, possibly as a result of cerebellar inhibition. The alertness of the patient during testing and the possible use of vestibular-suppressant medications should be checked.

Rotational testing also suggests an ongoing VOR asymmetry in agreement with the presence of post-head-shake nystagmus on physical examination. Posturography testing suggests an inability to use vestibular information to maintain upright balance and is consistent with the patient's inability to stand on a com-

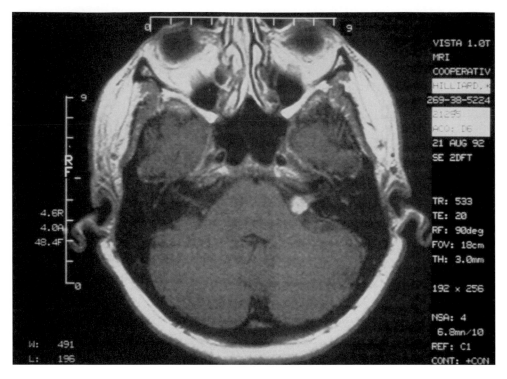

Figure Case 50–2 Axial T1-weighted magnetic resonance imaging scan with gadolinium enhancement of the brain showing a cerebellopontine angle neoplasm involving the left internal auditory canal consistent with an acoustic neuroma.

pliant foam pad with the eyes closed during physical examination. The normal ocular motor test and normal MRI of the brain suggest that there is no significant neurologic dysfunction. This agrees with the patient's normal neurologic examination aside from difficulty with upright balance.

The laboratory test results, in agreement with the physical exam, suggest uncompensated vestibular dysfunction.

Question 5: What are the possible causes for this patient's ongoing vestibular dysfunction and poor compensation?

Answer 5: The onset of new vestibular symptoms following stereotactic irradiation of an acoustic neuroma has been reported to occur in 29% of patients, typically beginning 6 months after treatment.[4] While the cause is not known with certainty, the symptoms may be due to aberrant activity in the vestibular nerve or vestibular labyrinth. The aberrant activity could be caused either by ongoing radiation-induced neuritis causing axonal demyelination and neural fibrosis or by metabolic changes within the inner ear. These effects could be caused by radiation-induced vasculitis or by direct effects on the eighth cranial nerve or inner ear. Other causes of impaired compensation (see Case 3) include a central nervous system abnormality, involvement of the contralateral vestibular system, causing a bilateral vestibular loss, multiple sensory deficits, a sedentary lifestyle, and vestibular-suppressant medications.

DIAGNOSIS/DIFFERENTIAL DIAGNOSIS

This patient was given a diagnosis of impaired vestibular compensation as a result of aberrant peripheral vestibular function.

TREATMENT/MANAGEMENT

Question 6: What are the treatment options for this patient?

Answer 6: Treatment options for this patient include a trial of a vestibular-suppressant medication, a trial of vestibular rehabilitation, and ablation of the left labyrinth. In general, the use of vestibular-suppressant medications in a patient with bilaterally reduced vestibular-sensitivity is not likely to be effective and may worsen the symptoms. However, in the special situation where aberrant peripheral vestibular function is suspected to be causing a centrally mediated reduction in overall vestibular sensitivity, the use of a benzodiazepine-class suppressant might prove beneficial. A course of aggressive vestibular rehabilitation should be tried. Treatment with a low dose of a benzodiazepine in combination with vestibular rehabilitation might prove beneficial. Ablation of the left labyrinth should be considered if the patient fails to benefit from these interventions.

FOLLOW-UP

The patient was treated first with a course of vestibular rehabilitation and then with a combination of clonazepam, 0.25 mg orally once or twice daily, and vestibular exercises. At a follow-up evaluation visit 3 months later, the patient's symptoms were unchanged. The patient then underwent a transmastoid labyrinthectomy. Postoperatively, her patient's symptoms gradually improved. Several months following surgery, the patient complained of dizziness only with rapid head movements and still noticed difficulty walking in dimly lit environments.

SUMMARY

A 68-year-old woman presented with dizziness 2 years following gamma knife treatment for an acoustic neuroma. Physical examination and laboratory tests suggested impaired vestibular compensation. The patient's symptoms, which also included disequilibrium, were not relieved by meclizine. Following an unsuccessful trial of vestibular rehabilitation and clonazepam therapy, the patient underwent a transmastoid labyrinthectomy. Postoperatively, her dizziness was much reduced, although she remained symptomatic with rapid head movements.

TEACHING POINTS

1. **The most common treatment of patients with acoustic neuroma is microsurgical excision of the tumor.** Other treatment options include observation, planned subtotal removal, and stereotactic irradiation. Se-

lection of the appropriate treatment option depends on many factors and should be individualized.

2. **Dizziness occurs more commonly after stereotactic irradiation in patients with normal pretreatment vestibular function.** Patients should be counseled regarding the occurrence of vestibular symptoms following stereotactic irradiation.

3. **Dizziness following stereotactic irradiation may be related to reduced or aberrant vestibular nerve activity.** Symptoms may persist as a result of impaired vestibular compensation.

4. **A treatment option for patients with presumed aberrant peripheral vestibular function is peripheral vestibular ablation.**

REFERENCES

1. Strasnick B, Glasscock ME, Haynes D, McMenomey SO, Minor LB: The natural history of untreated acoustic neuromas. Laryngoscope 104:1115–1119, 1994.
2. Wiet RJ, Zappia JJ, Hecht CS, O'Connor CA: Conservative management of patients with small acoustic tumors. Laryngoscope 105:795–800, 1995.
3. Sekhar LN, Gormley WB, Wright DC: The best treatment for vestibular schwannoma (acoustic neuroma): Microsurgery or radiosurgery? Am J Otol 17(4):676–689, 1996.
4. Lunsford LD, Linskey ME, Flickinger JC: Stereotactic radiosurgery for acoustic nerve sheath tumors. In: Tos M, Thompson J (eds). Proceedings of the First International Conference on Acoustic Neuroma. Amsterdam: Kugler, 1992, pp 279–287.

Superior Semicircular Canal Dehiscence Syndrome— Tullio's Phenomenon

W hat is controversial about the superior semicircular canal dehiscence syndrome? This diagnostic entity has been described only recently and is not fully understood. Questions remain regarding how to establish the diagnosis and what treatment, if any, is appropriate.

HISTORY

A 30-year-old woman complained of disequilibrium and intermittent dizziness. Symptoms began several years prior to evaluation but recently became noticeably worse following a ski vacation. The dizziness seemed to be associated with loud sounds, especially when they approached from her right. Along with her dizziness, the patient noticed difficulty with vision because of an apparent movement of visual objects. Another type of dizziness occurred with coughing, sneezing, and straining at stool. With this latter dizziness, the patient did not notice any alterations in her vision. She did not complain of hearing loss, tinnitus, or ear fullness. Her past medical history was negative. She had used meclizine for her symptoms without relief and was currently using no medications.

Question 1: Based on the patient's history, what are the diagnostic considerations? What is the significance of the patient's sensitivity to loud sounds? What is the significance of her sensitivity to coughing, sneezing, and bowel movements?

Answer 1: This patient's history suggests a vestibular abnormality based on the combination of dizziness and visual disturbance. The most prominent feature of the patient's history is the elicitation of dizziness both with loud sounds and with activities that increase intrathoracic pressure. Moreover, the patient experienced abnormal vision in response to loud sounds, which suggests the presence of sound-induced abnormal eye movements.

Dizziness in response to sound has been termed the *Tullio phenomenon*. The Tullio phenomenon has been associated with Meniere's syndrome, congenital ear anomalies, infectious etiologies such as syphilis, chronic ear pathology, trauma, perilymphatic fistula, and fenestration surgery.[1] The patient's sensitivity to changes in intrathoracic pressure is of uncertain cause but can be associated with the same etiologies that cause the Tullio phenomenon. The patient's history does not suggest Meniere's syndrome or an infectious etiology. She had not suffered trauma or undergone ear surgery.

PHYSICAL EXAMINATION

Neurologic examination was normal, with the exception of difficulty performing tandem walking. Neurotologic examination revealed no spontaneous nystagmus, no post-headshake nystagmus, a normal head thrust, a negative Dix-Hallpike test, increased sway without falling when asked to stand on a compliant foam surface with the eyes closed, and a negative stepping test. With tragal stimulation on the right, Valsalva maneuver, or pneumatic otoscopy on the right, the patient experienced her typical pressure-induced dizziness. Simultaneous observation of the patient's eye movements using infrared goggles revealed abnormal eye movements during pneumatic otoscopy but no abnormal eye movements during tragal stimulation or Valsalva maneuver. The abnormal eye movement observed was a vertical-torsional eye deviation without nystagmus.

Question 2: Based on the patient's physical examination, what are the likely diagnoses? What is the Hennebert symptom and the Hennebert sign? What is the significance of the patient's positive Hennebert symptom and sign?

Answer 2: The patient's physical examination suggests a right-sided peripheral vestibular ailment that has produced pressure sensitivity and sound sensitivity. A perilymphatic fistula is the most likely diagnosis, although the other conditions noted above must be considered. The vertical-torsional eye movement induced by pneumatic otoscopy suggests involvement of one of the vertical semicircular canals on the right. This patient had both a positive Hennebert symptom and a positive Hennebert sign, that is, pressure-induced dizziness and pressure-induced eye movements, respectively. Hennebert's symptom and sign originally were believed to be pathognomonic for syphilitic osteitis of the temporal bone. Hennebert's sign can be positive in Meniere's disease, where it is thought to be due to vestibular fibrosis causing the otolith organs to contact the undersurface of the stapes,[2] in the presence of a perilymphatic fistula and can occur after stapedectomy.

LABORATORY TESTING

Videonystagmography revealed no spontaneous or gaze-evoked nystagmus, normal positional testing, and normal caloric responses.

Rotational testing revealed a directional preponderance.

Posturography reveal increased postural sway in a nonspecific pattern.

Audiometric testing revealed a mild low-frequency sensorineural hearing loss in the right ear.

Question 3: Based on the additional information available from laboratory testing, what is the likely diagnosis? Should additional testing be considered?

Answer 3: Laboratory testing suggests that the horizontal semicircular canals respond normally. However, the directional preponderance on rotational testing suggests an ongoing vestibulo-ocular imbalance. Audiometric testing suggests a right-sided abnormality consistent with the patient's complaints of dizziness when exposed to loud noises on the right. To better define the anatomy of the right labyrinth, the patient should undergo a specialized CT scan of the temporal bone.

ADDITIONAL LABORATORY TESTING

A CT scan of the temporal bones that was optimized for visualizing the superior semicircular canal revealed a dehiscence of the right superior semicircular canal. Figure Case 51–1 illustrates diagrammatically the finding seen on the CT scan.

Question 4: What is dehiscence of the superior semicircular canal?

Answer 4: Dehiscence of the superior semicircular canal is a recently described finding in which the bone overlying the rostral aspect of the superior semicircu-

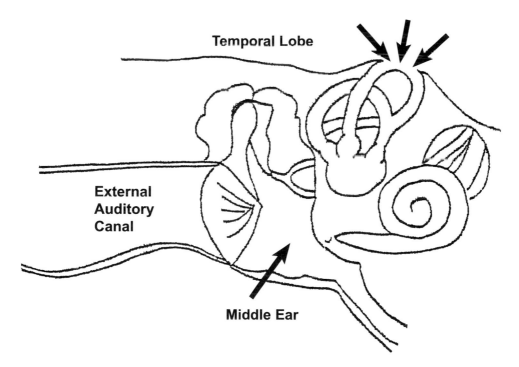

Figure Case 51–1 Diagrammatic illustration of dehiscence of the right superior semicircular canal. (*Source*: With permission from Smullen JL, et al: Superior semicircular canal dehiscence: A new cause of vertigo. J La State Med Soc 151:397–400, 1999.[5])

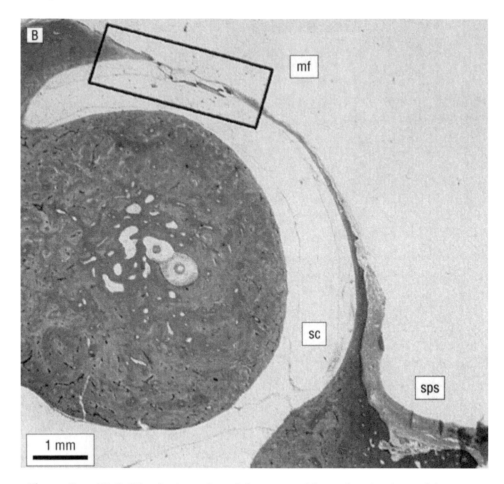

Figure Case 51–2 Histologic section of the temporal bone showing bony dehiscence of the superior semicircular canal. mf = middle fossa floor; sc = semicircular canal; sps = superior petrosal sinus. (*Source*: With permission from Carey JP et al: Dehiscence or thinning of the bone overlying the superior semicircular canal in a temporal bone study. Arch Otolaryngol Head Neck Surg 126:137–147, 2000.[6])

lar canal is thin or absent.[3] This is a variant of a semicircular canal fistula (Fig. Case 51–2).

Question 5: What is the mechanism for the signs and symptoms seen with dehiscence of the superior semicircular canal?

Answer 5: The signs and symptoms seen in patients with dehiscence of the superior semicircular canal probably relate to the transmission of pressure from the external auditory canal into the vestibular labyrinth.[4] This patient's complaints of visual motion when exposed to loud sounds and her abnormal eye movements during pneumatic otoscopy probably relate to inappropriate stimulation of the vestibular hair cells of the right superior semicircular canal in response to sound or pressure.

TREATMENT

Question 6: What are the treatment options for a patient with dehiscence of the superior semicircular canal?

Answer 6: Treatment options for patients with dehiscence of the superior semi-circular canal include observation or surgical repair. Many patients are relieved to receive a diagnosis that explains their symptoms, and because the symptoms are rarely disabling, they may choose to do nothing further. Surgical repair can be offered to those troubled by the symptoms.

The patient requested surgical intervention. The repair was performed via a middle fossa craniotomy. The dehiscent segment was repaired by creating a rigid seal of the canal using bone pâte and covering the area with a chip of cortical bone to separate the canal from the dura of the temporal lobe.

FOLLOW-UP

Three months following surgery, the patient reported no further episodes of sound sensitivity or symptoms associated with increased intrathoracic pressure. However, she continued to suffer from mild disequilibrium.

SUMMARY

A 30-year-old woman complained of disequilibrium and intermittent dizziness associated with loud sounds, coughing, sneezing, and straining at stool. The patient's physical examination suggested a right sided peripheral vestibular ailment that produced pressure sensitivity and sound sensitivity consistent with a peri-lymphatic fistula. A CT scan of the temporal bones revealed a dehiscence of the right superior semicircular canal. Surgical repair was performed to re-create a rigid seal of the semicircular canal. Sound and pressure sensitivity remitted, but mild disequilibrium persisted.

TEACHING POINTS

1. **Dizziness in response to sound is termed the *Tullio phenomenon*.** The Tullio phenomenon has been associated with Meniere's syndrome, congenital ear anomalies, syphilitic osteitis of the temporal bone, chronic ear pathology, trauma, perilymphatic fistula, and stapes surgery.
2. **Pressure-induced dizziness is termed *Hennebert's symptom*,** and pressure-induced eye movements is termed *Hennebert's sign*. Hennebert's symptom and sign are nonspecific indicators of a peripheral vestibular disorder. They can be positive in leutic involvement of the inner ear; in Meniere's disease, where it is thought to be due to vestibular fibrosis causing the saccule to contact the undersurface of the stapes; in the presence of a perilymphatic fistula; and can occur after stapedectomy.

3. **Dehiscence of the superior semicircular canal is to a recently described finding in which the bone overlying the rostral aspect of the superior semicircular canal is thin or absent.**
4. **Treatment options for patients with dehiscence of the superior semicircular canal include observation and surgical repair.**

REFERENCES

1. Watson SRD, Halmagyi M, Colebatch JG: Vestibular hypersensitivity to sound (Tullio phenomenon). Neurology 54:722–728, 2000.
2. Nadol JB: Positive "fistula sign" with an intact tympanic membrane. Arch Otolaryngol 100:273–278, 1974.
3. Minor LB, Solomon D, Zinreich J, Zee DS: Sound- and/or pressure-induced vertigo due to bone dehiscence of the superior semicircular canal. Arch Otolaryngol Head Neck Surg 124(3):249–258, 1998.
4. Hirvonen TP, Carey JP, Liang CJ, Minor LB: Superior canal dehiscence. Mechanisms of pressure sensitivity in a chinchilla model. Arch Otolaryngol Head Neck Surg 127:1331–1336, 2001.
5. Smullen JL, Andrist EC, Gianoli GJ: Superior semicircular canal dehiscence: A new cause of vertigo. J La State Med Soc 151:397–400, 1999.
6. Carey JP, Minor LB, Nager GT: Dehiscence or thinning of the bone overlying the superior semicircular canal in a temporal bone study. Arch Otolaryngol Head Neck Surg 126:137–147, 2000.

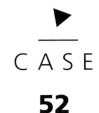

Perilymphatic Fistula

What is controversial about perilymphatic fistula? The presence of a peri-lymphatic fistula is often impossible to confirm or rule out. Thus, it is usually difficult to determine definitively which patients have such a diagnosis. This diagnostic uncertainty leads to difficulties in appropriate management. Specifically, should patients whose history suggests a perilymphatic fistula undergo exploratory surgery?

HISTORY

A 42-year-old female social worker presented with a chief complaint of dizziness that she described as a sense of lightheadedness that worsened with rapid head movements. Dizziness was present daily and was exacerbated by bending, coughing, and sneezing, and occasionally by bowel movements. The patient also reported hearing loss and tinnitus in the left ear. She dated the onset of her symptoms to head trauma sustained 14 months earlier during a family dispute. The patient was reluctant to provide details of this event. She had no significant past medical history other than the head trauma and was not using any medications prior to her dizziness. The family history was noncontributory. The patient's evaluation by her primary care physician included a normal CT scan. Meclizine was prescribed and provided some benefit, but the patient continued to be symptomatic.

Question 1: Based on the patient's history, what are the diagnostic considerations in this case?

Answer 1: Although this patient does not report episodic vertigo, her complaint of dizziness worsened by head movements is suggestive of a peripheral vestibular disorder. The associated unilateral auditory symptoms suggest involvement of the inner ear as well. Because her symptoms followed head trauma, diagnostic considerations include labyrinthine concussion, posttraumatic endolymphatic hydrops, and perilymphatic fistula. The symptoms worsened with Valsalva maneuvers, which is particularly suggestive of perilymphatic fistula.

PHYSICAL EXAMINATION

The patient had full extraocular movements but was noted to have an exophoria, that is, a latent ocular lateral misalignment when fusion was broken. There was no nystagmus. She had decreased pinprick sensation on the left side of her face that did not follow a dermatomal pattern but, according to the patient, corresponded to the region injured in the trauma 14 months prior to evaluation. She had normal strength and extremity sensation and normal coordination. Her gait was normal except for slight difficulty with tandem walking. Romberg's test was negative.

On otologic examination, the left eardrum had a normal appearance, but within the middle ear space the incus appeared to be dislocated. The long process of the incus had moved laterally and anteriorly from its normal position. The right ear appeared normal. On tuning fork examination, the Rinne test was negative on the left and positive on the right. Weber's test revealed lateralization to the left. On neurotologic examination, there was no nystagmus using infrared glasses. The head thrust was normal. There was no post-head-shaking nystagmus or positional nystagmus. On pneumatic otoscopy the eardrum was freely mobile, and with repeated pressure changes the patient began to feel dizzy and nauseous. No nystagmus was observed during pneumatic otoscopy, tragal stimulation, or Valsalva maneuvers. The patient had great difficulty standing on a compliant foam surface with her eyes open and could not stand on foam at all with her eyes closed.

Question 2: Based on the history and physical examination, what is this patient's likely diagnosis and what further laboratory testing is indicated?

Answer 2: This patient has a posttraumatic peripheral vestibulopathy that may be caused by labyrinthine concussion or perilymphatic fistula and traumatic ossicular chain disruption. The tuning fork examination and otoscopy suggest the presence of a conductive hearing loss on the left, probably as a result of dislocation of the incus. The association of ongoing dizziness and traumatic dislocation of the incus raises the possibility of additional ossicular dislocation involving the stapes and possible perilymphatic fistula involving the oval window. Appropriate laboratory testing includes audiometry and vestibular laboratory studies to document the character and extent of injury and to serve as a baseline should the patient require surgery for repair of the ossicular chain dislocation or perilymphatic fistula.

LABORATORY TESTING

Videonystagmography: Ocular motor function was normal. There was no spontaneous or positional nystagmus. Caloric testing revealed a borderline normal left reduced vestibular response of 21%.

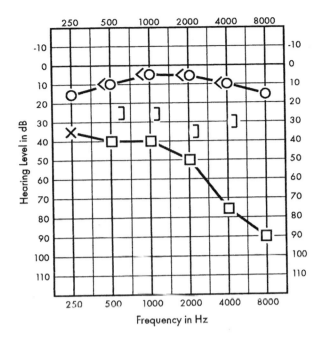

Figure Case 52–1 Audiogram.

Rotational testing revealed a left directional preponderance.

Posturography indicated excessive sway on conditions 4, 5, and 6, that is, a surface dependence pattern.

An audiogram revealed normal hearing in the right ear. The left ear had a mixed conductive and sensorineural hearing loss with preserved word recognition (Case Fig. 52–1).

DIAGNOSIS/DIFFERENTIAL DIAGNOSIS

Question 3: Based on the additional information from laboratory testing, what is the patient's likely diagnosis and what course of management should be taken?

Answer 3: The presence of a conductive hearing loss on audiologic testing supports the impression of a traumatic ossicular chain disruption. The sensorineural portion of the hearing loss raises the possibility that the cochlea also was damaged. The sensorineural hearing loss could have been caused by labyrinthine concussion or perilymphatic fistula. The results of vestibular testing support the presence of ongoing vestibular system dysfunction, and the unilateral caloric weakness supports a peripheral vestibulopathy as the cause. The vestibular symptoms and signs could be the result of either a perilymphatic fistula or labyrinthine concussion.

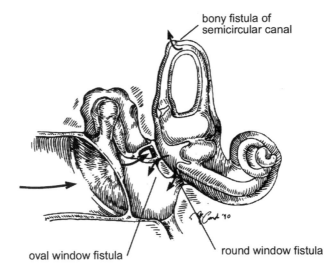

bony fistula of
semicircular canal

oval window fistula

round window fistula

Figure Case 52–2 Schematic drawing of the middle and inner ears showing common sites of perilymphatic fistulas. Curved arrows highlight the movement of perilymph through the round window membrane, the oval window, and a semicircular canal fistula. (*Source*: Modified with permission from Glasscock ME et al: Handbook of Vertigo. New York: Raven Press, 1990, p 17.[10])

Surgical exploration of the middle ear is indicated to restore hearing by reconstructing the ossicular chain and to rule out a perilymphatic fistula as a cause of the continuing vestibular symptoms.

Question 4: What is a perilymphatic fistula?

Answer 4: A perilymphatic fistula is an abnormal connection between the middle and inner ear spaces, specifically between the air-filled middle ear and the perilymphatic space of the inner ear.[1] A perilymphatic fistula can occur through the bony labyrinth (so-called bony fistula); through the oval window (so-called oval window fistula); or through the round window (so-called round window fistula) (Case Fig. 52–2).

Question 5: What are the common presenting symptoms and signs of perilymphatic fistula?

Answer 5: Common presenting symptoms and signs of perilymphatic fistula include sensorineural hearing loss that is often fluctuating, but may be constant or progressive, and tinnitus.[2] Vestibular symptoms are usually nonspecific and include mild unsteadiness and disequilibrium. Occasionally, patients with perilymphatic fistula report vertigo, especially during Valsalva maneuvers (coughing, sneezing, bending, lifting, or straining at stool). Perilymphatic fistula should be considered in patients (usually children) with a history of recurrent meningitis or progressive sensorineural hearing loss following an episode of otitis media.[3] Although it is possible that perilymphatic fistula can cause a pure vestibular syndrome without auditory or aural symptoms, the prevalence of this entity is controversial. Because it is not possible to diagnose a perilymphatic fistula solely on the basis of vestibular symptoms, most clinicians require a history of a traumatic inciting event and clear lateralization, for example, by the presence of hearing loss, to consider the diagnosis of a perilymphatic fistula.

Question 6: What are the causes of perilymphatic fistula?

Answer 6: Perilymphatic fistula can be iatrogenic, traumatic, erosive, spontaneous, or congenital. Iatrogenic fistulas are most commonly associated with surgery involving the stapes, in particular stapedectomy in patients with otosclersosis and during ossicular chain reconstruction. Traumatic perilymphatic fistula can be a result of direct penetrating injury; indirect injury following blunt head trauma, which probably accounts for this patient's perilymphatic fistula; or barotrauma.[4-6] Erosive perilymphatic fistula usually is caused by chronic middle ear and mastoid infection with an associated cholesteatoma (see Case 18) or, rarely, neoplasia. Spontaneous perilymphatic fistulas are highly controversial unless a congenital inner ear malformation is present.[7] Perilymphatic fistula related to a congenital inner ear malformation can occur spontaneously or, more commonly, after minor head trauma or forced Valsalva maneuver.

This patient was given a diagnosis of posttraumatic perilymphatic fistula.

TREATMENT/MANAGEMENT

A suspected perilymphatic fistula can be initially treated with a period of bed rest and reduced activity. Persistence of symptoms or deterioration of hearing are indications for surgical middle ear exploration. Because this patient also had evidence of ossicular chain dislocation, a middle ear exploration was performed without delay.

Middle ear exploration is usually performed under local anesthesia. Using an operating microscope, the tympanic membrane is reflected open, and the ossicular chain and oval and round window membranes are inspected directly. Perilymphatic fistula can be confirmed by visualizing a tear, rupture, or fracture of one of the inner ear membranes. In the past, the observation of clear fluid "pooling" around the inner ear membranes had been considered evidence of a perilymphatic fistula. However, it is now known that this sign is highly inaccurate. Specific assays for detecting perilymph have been studied, the most promising being the beta-2 transferrin assay, but have not yet been proven to be clinically reliable.[8,9]

In this patient, the incus was found to be severely dislocated; the annular ligament of the stapes was torn, and the stapes was partially subluxed into the vestibule. Repair was performed by first removing the incus. The stapes was then lifted back into its proper position, and a fascial graft was used to seal the ruptured annular ligament. The incus was then repositioned in the middle ear to reconstruct the ossicular chain.

After this procedure, the patient had complete restoration of the conductive component of her hearing loss, and she has had no further vertigo.

SUMMARY

A 42-year-old woman complained of dizziness following blunt head trauma. The patient had associated mild hearing loss and tinnitus in the left ear. Examination suggested damage to the ossicular chain and possible perilymphatic fistula. Laboratory testing demonstrated a mixed conductive and sensorineural hearing loss and a vestibular reduction on the left. The patient underwent middle ear exploration with repair of an oval window fistula and ossicular chain reconstruction.

TEACHING POINTS

1. **Peripheral vestibular-related symptoms following head trauma can be caused by labyrinthine concussion, posttraumatic endolymphatic hydrops, and perilymphatic fistula.**
2. **A perilymphatic fistula is an abnormal connection between the middle and inner ear spaces.** It can result from a fistula of the bony labyrinth, a rupture of the oval window, or a rupture of the round window.
3. **Symptoms and signs of perilymphatic fistula include sensorineural hearing loss that is often fluctuating, but can be constant or progressive, and tinnitus.** Vestibular symptoms are usually nonspecific, including mild unsteadiness and disequilibrium. Occasionally, patients with perilymphatic fistula report vertigo, especially during Valsalva maneuvers (coughing, sneezing, bending, lifting, or straining at stool).
4. **The causes of perilymphatic fistula include iatrogenic, traumatic, erosive, congenital, and spontaneous varieties.** The occurrence of spontaneous perilymphatic fistula is highly controversial unless a congenital inner ear malformation is present. Perilymphatic fistula should be considered in patients (usually children) with a history of recurrent meningitis or progressive sensorineural hearing loss following an episode of otitis media.
5. **The treatment of a suspected perilymphatic fistula includes a trial of bed rest and reduced activity to allow natural healing of the fistula.** Persistence of symptoms or deterioration of hearing are indications for surgical middle ear exploration. The purposes of surgical exploration are to confirm the presence of a fistula and to repair the fistula using fascial grafts.

REFERENCES

1. Bhansali SA: Perilymph fistula. Ear Nose Throat 68:11–26, 1989.
2. Hughes GB, Sismanis A, House JW: Is there consensus in perilymph fistula management? Otolaryngol Head Neck Surg 102:111, 1990.
3. Bluestone CD: Otitis media and congenital perilymphatic fistula as a cause of sensorineural hearing loss in children. Pediatr Infect Dis J 7:S141–S145, 1988.
4. Emmett JR, Shea JJ: Traumatic perilymph fistula. Laryngoscope 90:1513–1520, 1980.
5. Glasscock ME, McKennan KX, Levine SC: Persistent traumatic perilymph fistulas. Laryngoscope 97:860–864, 1987.
6. Pullen FW: Perilymphatic fistula induced by barotrauma. Am J Otol 13:270–272, 1992.
7. Schuknecht HF: Mondini dysplasia: A clinical and pathological study. Ann Otol Rhinol Laryngol 89(Suppl):3–23, 1980.
8. Bassiouny M, Hirsch BE, Kelly RH, Kamerer DB, Cass SP: Beta 2 transferrin application in otology. Am J Otol 13:552–555, 1992.
9. Skedros DG, Cass SP, Hirsch BE, Kelly RH: Sources of errors in use of beta 2 transferrin analysis for diagnosing perilymphatic and cerebral spinal fluid leaks. Otolaryngol Head Neck Surg 109:861–864, 1993.
10. Glasscock, ME, Cueva RA, Thedinger BA: Handbook of Vertigo. New York: Raven Press, 1990.

Cervicogenic Dizziness

W hat is controversial about cervicogenic dizziness? There is controversy regarding the very existence of cervicogenic dizziness, or cervical vertigo. Thus, questions abound regarding how such a diagnosis can be established and how such patient should be treated.

HISTORY

A 49-year-old male delivery van driver presented with the chief complaint of dizziness and lightheadedness during the previous 5 months. The patient had symptoms that fluctuated daily. Head movements exacerbated his symptoms, as did being in large rooms or complex visual environments. The patient had no complaints of hearing loss or tinnitus and no neurologic complaints. He dated the onset of symptoms to an automobile accident in which he was struck from the rear, causing him to experience a flexion-extension "whiplash" injury of the neck. The patient did not strike his head or lose consciousness during the accident. His symptoms were worse on the days when he experienced neck pain or neck muscle spasm. There was no significant past medical history. The family history was noncontributory.

Question 1: Based on the patient's history, what is the likely diagnosis?

Answer 1: Exacerbation of the patient's symptoms with head movement suggests a balance abnormality, possibly vestibular in origin. The patient also appears to be suffering from space and motion discomfort. The close association of his symptoms with neck pain and their onset following a neck injury suggests that this patient's complaints are likely to be a result of cervicogenic dizziness, also known

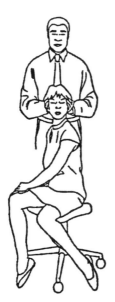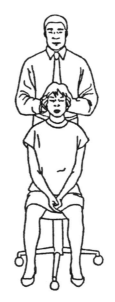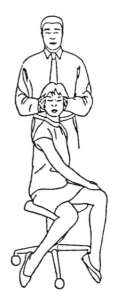

Figure Case 53–1 Head-fixed, body-turned maneuvers. With the patient on a swivel chair, the examiner stabilizes the head while the patient turns the body in such a way that the torso rotates with respect to the head, thereby stimulating the neck without stimulating the labyrinth. (*Source*: With permission from Fitz-Ritson D: Assessment of cervicogenic vertigo. J Manipulative Physiol Ther 14(3):193–198, 1991, p 195.[11])

as *cervical vertigo.*[1,2] Cervicogenic dizziness is a controversial diagnosis that is often considered when patients have dizziness and disequilibrium in association with neck pain. Other diagnostic considerations include benign paroxysmal positional vertigo, posttraumatic endolymphatic hydrops, peripheral vestibulopathy of uncertain etiology, or a central nervous system abnormality, structural or otherwise, that is now manifesting as dizziness either independent of or exacerbated by the motor vehicle accident.

PHYSICAL EXAMINATION

General, neurologic, and otologic examinations were normal, with the exception of decreased range of motion of the neck and a complaint of disequilibrium when turning the head, especially when attempting to bring the chin to the shoulder in either direction. Head-fixed, body-turned maneuvers (Case Fig. 53–1) were performed with infrared glasses with the head held still and the body turned while the patient sat on a swivel chair. He experienced dizziness and was noted to have several beats of right-beating nystagmus during rotation of the body to the left while he was looking straight ahead.

Question 2: Based on the history and physical examination, what is this patient's likely diagnosis? What laboratory tests would be helpful in establishing a diagnosis?

Answer 2: This patient's history and physical examination are suggestive of cervicogenic dizziness with an abnormal cervico-ocular reflex. Given the uncertainty of this diagnosis and the controversial nature of cervicogenic dizziness, both brain imaging and quantitative vestibular testing are warranted.

LABORATORY TESTING

Videonystagmography: Ocular motor function was normal.

An MRI scan of the brain was normal.

Right-beating nystagmus during head-fixed, body-turned maneuvers was recorded with the body turned to the left. This was seen in both the lying and seated positions.

Question 3: What is the cervico-ocular reflex? What is a possible explanation for this patient's disequilibrium?

Answer 3: The cervico-ocular reflex is an eye movement response to relative movement of the head with respect to the torso, that is, neck movement. The reflex is based upon afferent activity from the neck rather than from the labyrinth. Relative movement between the head and the torso alters the neural activity relayed to the vestibular nuclei regarding head position. These afferents primarily comprise neck muscle proprioceptive fibers.[3] This innervation may arise from joint afferents in the neck.[3] Also, other nerves may arise from facet joints in the cervical spine. The cervico-ocular reflex is thought to be of minimal importance in normal individuals, because quantitative testing of the reflex has revealed minimal eye movements as a result of relative motion between the head and torso with the head fixed in space.[4-6] However, numerous case reports attest to the dizziness and disequilibrium experienced by patients who have sustained neck injuries, and some patients have demonstrated nystagmus during the head-fixed, body-turned maneuver.[7] Also, anesthetizing one side of the neck produces acute disequilibrium and imbalance.[8] Vibration of the neck in patients with a unilateral vestibular lesion also suggests an increase in signals from the neck.[9] This patient appears to have a heightened cervico-ocular reflex when the body is turned to the left, so that clearly visible nystagmus was generated.

Question 4: What is the significance of this patient's episodic neck muscle spasm and its association with symptoms of dizziness?

Answer 4: The cause-and-effect relationship between the patient's neck muscle spasm and his symptoms of dizziness is uncertain. As described above, abnormal afferent activity from the neck could lead to dizziness as a result of the central nervous system receiving aberrant information regarding the position of the head in space. Such aberrant information could be made more unreliable by neck muscle spasm. Conversely, the vestibulo-colic and cervico-colic reflexes (see Chapter 1), which are designed to help stabilize the head in space, could be leading to excessive neck muscle activity when the patient is experiencing a vestibular imbalance. Thus, patients with cervicogenic dizziness may experience a "vicious cycle" of excessive neck muscle activity exacerbating their dizziness, which subsequently exacerbates their neck discomfort.

Question 5: What types of injuries can cause cervicogenic dizziness?

Answer 5: Cervicogenic dizziness has been reported in flexion-extension injuries often related to motor vehicle accidents, severe cervical arthritis, herniated cervical disks, and trauma, especially blunt trauma to the top of the head.[10]

DIAGNOSIS/DIFFERENTIAL DIAGNOSIS

This patient was given the diagnosis of cervicogenic dizziness.

TREATMENT/MANAGEMENT

Cyclobenzaprine was prescribed as a muscle relaxant to be used on an as-needed basis. A soft cervical collar was also prescribed for the patient, and he was admonished not to use the collar for more than 1 to 2 hours per day so that he did not lose neck muscle strength and continued to stimulate neck proprioception. This patient was treated with physical therapy to improve range of motion of the neck and to reduce neck muscle spasm and discomfort. These treatment interventions provided significant relief, but he remained symptomatic, especially if he was required to turn his head repeatedly for several hours—for instance, while driving an automobile for long distances.

SUMMARY

A 49-year-old man presented with the chief complaint of dizziness whose onset was associated with a flexion-extension injury during a motor vehicle accident. Examination revealed nystagmus during head-fixed, body-turned maneuvers, suggesting the diagnosis of cervicogenic dizziness. The patient was treated with physical therapy, muscle relaxants, and a soft cervical collar and gained symptomatic relief.

TEACHING POINTS

1. **Cervicogenic dizziness is a controversial diagnosis that refers to dizziness and disequilibrium thought to be caused by abnormal afferent activity from the neck.** The close temporal association of symptoms of dizziness and neck pain following a neck injury should suggest a diagnosis of cervicogenic dizziness. Cervicogenic dizziness can be seen in association with flexion-extension (whiplash) injuries, severe cervical arthritis, herniated cervical disks, and head trauma, especially blunt trauma to the top of the head.
2. **The cervico-ocular reflex, an eye movement response to neck movement, is thought to be of minimal importance in normal individuals.** However, a patient who has sustained a neck injury may have an abnormal or exaggerated cervico-ocular reflex that causes dizziness or disequilibrium when the head is turned.
3. **Neck muscle spasm and pain are often associated with symptoms of dizziness. The cause-and-effect relationship between these two symptoms is uncertain.** In fact, patients with cervicogenic dizziness may experience a "vicious cycle" of excessive neck muscle activity exacerbating their dizziness, which subsequently exacerbates their neck discomfort.

4. **Treatment of cervicogenic dizziness includes muscle relaxants and physical therapy to improve range of motion of the neck and to reduce neck muscle spasm and discomfort.** Use of a cervical collar should be limited to 1 to 2 hours per day.

REFERENCES

1. Ryan GMS, Cope S: Cervical vertigo. Lancet 2:1355–1358, 1955.
2. Jongkees LBW: Cervical vertigo. Laryngoscope 79:1473–1484, 1969.
3. Neuhuber WL, Zenker W: Central distribution of cervical primary afferents in the rat, with emphasis on proprioceptive projections to vestibular, perihypoglossal, and upper thoracic spinal nuclei. J Comp Neurol 280:231–253, 1989.
4. Huygen PLM, Verhagen WIM, Nicolasen MGM: Cervico-ocular reflex enhancement in labyrinthine-defective and normal subjects. Exp Brain Res 87:457–464, 1991.
5. Barlow D, Freedman W: Cervico-ocular reflex in the normal adult. Acta Otolaryngol 89:487–496, 1980.
6. Bronstein A, Hood J: The cervico-ocular reflex in normal subjects and patients with absent vestibular function. Brain Res 373:399–408, 1986.
7. Oosterveld WJ, Kortschot HW, Kingma GG, de Jong HA, Saatci MR: Electronystagmographic findings following cervical whiplash injuries. Acta Otolaryngol (Stockh) 111:201–205, 1991.
8. De Jong PTV, Vianney de Jong JMB, Cohen B, Jongkees BW: Ataxia and nystagmus induced by injection of local anesthetics in the neck. Ann Neurol 1:240–246, 1977.
9. Strupp M, Arbusow V, Dieterich M, Sautier W, Brandt T: Perceptual and oculomotor effects of neck muscle vibration in vestibular neuritis. Ipsilateral somatosensory substitution of vestibular function. Brain 121:677–685, 1998.
10. Wrisley DM, Sparto PJ, Whitney SL, Furman JM: Cervicogenic dizziness. J Orthop Sports Phys Ther 30(12):755–766, 2000.
11. Fitz-Ritson D: Assessment of cervicogenic vertigo. J Manipulative Physiol Ther 14(3):193–198, 1991.

Chronic Fatigue Syndrome

W hat is controversial about chronic fatigue syndrome? Chronic fatigue syndrome is a descriptive diagnosis of a condition whose etiology is unknown. In addition to the diagnostic imprecision, it is unknown whether or not the balance system, particularly the vestibular system, is involved in this disorder. There is no agreed-upon treatment for chronic fatigue syndrome.

HISTORY

A 28-year-old male accountant complained of a constant sense of lightheadedness, dizziness, and spatial disorientation that he dated to a flu-like illness accompanied by fever, chills, and a sore throat 9 months before evaluation. He did not experience vertigo or disequilibrium. Symptoms of disequilibrium were first noticed several weeks after the illness. These were accompanied by a sense of fatigue and decreased "energy" that caused him to reduce his daily activities significantly, as well as difficulty concentrating. The symptoms fluctuated little on a day-to-day basis, but the patient noted that they were exacerbated by exertion. He did not describe true vertigo or exacerbation of symptoms with rapid head movement. He had a sense of weakness in the legs and pain in the joints. He complained of poor-quality sleep. There was no significant past medical history. The family history was negative for neurologic or otologic disease.

The patient's primary care physician had performed an MRI scan, which was normal. The patient had reduced his workload as an accountant from full time to part time.

Question 1: Based on the patient's history, what are the diagnostic considerations?

Answer 1: This patient's history is quite nonspecific and gives little indication of a vestibular disorder, especially a peripheral vestibular abnormality. A non-vestibular cause of dizziness should be considered. The role of the patient's flu-like illness is uncertain.

PHYSICAL EXAMINATION

Neurologic examination was normal, with the exception of a slightly wide-based gait. The patient's sway during Romberg's test was somewhat increased, but he did not fall. He also swayed but did not fall while standing on a compliant foam surface with his eyes either open or closed. Otologic and neurotologic examinations were normal.

Question 2: How does the physical examination add to the diagnostic considerations? What laboratory testing, if any, would be helpful in establishing a diagnosis?

Answer 2: The physical examination provides little additional information regarding diagnostic possibilities. Laboratory testing may provide additional help in establishing a diagnosis. Vestibular laboratory testing in particular is appropriate because of this patient's complaint of spatial disorientation and disequilibrium. Screening blood studies are appropriate. The patient's complaint of chronic fatigue and decreased energy level suggests the possibility of a persistent viral infection, such as with the Epstein-Barr virus.

LABORATORY TESTING

Videonystagmography: Ocular motor function was normal. There was no static or paroxysmal positional nystagmus. Caloric irrigations were normal.

Rotational testing was normal.

Posturography indicated excessive postural sway in a nonspecific pattern.

Blood studies including a complete blood count, an erythrocyte sedmentation rate, serum chemistry including calcium, thyroid function tests, and an antinuclear antibody titer were normal.

DIAGNOSIS/DIFFERENTIAL DIAGNOSIS

Question 3: Based on the additional information from laboratory studies, what are the diagnostic possibilities?

Answer 3: This patient's laboratory tests suggest a nonspecific disorder that may or may not involve the vestibular system, considering the isolated nonspecific abnormalities on posturography. Possibly, the patient's flu-like illness 9 months before evaluation triggered his persistent symptoms, which are in some way related to his previous viral infection.

Question 4: What is chronic fatigue syndrome? What are the balance symptoms associated with this syndrome?

Table Case 54–1 Revised Centers for Disease Control Criteria for Chronic Fatigue Syndrome

A case of chronic fatigue syndrome is defined by the presence of:
1. Clinically evaluated, unexplained, persistent or relapsing fatigue that is of new or definite onset; is not the result of ongoing exertion; is not alleviated by rest; and results in substantial reduction in previous levels of occupational, education, social, or personal activities
and
2. *Four or more* of the following symptoms that persist or recur during six or more consecutive months of illness and that do not predate the fatigue:
   - Self-reported impairment in short term memory or concentration
   - Sore throat
   - Tender cervical or axillary nodes
   - Muscle pain
   - Multijoint pain without redness or swelling
   - Headaches of a new pattern or severity
   - Unrefreshing sleep
   - Post-exertional malaise lasting ≥24 hours

Source: Adapted with permission from Fukuda K et al: The chronic fatigue syndrome: A comprehensive approach to its definition and study. International Chronic Fatigue Syndrome Group. Ann Intern Med 121:953, 1994,[5] and UptoDate OnLine 9.3, November 15, 2001 (*www.uptodate.com*).[6]

Answer 4: Chronic fatigue syndrome is a controversial disorder characterized by fatigue, malaise, decreased "energy," and disequilibrium.[1,2] See Table Case 54–1. Some patients experience depression.[2] The cause is unknown. Two studies have documented nonspecific postural sway abnormalities in patients with chronic fatigue syndrome.[3,4] A vestibular origin for this disequilibrium is uncertain.[4]

This patient was given a diagnosis of chronic fatigue syndrome.

TREATMENT/MANAGEMENT

There is no known treatment for chronic fatigue syndrome. The patient was treated with vestibular rehabilitation. Several mild vestibular suppressants, including meclizine and diazepam, were prescribed, but they worsened the patient's symptoms. The patient did not benefit from a trial of amitriptyline. During an 18-month period following evaluation, the patient gradually recovered from his symptoms and was able to return to his work as an accountant on a full-time basis.

SUMMARY

A 28-year-old male accountant presented with a constant sense of dizziness, disequilibrium, and lightheadedness that had persisted for 9 months. The patient dated the onset of his symptoms to a flu-like illness unaccompanied by vertigo. The physical examination revealed only increased postural sway during standing. The MRI scan was normal. Vestibular laboratory testing indicated increased postural sway without obvious vestibular system involvement. Blood studies indicated an elevated Epstein-Barr virus titer consistent with a previous infection. The patient was given the diagnosis of chronic fatigue syndrome. The significance of the elevated Epstein-Barr virus titer was considered questionable. Treatment consisted of a trial of vestibular-suppressant medications, which were not helpful, and balance therapy. The patient gradually improved during the 18 months following evaluation.

TEACHING POINTS

1. **Chronic fatigue syndrome is a controversial disorder characterized by fatigue, malaise, decreased "energy," and, not uncommonly, disequilibrium.**
2. **Disequilibrium associated with chronic fatigue syndrome is of uncertain etiology. Nonspecific postural sway abnormalities are commonly observed that do not aid in the localization of this disorder.**
3. **The cause of chronic fatigue syndrome is unknown.** Although it has been suggested that patients with chronic fatigue syndrome are more likely to have elevated Epstein-Barr virus titers, this finding has not been substantiated in the literature.
4. **Treatment of chronic disequilibrium associated with chronic fatigue syndrome consists of a trial of vestibular-suppressant medications and vestibular rehabilitation (see Case 17 for the treatment of nonspecific vestibulopathy).** Gradual improvement with periods of waxing and waning of symptoms may be expected.

REFERENCES

1. Schluederberg A, Struas SE, Peterson P, Blumenthal S, Komaroff AL, Spring SB, Landay A, Buchwald D: Chronic fatigue syndrome research. Ann Intern Med 117:325–331, 1992.
2. Komaroff AL: Clinical presentation of chronic fatigue syndrome. In: Bock GR, Whelan J (eds). Chronic Fatigue Syndrome. New York: Wiley, 1993, pp 43–61.
3. Furman JM: Testing of vestibular function: An adjunct in the assessment of chronic fatigue syndrome. Rev Infect Dis 13(Suppl 1):S109–S111, 1991.
4. Ash-Bernal R, Wall C 3rd, Komaroff AL, Bell D, Oas JG, Payman RN, Fagioli LR: Vestibular function test anomalies in patients with chronic fatigue syndrome. Acta Otolaryngol (Stockh) 115(1):9–17, 1995.
5. Fukuda K, Straus SE, Hickie I, Sharpe MC, Dobbins JG, Komaroff A: The chronic fatigue syndrome: A comprehensive approach to its definition and study. International Chronic Fatigue Syndrome Study Group. Ann Intern Med 121:953, 1994.
6. Straus SE, Gluckman SJ: Clinical features of chronic fatigue syndrome. UptoDate Online 9.3, November 15, 2001.

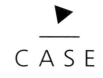

Driving and Dizziness

HISTORY

A 46-year-old female school bus driver was evaluated for dizziness that occurred intermittently during the preceding 18 months. Symptoms occurred
as often as several times each day or as infrequently as several times per week.
Dizziness consisted of episodes lasting for a few seconds to several minutes. These
episodes were characterized by a slight visual change causing double and blurred
vision. The patient also had episodic numbness. She noted a sense of lightheadedness, a sensation of movement, and gait instability with the episodes. There
was also occasional associated nausea and head pressure and circumoral paresthesias. The patient did not complain of blindness, weakness, clumsiness, confusion, or loss of consciousness. Her past medical history was significant for myo-
cardial infarction 8 years earlier, hypertension, and a remote history of migraine
headaches, although none for approximately 20 years. Current medications included an antihypertensive agent and a cholesterol-lowering agent. The patient
smoked one pack of cigarettes per day and did not use alcohol.

Question 1: Based on the patient's history, what is the diagnosis?

Answer 1: This patient's history does not suggest a definitive diagnosis. Rather, it
suggests a nonspecific disorder that may be vestibular or nonvestibular in origin.
The patient's history of migraine headaches suggests the possibility of migraine-
related vestibulopathy, but the patient has been headache free for 20 years.

PHYSICAL EXAMINATION

Neurologic and otologic examinations were normal. Neurotologic examination also was normal, including a search for spontaneous nystagmus, a normal head thrust, a negative Dix-Hallpike test, and normal stability on a foam pad.

LABORATORY TESTING

Videonystagmography: Ocular motor, postural, and caloric tests were normal. Rotational testing revealed a moderately reduced magnitude of responses without asymmetry. Posturography testing and audiometry were normal. MRI scan of the brain was normal, as were noninvasive carotid studies.

Question 2: Based on the history, physical examination, and laboratory tests, what are the diagnostic possibilities for this patient?

Answer 2: The additional information provided by the physical examination and laboratory tests still does not provide an obvious diagnosis. The patient's presentation remains consistent with nonspecific dizziness of uncertain etiology, possibly related to a vestibular disorder.

DIAGNOSIS/DIFFERENTIAL DIAGNOSIS

This patient was given a diagnosis of nonspecific vestibulopathy.

TREATMENT

Question 3: What are the treatment options for this patient?

Answer 3: Treatment options include further investigation of her dietary habits with counseling to encourage adoption of a low-salt diet and education regarding dietary migraine triggers, reduction and avoidance of nicotine and overuse of caffeine, use of a low-dose vestibular-suppressant on an as-needed basis, and medical treatment for migraine-related vestibulopathy, for example, with a tricyclic antidepressant.

The patient underwent dietary counseling and was prescribed imipramine, 10 mg orally at hour of sleep.

Question 4: Under what circumstances might a patient with a vestibular disorder have difficulty operating a motor vehicle and why?

Answer 4: A patient with a vestibular abnormality might be expected to have difficulty operating a motor vehicle because of the combination of active and passive head movements used while driving. Thus, a patient with a vestibular disorder may have increased difficulty driving on very curved roads and exit ramps, even at posted speeds, and while driving in ramped or circular parking garages. A patient with a vestibular disorder also may be challenged by the visual–vestibular interaction associated with driving. When one looks at objects outside of the vehicle, the visual and vestibular systems act in concert, whereas when one looks

disorders may have increased difficulty operating motor vehicles even while driving under ideal conditions.

3. **Certain vestibular disorders are more worrisome than others for patients driving a motor vehicle, such as Tumarkin's otolithic crisis and chronic constant dizziness.**

4. **In Pennsylvania, physicians are not required to report individuals with dizziness, disequilibrium, or vestibular disorders.** Reporting guidelines in countries other than the United States may differ.

5. **The appropriate instructions regarding driving for a patient with dizziness are controversial but should probably be different for driving commercial vehicles compared to passenger vehicles.**

6. **Patients with chronic dizziness reduce their amount of driving.** However, most patients continue to drive even if their doctor warns them that it would be dangerous to do so.

REFERENCES

1. Sindwani R, Parnes LS, Goebel JA, Cass SP: Approach to the vestibular patient and driving. A patient perspective. Otolaryngol Head Neck Surg 121:13–17, 1999.
2. Moser M: An objective testing method to determine driving ability. Acta Otolaryngol (Stockh) 99:326–329, 1985.
3. Gimse R, Bjorgen IA, Straume A: Driving skills after whiplash. Scand J Psych 38:165–170, 1997.
4. Annex A. Title 67: Transportation, Part I. Department of Transportation, Subpart A. Vehicle Code Provisions, Article IV. Licensing, Chapter 83, Physical and Mental Criteria Including Vision Standards Relating to the Licensing of Drivers, Motor Vehicle Operations, Harrisburg: Pennsylvania Department of Transportation, p. 7.
5. Mckiernan D, Jonathan D: Driving and vertigo. Clin Otolaryngol Allied Sci 26(1):1–3, 2001.
6. Hoffman HJ, Ko C, Sklare DA: How is the frequency of driving an automobile affected by chronic (3+ months) problems with imbalance and/or dizziness? Presented at the American Public health Association National Meeting, October 2001.

Malingering

What is controversial about malingering? Whether a patient is willfully attempting to deceive the physician, is manifesting a conversion disorder, or has a highly unusual nonphysiologic presentation is often uncertain. Determining the patient's status is often important both medically and legally.

HISTORY

A 34-year-old male construction worker complained of dizziness for 3 months. The patient dated the onset of symptoms to a head injury that occurred on the job. While he was wearing his hardhat, a small piece construction equipment weighing about 2 pounds fell several feet and struck him on top of the head. The patient had no loss of consciousness and was able to continue working that day. The next day, he did not report for work and presented to a local emergency room complaining of dizziness. His evaluation, including a CT scan of the head, disclosed no apparent abnormality, and he was released. The patient returned to work the next day but could not tolerate the increased dizziness that his work provoked. He has not worked since that time. His primary care physician prescribed a nonsteroidal anti-inflammatory agent, but the patient remained symptomatic. The patient's dizziness was characterized by a constant sense of lightheadedness that was exacerbated by exertion. He did not complain of visual motion sensitivity, worsening of symptoms with rapid head movement, or gait instability. His past medical history was negative, except for a concussion with loss of consciousness for several minutes 10 years earlier that was sustained in a motor vehicle accident. The patient was using no medications, smoked one pack of cigarettes per day, and consumed alcohol occasionally without worsening of his dizziness.

Question 1: What diagnostic entities should be considered?

Answer 1: The patient's symptoms are nonspecific and are not highly suggestive of a vestibular abnormality. The head trauma was mild and probably was not associated with a labyrinthine concussion, but this must be considered. A postconcussion syndrome also should be considered, although the patient did not lose consciousness and did not complaint of headache.

PHYSICAL EXAMINATION

The neurologic examination was normal, except that the patient demonstrated excessive sway during Romberg testing without falling. Otologic examination was normal. Neurotologic examination revealed no spontaneous nystagmus, a normal head thrust, negative Dix-Hallpike testing, and excessive sway without falling while standing on a foam pad both with eyes open and with eyes closed. During the stepping test, the patient had no clear rotation.

Question 2: What is malingering? Which audiovestibular measures can be used to help assess for malingering?

Answer 2: Malingering has been defined as "The false and fraudulent simulation or exaggeration of physical or mental disease or defect, performed in order to obtain money or drugs, to evade duty or criminal responsibility, or for other reasons that may be readily understood by an objective observer from the individual's circumstances, rather than from learning the individual's psychology."[1]

Some audiovestibular tests are objective and require minimal patient cooperation, such as an assessment of nystagmus during ocular motor screening, positional testing, caloric testing, and rotational testing. Posturography requires much cooperation and can yield results that suggest malingering or lack of cooperation on the part of the patient. Several studies have asked persons to feign, that is, simulate, posturographic abnormalities.[2–4] These persons produced posturography patterns that looked aphysiologic.[5] However, an aphysiologic pattern on posturography does not necessarily indicate malingering, since aphysiologic patterns have been found both in patients with psychiatric disorders and in suspected malingerers.[5]

Audiologists are trained to detect inconsistent responses during hearing tests that suggest possible factitious hearing loss. Several special audiometric tests, such as Stenger's test, can be used to uncover factitious hearing. Two particular abnormalities of posture and gait, astasia-abasia and camptocornia, have been linked to psychiatric disorders.[6] A study by Gianoli et al.[7] determined that patients with the potential for secondary gain had a lower percentage of abnormalities on electronystagmography and an aphysiologic sway pattern on posturography.

LABORATORY TESTING

Videonystagmography: Ocular motor, postural, and caloric tests were normal. Rotational testing was normal. Posturography revealed excessive sway during sensory conditions 1, 2, and 3 but not 4, 5, and 6, that is, an aphysiologic pattern.

Audiometric testing revealed a bilateral high-frequency sensorineural hearing loss consistent with noise-induced hearing loss.

MRI scan of the brain was normal.

Question 3: Based on the additional information from the physical examination and laboratory tests, what is the differential diagnosis? Is this patient malingering?

Answer 3: No definite diagnosis can be made based on the additional information from the physical examination and laboratory tests. The abnormal posturography showed an aphysiologic pattern. Given the patient's unwillingness or inability to return to work, malingering must be suspected but cannot be confirmed. The patient had no abnormalities of posture and gait aside from excessive sway on Romberg testing and no evidence of a factitious hearing loss. His laboratory tests were normal, aside from posturography, which further supports possible malingering.

DIAGNOSIS/DIFFERENTIAL DIAGNOSIS

This patient was given a diagnosis of dizziness of uncertain etiology. Malingering was considered possible but could not be confirmed.

TREATMENT

Question 4: What treatment, if any, would be appropriate for this patient?

Answer 4: It is difficult to recommend treatment for patients with poorly defined symptoms who may be malingering. The patient was sent to a physical therapist for a functional balance assessment (see Chapter 6) and a course of vestibular rehabilitation.

FOLLOW-UP

The patient was retested on posturography as part of the physical therapy assessment 1 week later. Again the results were unusual. The patient had excessive sway on conditions 1 and 2 but had normal sway patterns on conditions 3 to 6, indicating inconsistencies with the first posturography test that also demonstrated an aphysiologic pattern. The patient continued to have difficulty standing on the foam pad with eyes open and closed. The Dynamic Gait Index score was 23 out of 24, the Dizziness Handicap Inventory score was 84, and the Activities-specific Balance Confidence score was 65% (see Chapter 6). The patient's perceived dizziness on a 0–100 scale was 90, and he stated that his dizziness was constant. The patient was given a home exercise program to address his balance dysfunction during standing. He was seen on follow-up on two occasions for vestibular rehabilitation. The patient's scores on both objective and subjective functional balance assessment measures remained unchanged, and vestibular rehabilitation was discontinued.

The patient subsequently filed a disability claim that was denied. The patient planned to enlist the aid of an attorney and to appeal the negative decision

SUMMARY

A 34-year-old construction worker complained of dizziness following minor head trauma without loss of consciousness. During assessment, he evidenced excessive sway during Romberg testing and an aphysiologic pattern during posturography, suggesting the possibility of malingering. No definitive diagnosis could be reached. The patient did not return to work and filed a disability claim.

TEACHING POINTS

1. Malingering has been defined as "The false and fraudulent simulation or exaggeration of physical or mental disease or defect, performed in order to obtain money or drugs, to evade duty or criminal responsibility, or for other reasons that may be readily understood by an objective observer from the individual's circumstances, rather than from learning the individual's psychology."[1].
2. Some audiovestibular tests are objective and require minimal patient cooperation, whereas posturography requires much cooperation.
3. Posturography can yield results that suggest malingering or a lack of cooperation on the part of the patient.
4. An aphysiologic pattern on posturography does not necessarily indicate malingering since aphysiologic patterns have been found in patients with psychiatric disorders and suspected malingering.
5. Audiometric testing using one of several tests, such as Stenger's test, can uncover a factitious hearing loss.

REFERENCES

1. Gorman WF: Defining malingering. J Forensic Sci 27(2):401–407, 1982.
2. Uimonen S, Laitakari K, Kiukaanniemi H, Sorri M: Does posturography differentiate malingerers from vertiginous patients? J Vestib Res 5(2):117–124, 1995.
3. Goebel JA, Sataloff RT, Hanson JM, Nashner LM, Hirshout DS, Sokolow CC: Posturographic evidence of nonorganic sway patterns in normal subjects, patients, and suspected malingers. Otolaryngol Head Neck Surg 117:293–302, 1997.
4. Krempl GA, Dobie RA: Evaluation of posturography in the detection of malingering subjects. Am J Otol 19:619–627, 1998.
5. Cevette MJ, Puetz B, Marion MS, Wertz ML, Muenter MD: Aphysiologic performance on dynamic posturography. Otolaryngol Head Neck Surg 112:676–688, 1995.
6. Sinel M, Eisenberg MS: Two unusual gait disturbances: Astasia abasia and camptocormia. Arch Phys Med Rehabil 71:1078–1080, 1990.
7. Gianoli G, McWilliams S, Soileau J, Belafsky P: Posturographic performance in patients with the potential for secondary gain. Otolaryngol Head Neck Surg 122:11–18, 2000.

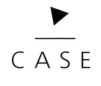

Vascular Cross-Compression Syndrome of the Eighth Cranial Nerve

What is controversial about vascular cross-compression syndrome of the eighth cranial nerve? The existence of vascular cross compression of the eighth cranial nerve by large loops of the anterior inferior cerebellar artery in the internal auditory canal is well known. However, the clinical significance of small arteries and veins juxtaposed to the eighth cranial nerve is uncertain. Thus, establishing such a diagnosis and recommending treatment is challenging.

HISTORY

A 50-year-old man presented with a chief complaint of disequilibrium that was more or less constant but was particularly exacerbated by lying on his right side. The patient experienced a sense of motion while lying on his right side that was not paroxysmal. It lasted as long as he maintained that position and become worse until he could no longer stay in that position. The patient did not complain of hearing loss but did note occasional noise and occasional sharp pain in his right ear. He had suffered from these symptoms for 2 years, and the onset had been gradual. His past history was significant for a 3-day episode of flu-like symptoms and vertigo 5 years before evaluation that was diagnosed as labyrinthitis. Several weeks after that episode of vertigo, the patient's symptoms had completely resolved and he became asymptomatic for approximately 3 years. There was no other past medical history of significance. He had used multiple medications including meclizine, diazepam, promethazine, lioresal, carbamazepine, and amitriptyline with minimal or no benefit. The patient had been treated for presumed endolymphatic hydrops with a combination of hydrochlorothiazide and triamterene and a salt-restricted diet with no benefit. There was a family history of trigeminal neuralgia in the patient's mother. The patient was extremely troubled by his symptoms and had discontinued his work as an accountant.

Question 1: Based on the patient's history, what are the diagnostic possibilities?

Answer 1: This patient's history is unusual. The symptoms are positional but are not characterized by vertigo and are not paroxysmal. Thus, benign paroxysmal positional vertigo is unlikely. However, the patient's history is consistent with a peripheral vestibular ailment because of the ear pain, tinnitus, and past history of an acute vestibular syndrome. The vestibular abnormality is probably on the right, considering the laterality of the otologic symptoms and the exacerbation while lying on the right side. Experience has shown that patients who can identify a side that elicits symptoms when dependent often have their abnormality on the ipsilateral side. The patient's history does not, however, fit into a common diagnostic category. Physical examination and laboratory testing may help to establish a diagnosis.

PHYSICAL EXAMINATION

The patient's general examination was normal. Neurologic examination was normal, with the exception of mild instability during tandem walking. Otologic examination was normal. Neurotologic examination revealed no spontaneous nystagmus and normal Dix-Hallpike maneuvers. Static positional testing using infrared goggles revealed that the patient had a strong sense of disequilibrium while lying on his right side and a weak left-beating nystagmus. The patient could not maintain balance while standing on a compliant foam surface with the eyes closed.

LABORATORY TESTING

Videonystagmography: Ocular motor function was normal. There was a low-amplitude left-beating nystagmus in the head-right and right-lateral positions of 4 degrees per second. There was a 22% right reduced vestibular response during caloric testing.

Rotational testing was normal

Posturography indicated excessive sway on conditions 5 and 6, that is, a vestibular pattern.

An audiogram revealed a mild high-frequency sensorineural hearing loss in the right ear, with normal hearing in the left ear. Word recognition was excellent bilaterally, with normal acoustic reflexes. Brainstem auditory-evoked responses were normal bilaterally.

An MRI scan of the brain was normal.

DIAGNOSIS/DIFFERENTIAL DIAGNOSIS

Question 2: Based on the patient's history, physical examination, and laboratory studies, what is the differential diagnosis?

Answer 2: This patient is likely to have a peripheral vestibulopathy on the right, possibly as a result of the viral syndrome and "labyrinthitis" 5 years before evaluation, which was probably a viral vestibular neuritis. The patient has evidence of an ongoing vestibulospinal abnormality and a very-low-amplitude positional nystagmus, all consistent with an ongoing vestibular system abnormality. The precise diagnosis cannot be stated with certainty. In light of the patient's family history of trigeminal neuralgia and personal history of atypical ear pain associated with chronic dizziness, the possibility of a vascular cross-compression syndrome affecting the eighth cranial nerve should be considered.[1] The clinical description of this condition is controversial, with no agreed-on set of diagnostic criteria.[2] Indeed, for some experts, this condition does not even exist. However, recent histopathologic evidence suggests that small regions of the vestibular nerve can become demyelinated following an insult such as a viral infection, and these regions could then become susceptible to irritation by adjacent blood vessels.[3,4] An example of a vascular loop seen on MRI is shown in Figure Case 57–1. Note

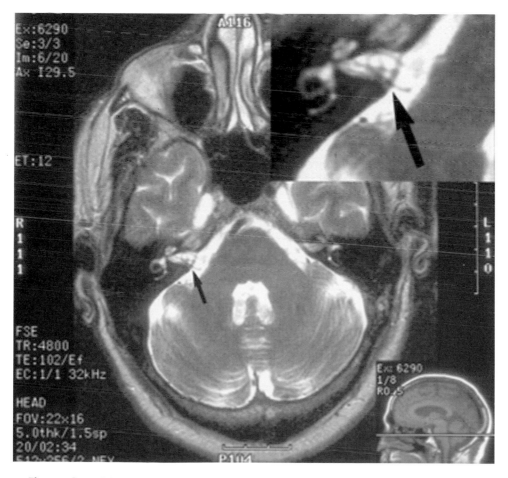

Figure Case 57–1 T2 weighted axial MRI of the brain. The arrow points to a vascular loop contacting the eighth cranial nerve in the right internal auditory canal.

that the patient discussed in the present case had a normal MRI. Vascular cross-compression syndrome of the eighth cranial nerve has been called *disabling positional vertigo* by Jannetta[5] and *vestibular paroxysmia* by Brandt and Dieterich.[6]

This patient was given the diagnosis of vascular cross-compression syndrome of the eighth cranial nerve.

TREATMENT/MANAGEMENT

Question 3: What treatments have been advocated for patients diagnosed with suspected vascular cross-compression syndrome of the eighth cranial nerve?

Answer 3: Treatment of suspected vascular compression syndrome of the eighth cranial nerve includes medications known to be effective for other disorders thought to result from vascular compression, such as tic douloureux and glossopharyngeal neuralgia. These agents include carbamazepine,[6] baclofen, and gabapentin. Other medications that are often prescribed for this condition include vestibular suppressants such as diazepam. Surgical treatment has been advocated for suspected vascular cross-compression syndrome of the eighth cranial nerve using microvascular decompression.[5] We suggest a trial of medical therapy before considering surgery.

This patient was treated with gabapentin and was much improved symptomatically.

SUMMARY

A 50-year-old man presented with the chief complaint of a sense of disequilibrium that was exacerbated by prolonged recumbency with the right side down. The patient's past history was significant for an acute vestibular syndrome probably of viral origin 5 years previously. The patient had no signs or symptoms of paroxysmal positional nystagmus. Audiometric and vestibular testing suggested a right-sided peripheral vestibular lesion. MRI scan was negative. The patient was given a diagnosis of possible vascular cross-compression syndrome of the eighth cranial nerve. He was treated with gabapentin, and his symptoms resolved almost completely.

TEACHING POINTS

1. **Small regions of the vestibular nerve can become demyelinated following an insult such as a viral infection, and these regions can then become susceptible to irritation by adjacent blood vessels.**
2. **Vascular cross-compression syndrome of the eighth cranial nerve, which has been called *disabling positional vertigo* and *vestibular paroxysmia*, refers to a cochleovestibular syndrome caused by compression of the eighth cranial nerve by blood vessels within the cerebellopontine angle.**
3. **The clinical description of vascular cross-compression syndrome of the eighth cranial nerve is controversial, with no agreed-on set of di-**

agnostic criteria. Features of this syndrome include dizziness associated with head movements or particular head positions, tinnitus, hearing loss, and ear pain. A history of symptoms consistent with a vascular compression syndrome such as trigeminal neuralgia supports the diagnosis of vascular cross-compression syndrome of the eighth cranial nerve.

4. **Treatment of vascular cross-compression syndrome of the eighth cranial nerve includes pharmacotherapy with carbamazepine, baclofen, or gabapentin.** Surgical treatment consists of microvascular decompression. We advocate a trial of medical therapy before referring a patient for a surgical opinion.

REFERENCES

1. Moller MB, Moller AR, Jannetta PJ, Jho HD, Sekhar LN: Microvascular decompression of the eighth nerve in patients with disabling positional vertigo: Selection criteria and operative results in 207 patients. Acta Neurochir (Wien) 125:75–82, 1993.
2. Ryu H, Yamamoto S, Sugiyama K, Nozue M: Neurovascular compression syndrome of the eighth cranial nerve. What are the most reliable diagnostic signs? Acta Neurochir (Wien) 140:1279 1286, 1998.
3. Schwaber MK, Whetsell WO: Cochleovestibular nerve compression syndrome. II. Vestibular nerve histopathology and theory of pathophysiology. Laryngoscope 102:1030–1036, 1992.
4. Colletti V, Fiorino FG, Carner M, Turazzi S: Vestibular neurectomy and microvascular decompression of the cochlear nerve in Meniere's disease. Skull Base Surg 4:65–71, 1994.
5. Jannetta PJ, Moller MB, Moller AR. Disabling positional vertigo. N Engl J Med 310:1700–1705, 1984
6. Brandt TH, Dieterich M: Vestibular paroxysmia (disabling positional vertigo). Neuro-Opththalmology 14:359-369, 1994.

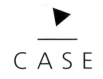
Bilateral Meniere's Disease

What is controversial about the treatment of bilateral Meniere's disease? Establishing the diagnosis of bilateral Meniere's disease can be complicated because each of the two ears can be involved at the same time or at different times, with similar or different degrees of severity. Treatment considerations are challenging because of the various combinations of bilateral auditory and vestibular impairment.

HISTORY

A 63-year-old man complained of vertigo and progressively worsening unsteadiness and disequilibrium. The patient reported a 20-year history of unilateral Meniere's disease but indicated that his current complaints included both recurrent vertigo and symptoms that were very different from recurrent vertigo. He noted that he had new gait instability with veering to both the right and the left, which was worse in the dark or while walking on soft (compliant) or uneven surfaces. In addition to unsteadiness, the patient reported difficulty with his vision, especially when attempting to focus on traffic signals or when walking or driving an automobile. He was unable to work at his usual occupation as an electrician.

In addition to his balance complaints, the patient reported recent worsening of his hearing. He had first noted episodic loss of hearing in his right ear approximately 20 years ago at about the time when he first began having attacks of vertigo. At first, his hearing improved between spells of vertigo, but over time the loss of hearing became permanent. The patient's hearing seemed stable during the preceding 3 years. However, during the last few months, he had noticed increasing difficulty with communication, especially understanding speech in the presence of background noise. He found that he had become increasingly reliant on lipreading.

Question 1: Based on the patient's history, what are the diagnostic considerations?

Answer 1: This patient has a history of Meniere's disease affecting the right ear. His recent history suggests a return of episodic vertigo that may be due to exacerbation of his right-sided vestibular abnormality. Alternatively, the patient may be suffering from an additional disorder affecting the left vestibular system or, less likely, the central nervous system. The patient's complaint of abnormal vision suggests possible oscillopsia caused by bilateral vestibular loss (see Case 4). Additionally, the patient's complaints of worsening hearing and difficulty with communication suggest possible bilateral cochlear involvement. Taken together, these aspects of the patient's history suggest bilateral otologic disease, probably bilateral Meniere's disease.

PHYSICAL EXAMINATION

Neurologic examination revealed full extraocular movements without nystagmus. The remainder of the neurologic examination was normal, except that the patient's gait had a wide base. Romberg's test was negative. Fluoroscopic examination was normal. Decreased hearing ability to finger rub was noted in both ears. On neurotologic examination, the patient had a low-amplitude right-beating nystagmus behind infrared goggles. On head thrust testing, refixation saccades were noted, with brisk head movements to both the right and the left. During ophthalmoscopy, a reduced VOR was noted. The dynamic visual acuity test was abnormal.[1] The patient was unable to stand on a compliant foam surface with the eyes closed without falling.

Question 2: Based on the additional information from the physical examination, what is the likely diagnosis?

Answer 2: The patient's physical examination suggests bilateral vestibular loss (see Case 4) as well as an ongoing VOR asymmetry. Specifically, the combination of oscillopsia, a bilaterally abnormal head thrust, abnormal VOR using ophthalmoscopy, and inability to stand on a compliant surface with the eyes closed suggests bilateral vestibular loss. The low-amplitude spontaneous vestibular nystagmus suggests a vestibulo-ocular asymmetry. Thus, the patient's physical examination lends further support to a diagnosis of bilateral ear disease.

LABORATORY TESTING

Videonystagmography: Ocular motor testing was normal, except for a low-amplitude right-beating spontaneous vestibular nystagmus. There was a direction-fixed right-beating static positional nystagmus. Caloric testing revealed absent responses to bithermal stimulation. In the right ear, there was no response to ice-water irrigation, with a low-amplitude right-beating nystagmus unaffected by thermal stimulation. In the left ear, there was a small but definite response to ice-water irrigation.

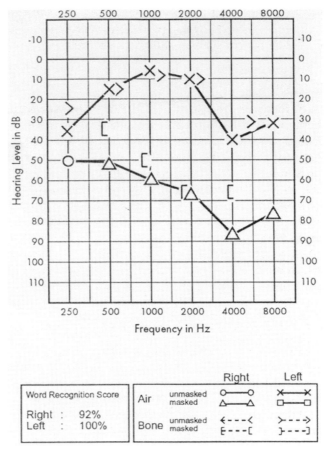

Figure Case 58–1 Audiogram.

Rotational testing revealed severely reduced responses, with a low-amplitude right-beating nystagmus seen during testing. Responses were evident during sinusoidal stimulation at frequencies above 0.5 Hz and following constant velocity rotation at 90 degrees per second.

Posturography indicated to excessive sway on conditions 5 and 6, that is, a vestibular loss pattern.

Audiometric testing indicated a bilateral asymmetric sensorineural hearing loss (Fig. Case 58–1). Electrocochleography of the left ear indicated an elevated summating potential to action potential ratio consistent with endolymphatic hydrops. Reliable potentials could not be obtained for the right ear.

An MRI scan of the brain was normal.

Question 3: Based on the patient's history, physical examination, and laboratory tests, what is the most likely diagnosis?

Answer 3: The patient's laboratory tests confirm bilateral otologic disease with severely reduced vestibular function bilaterally. Tests also confirm the mild vestibular ocular reflex asymmetry. Audiometric testing showing new hearing loss on the left side suggests active Meniere's disease in the left ear. Bilateral Meniere's disease remains the most likely diagnosis. The patient's history suggests that the long-standing right-sided otologic problem has been stable, with recent involvement of the left ear consistent with Meniere's disease.

Question 4: Why is this patient experiencing both episodic vertigo and oscillopsia and disequilibrium?

Answer 4: Each of the patient's episodes of vertigo is a result of an acute imbalance in peripheral vestibular function. Despite the fact that the patient has markedly reduced or absent vestibular responsiveness in the right ear from long-standing Meniere's disease, his new episodic loss of vestibular function in the left ear is provoking symptoms similar to those seen in individuals with unilateral vestibular involvement with an intact contralateral vestibular system. This phenomenon, known as *Becterew's phenomenon*, is characterized by behavioral manifestations in persons with acute unilateral peripheral vestibular disease with normal function contralaterally similar to those seen in persons with acute unilateral peripheral vestibular disease who have compensated for a previous contralateral vestibular deficit. In this patient, the complaints of oscillopsia and disequilibrium suggest that he is manifesting symptoms and signs of bilateral vestibular loss (see Case 4) superimposed on an episodic vestibular asymmetry.

Question 5: How often does Meniere's disease occur in both ears?

Answer 5: Estimates in the literature of the incidence of bilateral Meniere's disease range between 10% and 50%. The wide range of incidence rates largely reflects the criteria used to determine if Meniere's disease was present in the opposite ear and the duration of observation. A reasonable estimate is that 30% of patients with unilateral disease will develop symptoms of Meniere's disease in the opposite ear at some time in their lives.[2,3]

Question 6: Can bilateral Meniere's disease occur many years following the onset of unilateral Meniere's disease?

Answer 6: Yes, as exemplified by this patient, bilateral Meniere's disease can occur many years following the onset of unilateral Meniere's disease. However, bilateral disease will almost always manifest within 5 years of the initial presentation of unilateral disease, with most cases occurring within the first 2 years.

TREATMENT

Question 7: What treatments are appropriate for a patient with bilateral Meniere's disease?

Answer 7: Like patients with unilateral Meniere's disease, patients with bilateral Meniere's disease should be treated with a low-sodium diet and a diuretic. If this fails, oral immunosuppressive therapy for at least 6 weeks should be tried. Vestibular-suppressant medications and ablative surgical procedures should be avoided if possible. Endolymphatic sac decompression and shunting can be used when one of the ears can be clearly identified as the active offending ear.

Another treatment consideration for patients with bilateral Meniere's disease who do not respond to dietary sodium restriction and a diuretic is intramuscular streptomycin therapy. Intramuscular streptomycin reduces vestibular function bilaterally and thus can be used to treat vertigo caused by simultaneously active Meniere's disease in both ears, vertigo in a patient with bilateral Meniere's disease when the active ear cannot be determined, Meniere's disease in an only hearing ear, and Meniere's disease in the second ear when the first ear has been previously treated with an ablative procedure. Intramuscular streptomycin, like ablative surgical procedures, should be considered only in patients with disabling episodic vertigo who have not responded to conservative measures. It must be given in a controlled manner to produce a subtotal vestibular ablation, with the dose titrated to control episodes of acute vertigo while stopping short of complete bilateral loss of vestibular function.[4]

FOLLOW-UP

The patient was treated with a low-sodium diet and a diuretic. His symptoms persisted without change, and 2 months later the patient was treated with oral prednisone, starting at 60 mg per day for 2 weeks followed by an extended taper to 20 mg every other day for 6 weeks. He was also given dietary counseling to help control his salt intake. Additional testing for possible environmental and food allergies was requested. The episodes of vertigo decreased, but gait instability and hearing loss persisted. He was referred for a hearing aid evaluation and to vestibular rehabilitation for gait training and fall prevention counseling.

SUMMARY

Bilateral Meniere's disease was diagnosed in a patient with previously diagnosed long-standing unilateral Meniere's disease. Symptoms of acute vertigo and persistent gait instability and oscillopsia were present, suggesting a combination of acute recurrent unilateral vestibular disorder and bilateral vestibular loss. Audiologic and vestibular function testing confirmed the involvement of both ears. Intensive medical management reduced the severity of episodic vertigo, but bilateral deficits of both hearing and vestibular function persisted.

TEACHING POINTS

1. **Approximately 30% of patients with unilateral Meniere's disease will develop symptoms of Meniere's disease in the opposite ear at some time in their lives.**
2. **Bilateral Meniere's disease almost always will manifest within 5 years of the initial presentation of unilateral disease, with cases most occurring within the first 2 years.**
3. **Medical therapy is the first line of treatment.** Ablative procedures should be avoided if possible.
4. **Intramuscular streptomycin is an effective treatment for disabling vertigo in a patient with bilateral Meniere's disease refractory to conservative treatment.** It must be given in a controlled manner to prevent total vestibular ablation.

5. **Becterew's phenomenon is the occurrence of symptoms of acute vestibular imbalance in persons with acute unilateral peripheral vestibular disease who have compensated for a previous contralateral vestibular deficit.**

REFERENCES

1. Longridge NS, Mallison AI: A discussion of the dynamic illegible "E" test: A new method of screening for aminoglycoside vestibulotoxicity. Otolaryngol Head Neck Surg 92(6):671–676, 1984.
2. Wladislavosky-Waserman P, Facer GW, Mokri B, Kurland LT: Meniere's disease: A 30 year epidemiology and clinical study in Rochester, MN, 1951–1980. Laryngoscope 94:1098–1102, 1984.
3. Yazawa Y, Kitahara M: Bilateral endolymphatic hydrops in Meniere's disease: Review of temporal bone autopsies. Ann Otol Rhinol Laryngol 99:524–528, 1990.
4. Langman AW, Kemink JL, Graham MD: Titration streptomycin therapy for bilateral Meniere's disease. Ann Otol Rhinol Laryngol 99:923–926, 1990.

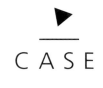

C A S E

59

Complementary and Alternative Therapies for Dizziness

What is controversial about complementary and alternative therapies for dizziness? By definition, complementary and alternative therapies are unproven. Further complicating the use of such therapies are potential interactions with other conventional treatments.

HISTORY

A 40-year-old woman presented with a complaint of dizziness. The patient was uncertain as to the date of onset. She related, however, that 2 years previously, she had been struck gently on the head by an overhead beam and had suffered from migraine headaches since that time. The dizziness seemed more prominent since then. The patient also reported a minor motor vehicle accident 6 years previously that resulted in *reflex sympathetic dystrophy* affecting her right lower extremity. The patient characterized her dizziness as lightheadedness and disequilibrium. She also complained of space and motion discomfort including unpleasant sensitivity to complex visual patterns and moving visual scenes. She was particularly bothered by grocery stores and shopping malls. The patient's past medical history was significant for strabismus with eye muscle surgery in childhood. She also described intermittent tachycardia of uncertain etiology. The patient was currently using no medications. Her family history was significant for a maternal aunt with migraine.

Question 1: Based on the patient's history, what are the diagnostic considerations?

Answer 1: The patient's history suggests a balance system abnormality but is nonspecific. Diagnostic considerations include migraine-related dizziness (see Cases

8, 21, 24) because of the patient's complaint of migraine headache and her family history of migraine; labyrinthine concussion because of the history of head trauma (see Case 11); anxiety-related dizziness (see Case 5) because of the patient's space and motion sensitivity; and visually related dizziness based on the patient's history of strabismus, that is, an ocular misalignment with no obvious cause. Note that space and motion discomfort is not specific for anxiety-related dizziness but may be seen in patients with vestibular disorders without anxiety. Also, note that the dizziness associated with strabismus is of uncertain cause.

ADDITIONAL HISTORY

The patient volunteered that since the onset of her dizziness she had tried many nonconventional therapies including vision therapy, herbal remedies, and electroacupressure. Unfortunately, none of these remedies provided significant long-term relief.

PHYSICAL EXAMINATION

The patient's general examination was normal. Neurologic examination was normal, with the exception of unsteady gait and a positive Romberg test; the patient fell backward. Otologic and neurotologic examinations were normal.

LABORATORY TESTING

Videonystagmography: Ocular motor, positional, and caloric tests were normal.
    Rotational testing revealed a mild right directional preponderance but only at the lowest frequency tested, 0.02 Hz.
    Audiometry was normal.
    MRI scan of the brain was normal.

Question 2: Based on the additional information from the physical examination and laboratory tests, what are the likely diagnostic considerations?

Answer 2: The patient's physical examination revealed gait instability and a positive Romberg test. Vestibular laboratory testing confirmed an ongoing vestibular ocular reflex asymmetry but did not provide localizing information. The diagnostic considerations noted above, namely, migraine-related and anxiety-related dizziness, still pertain. Labyrinthine concussion is unlikely given the mild nature of the head trauma and the absence of auditory symptoms. However, none of these diagnoses is definitive, and the patient may have a vestibular system abnormality that cannot be further defined.

DIAGNOSIS/DIFFERENTIAL DIAGNOSIS

The patient was given a diagnosis of vestibular system abnormality of uncertain etiology.

TREATMENT

Question 3: What treatments should be considered for this patient?

Answer 3: This patient has failed several nonconventional therapies. Because a definitive diagnosis cannot be reached, the patient should be treated for a non-specific vestibulopathy (Case 17).

The patient was referred for vestibular rehabilitation therapy and given a prescription for a low-dose clonazepam to be used on an as-needed basis.

FOLLOW-UP

The patient was seen in follow-up 3 months following her initial evaluation. Her symptoms were essentially unchanged, although she noted a slight benefit from clonazepam. The patient requested information regarding complementary and alternative therapies for dizziness other than those that she had already tried.

Question 4: What is a complementary or alternative therapy?

Answer 4: There is no single definition of a complementary or alternative therapy. The National Library of Medicine had previously defined alternative medicine as a nonorthodox therapeutic system that had no satisfactory scientific explanation for its effectiveness. (See The Alternative Medicine HomePage[1]). The Alternative Medicine HomePage states, "Since 1996, the National Library Medicine Medical Subject Headings Term Working Group, Office of Alternative Medicine, National Institutes of Health classifies alternative medicine as an unrelated group of non-orthodox therapeutic practices, often with explanatory systems that do not follow conventional biomedical explanations." The Alternative Medicine HomePage goes on to indicate that "Alternative therapies include, but are not limited to the following disciplines: folk medicine, herbal medicine, diet fads, homeopathy, faith healing, new age healing, chiropractic, acupuncture, naturopathy, massage, and music therapy." According to the National Institutes of Health, "The list of practices that are considered complementary and alternative medicine changes continually, as complementary and alternative medicine practices and therapies that are proven safe and effective become accepted as 'mainstream' health-care practices."[2]

ADDITIONAL FOLLOW-UP

The patient was provided with reading material and website addresses per the National Institutes of Health, National Center for Complementary and Alternative Medicine.[3]

Question 5: What are the categories of complementary and alternative medicine?

Answer 5: The National Institutes of Health recognizes five categories of complementary and alternative medical practices[2]: (*1*) alternative medical systems, (*2*) mind–body interventions, (*3*) biologically based treatments, (*4*) manipulative and body-based methods, and (*5*) energy therapies. Examples include Oriental medicine, Ayurvedic medicine, meditation, hypnosis, herbal therapy, orthomolecular therapy, manipulative therapy, massage therapy, therapeutic touch, and unconventional uses of electromagnetic fields.

Table Case 59–1 Complementary and
Alternative Therapies Advocated for
Patients with Dizziness*

Acupuncture
Acupressure/electroacupressure
Nutritional therapy (vitamins, minerals, trace elements)
Herbal remedies
  Ginger
  Ginko biloba
  Peppermint
  St. John's wort
  Vertigoheel
  Oto-Vite
  T-Bio
Colored lenses
Vision therapy
Aroma therapy
Magnets
Crystals
Massage therapy
Therapeutic touch

*Note that this is a partial list and that the inclusion of any of
the therapies in this table does not indicate the authors' en-
dorsement of the therapy.

Question 6: Which alternative therapies have been suggested for patients with dizziness?

Answer 6: Some of the therapies that had been advocated for patients with dizziness are listed in Table Case 59–1. Despite several studies in the medical literature and reports in lay material, no definitive answers are available regarding the usefulness of any of these treatments for dizziness (see, for example, Weiser et al., 1998.[4]) This is not surprising since once a treatment becomes recognized, it is no longer viewed as complementary or alternative. For example, the particle-repositioning maneuver for benign paroxysmal positional nystagmus was once considered an alternative therapy but is now recognized as standard practice.

Question 7: What are the possible hazards of complementary and alternative therapies for dizziness?

Answer 7: Many complementary and alternative therapies for dizziness are harmless, regardless of their efficacy. However, some of them may be hazardous for unknown reasons. Also, some of these therapies, such as herbal remedies, may interact with conventional therapies in unknown ways. For example, the dosage of herbal remedies may be uncertain, and such remedies may require an alteration in the choice or dosage of conventional medications.

SUMMARY

A 40-year-old woman presented with a complaint of dizziness whose date of onset was uncertain. There was a history of minor head trauma, migraine, reflex sympathetic dystrophy, and strabismus. The patient had tried many nonconventional therapies without significant long-term benefit. Physical examination revealed gait instability and a positive Romberg test. Laboratory testing revealed a mild vestibulo-ocular imbalance.

The patient was given a diagnosis of vestibular system abnormality of uncertain etiology. She was referred for vestibular rehabilitation therapy and given a prescription for a low-dose clonazepam to be used on an as-needed basis. At follow-up, the patient's symptoms were essentially unchanged. She requested information regarding complementary and alternative therapies for dizziness.

TEACHING POINTS

1. **Complementary and alternative medicine is an unrelated group of nonorthodox therapeutic practices, often with explanatory systems that do not follow conventional biomedical explanations.** Complementary and alternative therapies include, but are not limited to, the following disciplines: folk medicine, herbal medicine, homeopathy, faith healing, new age healing, chiropractic, acupuncture, naturopathy, massage, and music therapy. The list of practices that are considered complementary and alternative medicine changes continually as complementary and alternative medicinal practices and therapies that are proven safe and effective become accepted as mainstream health-care practices.
2. **The National Institutes of Health currently recognizes five categories of complementary and alternative medical practices: (1) alternative medical systems, (2) mind–body interventions, (3) biologically based treatments, (4) manipulative and body-based methods, and (5) energy therapies.** Examples include Oriental medicine, Ayurvedic medicine, meditation, hypnosis, herbal therapy, orthomolecular therapy, manipulative therapy, massage therapy, therapeutic touch, and unconventional uses of electromagnetic fields.
3. **Many types of complementary and alternative therapies have been advocated for patients with dizziness.** The usefulness of these treatments for dizziness is uncertain. This is not surprising since once a treatment becomes recognized, it is no longer viewed as complementary or alternative.
4. **Some complementary and alternative therapies may be hazardous or may interact with conventional therapies in unknown ways.**

REFERENCES

1. The Alternative Medicine HomePage: http://www.pitt.edu/~cbw/altm.html, 10.27.01.
2. The Combined Health Information Database: http//child.nih.gov/subfile/contribs/am.html, 10/27/01.
3. National Institutes of Health, National Center for Complementary and Alternative Medicine: http://nccam.nih.gov, 10/27/01.
4. Weiser M, Strosser W, Klein P: Homeopathic vs. conventional treatment of vertigo. A randomized double-blind controlled clinical study. Arch Otolaryngol Head Neck Surg 124:879–885, 1998.

Bibliography

Abel LA, Traccis S, Dell'Osso L, Daroff R, Troost B: Square wave oscillation. Neuro-ophthalmology 4:21–25, 1984.

Abu-Arafeh I, Russell G: Paroxysmal vertigo as a migraine equivalent in children: A population-based study. Cephalalgia 15(1):22–25, 1995.

Alvord LSS, Herr RD: ENG in the emergency room: Subtest results in acutely dizzy patients. J Am Acad Audiol 5:384–389, 1994.

Amarenco P, Hauw J-J: Cerebellar infarction in the territory of the anterior and inferior cerebellar artery. Brain 113:139–155, 1990.

Amarenco P, Rosengart A, DeWitt LD, Pessin MS, Caplan LR: Anterior inferior cerebellar artery territory infarcts. Arch Neurol 50:154–161, 1993.

American Council for Headache Education, Constantine LM, Scott S: Migraine: The Complete Guide. New York: Dell, 1994.

American Psychiatric Association: Diagnostic and Statistical Manual of Mental Disorders, ed 4. Washington, DC: American Psychiatric Association, 1994.

Annex A. Title 67: Transportation, Part I. Department of Transportation, Subpart A. Vehicle Code Provisions, Article IV. Licensing, Chapter 83, Physical and Mental Criteria Including Vision Standards Relating to the Licensing of Drivers, Motor Vehicle Operations, Harrisburg: Pennsylvania Department of Transportation, p 7.

Arenberg IK, Ackley RS, Ferraro J, Muchnik C: EcoG results in perilymphatic fistula: Clinical and experimental studies. Otolaryngol Head Neck Surg 99(5):435–443, 1988.

Ariyasu L, Byl FM, Sprague MS, Adour KK: The beneficial effect of methylprednisolone in acute vestibular vertigo. Arch Otolaryngol Head Neck Surg 116:700–703, 1990.

Ash-Bernal R, Wall C 3rd, Komaroff AL, Bell D, Oas JG, Payman RN, Fagioli LR: Vestibular function test anomalies in patients with chronic fatigue syndrome. Acta Otolaryngol (Stockh) 115(1):9–17, 1995.

Baguley DM, Beynon GJ, Grey PL, Hardy DG, Moffat DA: Audio-vestibular findings in meningioma of the cerebellopontine angle: A retrospective review. J Laryngol and Otol 111:1022–1026, 1997.

Balaban CD, Jacob RG: Background and history of the interface between anxiety and vertigo. J Anxiety Disorders 15:27–51, 2001.

Balaban CD, Thayer JF: Neurological bases for balance-anxiety links. J Anxiety Disorders 15:53–79, 2001.

Baloh RW: Dizziness, Hearing Loss, and Tinnitus: The Essentials of Neurotology. Philadelphia: FA Davis, 1984.

Baloh RW: Dizziness: Neurological emergencies. Neurol Clin North Am 16(2):305–321, 1998.

Baloh RW: Otological aspects of cerebrovascular disease. In: Tool JF (ed). Handbook of Clinical Neurology, Vol 11: Vascular Diseases, Part III. New York: Elsevier, 1989, pp 129–135.

Baloh RW, Henn V, Jager J: Habituation of the human vestibulo-ocular reflex by low frequency harmonic acceleration. Am J Otolaryngol 3:235, 1982.

Baloh RW, Honrubia V: Clinical Neurophysiology of the Vestibular System, ed 2. Philadelphia: FA Davis, 1990.

Baloh RW, Honrubia V: Clinical Neurophysiology of the Vestibular System, ed. 3. New York: Oxford University Press, 1999.

Baloh RW, Honrubia V, Jacobson K: Benign positional vertigo: Clinical and oculographic features in 240 cases. Neurology 37:371–378, 1987.

Baloh RW, Honrubia V, Yee RD, Hess K: Changes in the human vestibulo-ocular reflex after loss of peripheral sensitivity. Ann Neurol 16:222–228, 1984.

Baloh RW, Jacobson K, Honrubia V: Horizontal semicircular canal variant of benign positional vertigo. Neurology 43:2542–2549, 1993.

Baloh RW, Jacobson K, Honrubia V: Idiopathic bilateral vestibulopathy. Neurology 39:272–275, 1989.

Baloh RW, Jacobson KM, Socotch TM: The effect of aging on visual-vestibuloocular responses. Exp Brain Res 95:509–516, 1993.

Baloh RW, Jacobson K, Winder T: Drop attacks with Meniere's syndrome. Ann Neurol 28:384–387, 1990.

Baloh RW, Lopez I, Ishiyama A, Wackym PA, Honrubia V: Vestibular neuritis: Clinical–pathologic correlation. Otolaryngol Head Neck Surg 114:586–592, 1996.

Baloh RW, Spooner JW: Downbeat nystagmus: A type of central vestibular nystagmus. Neurology 31:304–310, 1981.

Baloh RW, Yee RD, Honrubia V: Eye movements in patients with Wallenberg's syndrome. Ann NY Acad Sci 374:600–614, 1981.

Baloh RW, Yue Q, Jacobson KM, Honrubia V: Persistent direction-changing positional nystagmus: Another variant of benign positional nystagmus? Neurology 45:1297–1301, 1995.

Baloh RW, Yue Q, Socotch TM, Jacobson KM: White matter lesions and disequilibrium in older people. I. Case-control comparisons. Arch Neurol 52(10):970–974, 1995.

Bance M, Mai M, Tomlinson D, Rutka J: The changing direction of nystagmus in acute Meniere's disease: Pathophysiological implications. Laryngoscope 101:197–201, 1991.

Barlow D, Freedman W: Cervico-ocular reflex in the normal adult. Acta Otolaryngol 89:487–496, 1980.

Barna GB, Hughes BP: Autoimmunity and otologic disease: Clinical and experimental aspects. Clin Lab Med 8:389, 1988.

Basser L: Benign paroxysmal vertigo of childhood. Brain 87:141–152, 1964.

Bassiouny M, Hirsch BE, Kelly RH, Kamerer DB, Cass SP: Beta 2 transferrin application in otology. Am J Otol 13:552–555, 1992.

Behrman S, Carroll JD, Janota I, Matthews WB: Progressive supranuclear palsy. Brain 92:663–678, 1969.

Belal A, Glorig A: Disequilibrium of ageing (presbyastasis). J Laryngol Otol 100:1037–1041, 1986.

Bergstrom B: Morphology of the vestibular nerve. II. The number of myelinated vestibular nerve fibers in man at various ages. Acta Otolaryngol 76:173–179, 1973.

Bhansali SA: Perilymph fistula. Ear Nose Throat 68:11–26, 1989.

Bickerstaff E: Basilar artery migraine. Lancet 1:15–17, 1961.

Bienhold H, Flohr H: Role of commissural connexions between vestibular nuclei in compensation following unilateral labyrinthectomy. J Physiol 284:178, 1978.

Birnbaum MH, Soden R, Cohen AH: Efficacy of vision therapy for convergence insufficiency in an adult male population. J Am Optometr Assoc 70:225–232, 1999.

Biscaldi GP, Mingardi M, Pollini G, Moglia A, Bossi MC: Acute toluene poisoning. Electroneurophysiological and vestibular investigations. Toxicol Eur Res 3:271–273, 1981.

Black FO, Effron MZ, Burns DS: Diagnosis and management of drop attacks of vestibular origin: Tumarkin's otolithic crisis. Otolaryngol Head Neck Surg 90:256–262, 1982.

Black FO, Sando I, Hildyard VH, Hemenway WG: Bilateral multiple otosclerotic foci and endolymphatic hydrops. Ann Otol Rhinol Laryngol 78:1062–1073, 1969.

Blakely BW, Goebel J: The meaning of the word "vertigo." Otolaryngol Head Neck Surg 125:147–150, 2001.

Bluestone CD: Otitis media and congenital perilymphatic fistula as a cause of sensorineural hearing loss in children. Pediatr Infect Dis J 7:S141–S145, 1988.

Brandt T: Background, technique, interpretation, and usefulness of positional and positioning testing. In: Jacobson GP, Newman CW, Kartush JM (eds). Handbook of Balance Function Testing. St Louis: Mosby Year Book, 1993, pp 123–155.

Brandt T, Daroff R: The multisensory physiological and pathological vertigo syndromes. Ann Neurol 7:195–203, 1980.

Brandt T, Daroff RB: Physical therapy for benign paroxysmal positional vertigo. Arch Otolaryngol 106:484–485, 1980.

Brandt TH, Dieterich M: Vestibular paroxysmia (disabling positional vertigo). Neuro-Opththalmology 14:359–369, 1994.

Breslau N, Davis GC, Andreski P: Migraine psychiatric disorders, and suicide attempts. An epidemiologic study of young adults. Psychiatry Res 37:11–23, 1991.

Breslau N, Schultz LR, Stewart WF, Lipton R, Welch KMA: Headache types and panic disorder: Directionality and specificity. Neurology 56:350–354, 2001.

Britton TC, Thompson PD, van der Kamp W, Thompson PD, van der Kamp W, Rothwell JC, Day BL, Findley LJ, Marsden CD: Primary orthostatic tremor: Further observation in six cases. J Neurol 239:209–217, 1992.

Bronstein AM, Hood JD: The cervico-ocular reflex in normal subjects and patients with absent vestibular function. Brain Res 373:399–408, 1986.

Bronstein AM, Rudge P: Vestibular involvement in spasmodic torticollis. J Neurol Neurosurg Psychiatry 49:290–295, 1996.

Brookhouse PE, Worthington DW, Kelly WJ: Noise-induced hearing loss in children. Laryngoscope 102:645–655, 1992.

Brown DH, McClure JA, Downar-Zapolski Z: The membrane rupture theory of Meniere's disease—is it valid? Laryngoscope 98:599–601, 1988.

Brown JJ, Baloh RW: Persistent mal de debarquement syndrome: A motion-induced subjective disorder of balance. Acta Otolaryngol 8:219–222, 1987.

Brownell B, Oppenheimer DR: An ataxic form of subacute presenile polioencephalopathy (Creutzfeldt-Jakob disease). J Neurol Neurosurg Psychiatry 28:350–361, 1965.

Buttner-Ennever JA (ed): Neuroanatomy of the Oculomotor System. Amsterdam: Elsevier, 1988.

Campbell K, Harker AL, Abbas PJ: Interpretation of electrocochleography in Meniere's disease and normal subjects. Ann Otol Rhinol Laryngol 101:497, 1992.

Cannon SC, Robinson DA: The final common integrator is in the prepositus and vestibular nuclei. In: Keller EL, Zee DS (eds). Adaptive Processes in Visual and Oculomotor Systems. Oxford: Pergamon Press, 1986, pp 307–312.

Caplan L: Top of the basilar syndrome. Neurology 30:72–79, 1980.

Carey JP, Minor LB, Nager GT: Dehiscence or thinning of the bone overlying the superior semicircular canal in a temporal bone study. Arch Otolaryngol Head Neck Surg 126:137–147, 2000.

Carl JR, Optiacan LM, Chu FC, Zee DS: Head shaking and vestibulo-ocular reflex in congenital nystagmus. Invest Ophthalmol Vis Sci 26:1043–1050, 1985.

Casano RA, Johnson DF, Bykhovskaya Y, Torricelli F, Bigozzi M, Fischel-Ghodsian N: Inherited susceptibility to aminoglycoside ototoxicity: Genetic heterogeneity and clinical implications. Am J Otol 20:151, 1999.

Cass SP: Role of medications in otological vertigo and balance disorders. Semin Hearing 12:257–269, 1991.

Cass SP, Borello-France D, Furman JT: Functional outcome of vestibular rehabilitation in patients with abnormal sensory-organization testing. Am J Otol 40(2):248–260, 1997.

Cass SP, Furman JM, Ankerstjerne JKP, Balaban C, Yetiser S, Aydogan B: Migraine-related vestibulopathy. Ann Otol Rhinol Laryngol 106:182–189, 1997.

Causse JR, Uriel J, Berges J, Shambaugh GE Jr, Bretlau P, Causse JB: The enzymatic mechanism of the otospongiotic disease and NaF action on the enzymatic balance. Am J Otol 3:297, 1982.

Cawthorne TE: Vestibular injuries. Proc R Soc Med 39:270–273, 1945.

Cevette MJ, Puetz B, Marion MS, Wertz ML Muenter MD: Aphysiologic performance on dynamic posturography. Otolaryngol Head Neck Surg 112:676–688, 1995.

Chambers BR, Gresty MA: The relationship between disordered pursuit and vestibulo-ocular reflex suppression. J Neurol Neurosurg Psychiatry 46:61–66, 1983.

Coats AC: Vestibular neuronitis. Acta Laryngol (Suppl) 251:5–28, 1969.

Cody DT, Baker HL: Otosclerosis: Vestibular symptoms and sensorineural hearing loss. Ann Otol 87:778–796, 1978.

Cogan DG, Freese CG: Spasm of the near reflex. Arch Ophthalmol 54:752–759, 1955.

Cogan DS: Syndrome of nonsyphilitic interstitial keratitis and vestibuloauditory symptoms. Arch Ophthalmol 33:144, 1945.

Cohen B, Matsuo V, Raphan T: Quantitative analysis of the velocity characteristics of optokinetic nystagmus and optokinetic after-nystagmus. J Physiol 270:321–344, 1977.

Cohen M, Groswasser Z, Barchadski R, Appel A: Convergence insufficiency in brain-injured patients. Brain Injury 3(2):187–191, 1989.

Colletti V, Fiorino FG, Carner M, Turazzi S: Vestibular neurectomy and microvascular decompression of the cochlear nerve in Meniere's disease. Skull Base Surg 4:65–71, 1994.

Collewijn H, Van der Steen J, Ferman L, Jansen TC: Human ocular counterroll: Assessment of static and dynamic properties from electromagnetic scleral coil recordings. Exp Brain Res 59:185–196, 1985.

Collins WE: Arousal and vestibular habituation. In: Kornhuber HH (ed). Vestibular System Part 2: Psychophysics, Applied Aspects and General Interpretations. Berlin: Springer-Verlag, 1974, pp 361–368.

Cooksey FS: Rehabilitation in vestibular injuries. Proc R Soc Med 39:275, 1945.

Corbett JJ, Jacobson DM, Thompson HS, Hart MN, Albert DW: Downbeating nystagmus and other ocular motor defects caused by lithium toxicity. Neurology 39(4):481–487, 1989.

Crampton GH (ed): Motion and Space Sickness. Boca Raton: CRC Press, 1990.

Cutrer FW, Baloh RW: Migraine-associated dizziness. Headache 32:300–304, 1992.

Dandy WE: Meniere's disease: Its diagnosis and methods of treatment. Arch Surg 16:1127, 1928.

Daum KM: Characteristics of convergence insufficiency. Am J Optom Physiol Optics 65(6):426–438, 1988.

Davidoff RA: Migraine: Manifestations, Pathogenesis, and Management. Philadelphia: FA Davis, 1995.

De Jong PTV, Vianney de Jong JMB, Cohen B, Jongkees BW: Ataxia and nystagmus induced by injection of local anesthetics in the neck. Ann Neurol 1:240–246, 1977.

De la Meilleure G, Dehaene I, Depondt M, Damman W, Crevits L, Vanhooren G: Benign paroxysmal positional vertigo of the horizontal canal. J Neurol Neurosurg Psychiatry 60:68–71, 1996.

Demer JL, Zee DS: Vestibulo-ocular and optokinetic deficits in albinos with congenital nystagmus. Invest Ophthalmol Vis Sci 25:739–745, 1984.

Dickins JRE, Smith JT, Graham SS: Herpes zoster oticus: Treatment with intravenous acyclovir. Laryngoscope 98:776–779, 1988.

Digre KB: Opsoclonus in adults. Arch Neurol 43:1165–1175, 1986.

Dimitri PS, Wall C, Oas JG, Rauch SD: Application of multivariate statistics to vestibular testing: Discriminating between Meniere's disease and migraine associated dizziness. J Vestib Res 11(1):53–65, 2001.

Dix MR, Hallpike CS: The pathology, symptomotology and diagnosis of certain common disorders of the vestibular system. Proc R Soc Med 45:341–354, 1952.

Dix MR, Hood JD: Vestibular habituation: Its clinical significance and relationship to vestibular neuronitis. Laryngoscope 80:226–232, 1970.

Drachman DA, Diamond ER, Hart CW: Posturally-evoked vomiting: Association with posterior fossa lesions. Ann Otol 86:97–101, 1977.

Drachman DA, Hart CW: An approach to the dizzy patient. Neurology 22:323–334, 1972.

Duncan P, Weiner DK, Chandler J, Studenski S: Functional reach: A new clinical measure of balance. J Gerontol 45:192–197, 1990.

Dunniway HM, Welling DB: Intracranial tumors mimicking benign paroxysmal positional vertigo. Otolaryngol Head Neck Surg 118:429–436, 1998.

Emmett JR, Shea JJ: Traumatic perilymph fistula. Laryngoscope 90:1513–1520, 1980.

Engstrom H, Ades HW, Engstrom B, Gilchrest D, Bourne G: Structural changes in the vestibular epithelia in elderly monkeys and humans. Adv Otorhinolaryngol 22:93–110, 1977.

Epley JM: The canalith repositioning procedure: For treatment of benign paroxysmal positional vertigo. Otolaryngol Head Neck Surg 107:399–404, 1992.

Estol C, Caplan LR, Pressin MS: Isolated vertigo: An uncommon manifestation of vertebrobasilar ischaemia. Cerebrovasc Dis 6(Suppl 2):161, 1996.

Eviatar L: Vestibular testing in basilar artery migraine. Ann Neurol 9:126–130, 1980.

Evidente VG, Adler CH, Caviness JN, Gwinn KA: Effective treatment of orthostatic tremor with gabapentin. Movement Disorders 13(5):829–831, 1998.

Ferbert A, Bruckmann H, Drummen R: Clinical features of proven basilar artery occlusion. Stroke 21(8):1135–1142, 1990.

Ferraro JA, Arenberg K, Hassanein S: Electrocochleography and symptoms of inner ear dysfunction. Arch Otolaryngol 111:71–74, 1985.

Fetter M, Dichgans J: Vestibular neuritis spares the inferior division of the vestibular nerve. Brain 119:755–763, 1996.

Fisher CM: Vertigo in cerebrovascular disease. Arch Otolaryngol 85:529–534, 1967.

Fitz-Ritson D: Assessment of cervicogenic vertigo. J Manipulative Physiol Ther 14(3):193–198, 1991.

Fitzgerald DC: Head trauma: Hearing loss and dizziness. J Trauma 40(3):488–496, 1996.

Flohr H, Luneburg U: Effects of ACTH on vestibular compensation. Brain Res 248:169–173, 1982.

Fluur E: A comparison between subjective and objective recording of ocular counterrolling as a result of tilting. Acta Otolaryngol 79:111–114, 1975.

Fukuda T: The stepping test. Acta Otolaryngol 50:95–108, 1959.

Fukuda K, Straus SE, Hickie I, Sharpe MC, Dobbins JG, Komaroff A: The chronic fatigue syndrome: A comprehensive approach to its definition and study. International Chronic Fatigue Syndrome Study Group. Ann Intern Med 121:953, 1994.

Furman JM: Nystagmus and the vestibular system. In: Podos SM, Yanoff M (eds). Textbook of Ophthalmology. New York: Gower Medical, 1993, pp 9.1–9.7.

Furman JM: Testing of vestibular function: An adjunct in the assessment of chronic fatigue syndrome. Rev Infect Dis 13(Suppl 1):S109–S111, 1991.

Furman JM, Balaban CD, Pollack IF: Vestibular compensation following cerebellar infarction. Neurology 48:916–920, 1997.

Furman JM, Becker JT: Vestibular responses in Wernicke's encephalopathy. Ann Neurol 26:669–674, 1989.

Furman JM, Cass SP: Laboratory testing. I. Electronystagmography and rotational testing. In: Baloh RW, Halmagyi M (eds). Disorders of the Vestibular System. New York: Oxford University Press, 1996, pp 191–210.

Furman JM, Cass SP: Benign paroxysmal positional vertigo. N Engl J Med 341.1590–1596, 1999.

Furman JM, Crumrine PK, Reinmuth OM: Epileptic nystagmus. Ann Neurol 27:686–688, 1990.

Furman JM, Durrant JD, Hirsch WL: Eighth nerve signs in a case of multiple sclerosis. Am J Otolaryngol 10:376–381, 1989.

Furman JM, Eidelman BH, Fromm GH: Spontaneous remission of paraneoplastic saccadic fixation instability. Neurology 38:499–501, 1988.

Furman JF, Jacob RG: A clinical taxonomy of dizziness and anxiety in the otoneurological setting. J Anxiety Disorders 15.9–26, 2001.

Furman JM, Jacob RG: Psychiatric dizziness. Neurology 48:1161–1166, 1997.

Furman JM, Kamerer DB: Rotational responses in patients with bilateral caloric reduction. Acta Otolaryngol (Stockh) 108.355–361, 1989.

Furman JF, Redfern MS: Effect of aging on the otolith-ocular reflex. J Vestib Res 11(2):91–103, 2001.

Gacek RR: Singular neurectomy update II: Review of 102 cases. Laryngoscope 101:855–862, 1991.

Gacek RR: Transection of the posterior ampullary nerve for relief of benign paroxysmal positional vertigo. Ann Otol Rhinol Laryngol 83:596–605, 1974.

Gacek RR, Gacek MR: Vestibular neuronitis. Am J Otol 20:553–554, 1999.

Ghez C: Vestibular paresis: A clinical feature of Wernicke's disease. J Neurol Neurosurg Psychiatry 32:132–139, 1969.

Gianoli G, McWilliams S, Soileau J, Belafsky P: Posturographic performance in patients with the potential for secondary gain. Otolaryngol Head Neck Surg 122:11–18, 2000.

Gilman S, Bloedel JR, Lechtenberg R (eds): Disorders of the Cerebellum. Contemporary Neurology Series. Philadelphia: FA Davis, 1981.

Gimse R, Bjorgen IA, Straume A: Driving skills after whiplash. Scand J Psychology 38:165–170, 1997.

Glasscock ME, Cueva RA, Thedinger BA: Handbook of Vertigo. New York: Raven Press, 1990.

Glasscock ME, McKennan KX, Levine SC: Persistent traumatic perilymph fistules. Laryngoscope 97:860–864, 1987.

Goebel JA, Sataloff RT, Hanson JM, Nashner LM, Hirshout DS, Sokolow CC: Posturographic evidence of nonorganic sway patterns in normal subjects, patients, and suspected malingers. Otolaryngol Head Neck Surg 117:293–302, 1997.

Goldstein JH, Schneekloth BB: Spasm of the near reflex: A spectrum of anomalies. Surv Ophthalmol 40:269–278, 1996.

Gomez CR, Cruz-Flores S, Malkoff MD, Sauer CM, Burch CM: Isolated vertigo as a manifestation of vertebrobasilar ischemia. Neurology 47(1):94–97, 1996.

Gomori AJ, Partnow MJ, Horoupian DS: The ataxic form of Creutzfeldt-Jakob disease. Arch Neurol 29:318–323, 1973.

Gorman WF: Defining malingering. J Forensic Sci 27:401–407, 1982.

Gracia F, Koch J, Aziz N: Downbeat nystagmus as a side effect of lithium carbonate: Case report. J Clin Psychiatry 46:292–293, 1985.

Grad A, Baloh RW: Vertigo of vascular origin. Arch Neurol 46:281–284, 1989.

Grenman R: Involvement of the audiovestibular system in multiple sclerosis. An otoneurologic and audiologic study. Acta Otolaryngol 420(Suppl):1–95, 1985.

Gresty MA, Barratt HJ, Page NG, Ell JJ: Assessment of vestibulo-ocular reflexes in congenital nystagmus. Ann Neurol 17:129–136, 1985.

Griffin JF, Wray SH, Anderson DP: Misdiagnosis of spasm of the near reflex. Neurology 26:1018–1020, 1976.

Griffith AJ: Biological and clinical aspects of autoimmune inner ear disease. Yale J Biol Med 65:17–28, 1992.

Gross EM, Bradford BD, Viirre ES, Nelson JR, Harris JP: Intractable benign paroxysmal positional vertigo in patients with Meniere's disease. Laryngoscope 110:655–659, 2000.

Gyntelberg F, Vesterhauge S, Fog P, Isager H, Zillstorff K: Acquired intolerance to organic solvents and results of vestibular testing. Am J Ind Med 9:363–370, 1986.

Hain TC, Fetter M, Zee DS: Head-shaking nystagmus in patients with unilateral peripheral vestibular lesions. Am J Otolaryngol 8:36–47, 1987.

Hain TC, Helminski JO, Reis IL, Uddin MK: Vibration does not improve results of the canalith repositioning procedure. Arch Otolaryngol Head Neck Surg 126:617–622, 2000.

Hall SF, Ruby RRF, McClure JA: The mechanics of benign paroxysmal vertigo. J Otolaryngol 8:151–158, 1979.

Halmagyi GM, Brandt T, Dieterich M, Curthoys IS, Stark RJ, Hoyt WF: Tonic controversive ocular tilt reaction due to unilateral mesodiencephalic lesion. Neurology 40:1503–1509, 1990.

Halmagyi GM, Curthoys I: A clinical sign of canal paresis. Arch Neurol 45:737–739, 1988.

Halmagyi GM, Lessell I, Curthoys IS, Lessell S, Hoyt WF: Lithium-induced downbeat nystagmus. Am J Ophthalmol 107:664–670, 1989.

Hamid M, Hughes G, Kinney S: Criteria for diagnosing bilateral vestibular dysfunction. In: Graham MD, Kemink JL (eds). The Vestibular System: Neurophysiologic and Clinical Research. New York: Raven Press, 1987, pp 115–118.

Harada Y (ed): The Vestibular Organs. Amsterdam: Kugler & Guedini, 1988.

Harbert F: Benign paroxysmal positional nystagmus. Arch Ophthal 84:298–302, 1970.

Harris JP: Immunologic mechanisms in disorders of the inner ear. Otolaryngol Head Neck Surg, Update 1 380–395, 1989.

Hart C, McKinley P, Peterson B: Compensation following acute unilateral total loss of peripheral vestibular function. In: Graham M, Kemink J (eds). The Vestibular System: Neurophysiologic and Clinical Research. New York: Raven Press, 1987, pp 187–192.

Heilman KM: Orthostatic tremor. Arch Neurol 41:880–881, 1984.

Herdman SJ (ed): Vestibular Rehabilitation, ed 2. Philadelphia: FA Davis, 2000.

Herr RD, Zun L, Matthews JJ: A directed approach to the dizzy patient. Ann Emerg Med 18(6):664/101–672/109, 1989.

Hillel AD: History of stapedectomy. Am J Otolaryngol 4:131–140, 1983.

Hirsch BE, Cass SP, Sekhar LN, Wright DC: Translabyrinthine approach to skull base tumors with hearing preservation. Am J Otol 14(6):533–543, 1993.

Hirsch BE, Durrant JD, Yetiser S, Kamerer DB, Martin WH: Localizing retrocochlear hearing loss. Am J Otol 17(4):537–546, 1996.

Hirsch BE, Weissman JL, Curtin HD, Kamerer DB: Magnetic resonance imaging of large vestibular aqueduct. Arch Otolaryngol Head Neck Surg 118:1124–1127, 1992.

Hirvonen TP, Carey JP, Liang CJ, Minor LB. Superior canal dehiscence. Mechanisms of pressure sensitivity in a chinchilla model. Arch Otolaryngol Head Neck Surg 127:1331–1336, 2001.

Hockaday JM (ed): Migraine in Childhood. London: Butterworths, 1988.

Hodgson MJ, Furman J, Ryan C, Durrant J, Kern E: Encephalopathy and vestibulopathy following short-term hydrocarbon exposure. J Occup Med 31:51–54, 1989.

Hoffman HJ, Ko C, Sklare DA: How is the frequency of driving an automobile affected by chronic (3+ months) problems with imbalance and/or dizziness? Presented at the American Public health Association national meeting, October 2001.

Hotson JR, Baloh RW: Acute vestibular syndrome. N Engl J Med 339:680–685, 1998.

House JW, Brackmann DE: Facial nerve grading system. Otolaryngol Head Neck Surg 93:146–147, 1985.

Hughes CA, Proctor L: Benign paroxysmal positional vertigo. Laryngoscope 107:607–613, 1997.

Hughes GB, Barna BP, Kinney SE, Calabrese LH, Nalepa NL: Predictive value of laboratory tests in "autoimmune" inner ear disease: Preliminary report. Laryngoscope 96:502–505, 1986.

Hughes GB, Sismanis A, House JW: Is there consensus in perilymph fistula management? Otolaryngol Head Neck Surg 102:111, 1990.

Hunt JR: Herpetic inflammations of the geniculate ganglion: A new syndrome and its aural complications. Arch Otol 36:371–381, 1907.

Huygen PLM, Verhagen WIM, Nicolasen MGM: Cervico-ocular reflex enhancement in labyrinthine-defective and normal subjects. Exp Brain Res 87:457–464, 1991.

Hyden D, Larsby B, Andersson H, Odkvist LM, Liedgren SR, Tham R: Impairment of visuo-vestibular interaction in humans. ORL J Otorhinolaryngol Relat Spec 45:262–269, 1983.

Igarashi M: Physical exercise and acceleration of vestibular compensation. In: Lacour M, Toupet M, Denise P, Christen Y (eds). Vestibular Compensation. Amsterdam: Elsevier, 1989, pp 131–144.

Ishiyama A, Ishiyama GP, Lopez I, Eversole LR, Honrubia V, Baloh RW: Histopathology of idiopathic chronic recurrent vertigo. Laryngoscope 106:1340–1346, 1996.

Ito M (ed): The Cerebellum and Neural Control. New York: Raven Press, 1984.

Jackler RK, De La Cruz A: The large vestibular aqueduct syndrome. Laryngoscope 99:1238–1243, 1989.

Jackler RK, Dillon WP: Computed tomography and magnetic resonance imaging of the inner ear. Otolaryngol Head Neck Surg 99:494–504, 1988.

Jackson CG, Glasscock ME, Davis WE: Medical management of Meniere's disease. Ann Otol 90:142–147, 1981.

Jacob RG, Furman JM, Balaban CD: Psychiatric aspects of vestibular disorders. In: Baloh RW, Halmagyi M (eds). Disorders of the Vestibular System. New York: Oxford University Press, 1996, pp 509–528.

Jacob RG, Furman JM, Durrant JD, Turner SM: Panic, agoraphobia, and vestibular dysfunction. Am J Psychiatry 153:503–512, 1996.

Jacob RG, Whitney SL, Detweiler-Shostak G, Furman JM: Vestibular rehabilitation for patients with agoraphobia and vestibular dysfunction: A pilot study. J Anxiety Disorders 15(1–2):131–146, 2000.

Jacob RG, Woody SR, Clark DB, Lilienfeld SO, Hirsch BE, Kucera GD, Furman JM, Durrant JD: Discomfort with space and motion: A possible marker of vestibular dysfunction assessed by the Situational Characteristics Questionnaire. J Psychopathol Behav Assess 15:299–324, 1993.

Jacobson GP, Newman CW: The development of the Dizziness Handicap Inventory. Arch Otolaryngol Head Neck Surg 116:424–427, 1990.

Jacobson GP, Newman CW: Handbook of Balance Function Testing. St. Louis: Mosby Year Book, 1993.

Jannetta PJ, Moller MB, Moller AR: Disabling positional vertigo. N Engl J Med 310:1700–1705, 1984.

"JC": Living without a balancing mechanism. N Engl J Med 246:458–460, 1952.

Jellinger K, Heiss WD, Deisenhammer E: The ataxic (cerebellar) form of Creutzfeldt-Jakob disease. J Neurol 207:289, 1974.

Jenkins HA, Furman JM, Gulya AJ, Honrubia V, Linthicum FH, Mirka A: Disequilibrium of aging. Otolaryngol Head Neck Surg 100:272–282, 1989.

Johnson G: Medical management of migraine-related dizziness and vertigo. Laryngoscope 108(1 pt 2):1–28, 1998.

Jongkees LBW: Cervical vertigo. Laryngoscope 79:1473–1484, 1969.

Kamei T, Kornhuber H: Spontaneous and head-shaking nystagmus in normals and in patients with central lesions. Can J Otolaryngol 3:372–380, 1974.

Kasai T, Zee DS: Eye–head coordination in labyrinthine-defective human beings. Brain Res 144:123–141, 1978.

Kasser SL, Rose DJ, Clark S: Balance training for adults with multiple sclerosis: Multiple case studies. Neurol Rep 23(1):5–12, 1999.

Katz J (ed): Handbook of Clinical Audiology. Baltimore: Williams & Wilkins, 1994.

Kayan A, Hood JD: Neuro-otological manifestations of migraine. Brain 107:1123–1142, 1984.

Kelly JP: Vestibular system. In: Kandel ER, Schwartz JH, Jessell TM (eds). Principles of Neural Science, ed 3. Norwalk, CT: Appleton & Lange, 1991, pp 584–596.

Kemink JL, Telian SA, Graham MD, Joynt L: Transmatoid labyrinthectomy: Reliable surgical management of vertigo. Otolaryngol Head Neck Surg 101:5–10, 1989.

Kluge M, Beyenburg S, Fernandez G, Elger CE: Epileptic vertigo: Evidence for vestibular representation in human frontal cortex. Neurology 55(12):1906–1908, 2000.

Kogeorgos J, Scott DF, Swash M: Epileptic dizziness. Br Med J 282:687–689, 1981.

Komaroff AL: Clinical presentation of chronic fatigue syndrome. In: Bock GR, Whelan J (eds). Chronic Fatigue Syndrome. New York: Wiley, 1993, pp 43–61.

Konrad HR: Intractable vertigo—When not to operate. Otolaryngol Head Neck Surg 95:482–484, 1986.

Korzec K, Sobol SM, Kubal W, Mester SJ, Winzelberg G, May M: Gadolinium-enhanced magnetic resonance imaging of the facial nerve in herpes zoster oticus and Bell's palsy: Clinical implication. Am J Otol 12:163–168, 1991.

Krejcova H, Bojar M, Jerabek J, Thomas J, Jirous J: Otoneurological symptomatology in Lyme disease. Adv Otorhinolaryngol 42:210–212, 1988.

Krempl GA, Dobie RA: Evaluation of posturography in the detection of malingering subjects. Am J Otol 19:619–627, 1998.

Kubala MJ, Millikan CH: Diagnosis, pathogenesis, and treatment of "drop attacks." Arch Neurol 11:107–113, 1964.

Lacour M, Toupet M, Denise P, Christen Y (eds): Vestibular Compensation: Facts, Theories and Clinical Perspectives. Proceedings of the International Symposium. Paris: Elsevier, 1988.

Lafarga M, Berciano MT, Suarez I, Viadero CF, Andres MA, Berciano J: Cytology and organization of reactive astroglia in human cerebellar cortex with severe loss of granule cells: A study of the ataxic form of Creutzfeldt-Jakob disease. Neuroscience 40:337–352, 1991.

Langman AW, Kemink JL, Graham MD: Titration streptomycin therapy for bilateral Meniere's disease. Ann Otol Rhinol Laryngol 99:923–926, 1990.

Lanzi G, Balottin U, Fazzi E, Tagliasacchi M, Manfrin M, Mira E: Benign paroxysmal vertigo of childhood: A long follow-up. Cephalalgia 14:458–460, 1994.

Lawrence M: Possible influence of cochlear otosclerosis on inner ear fluids. Ann Otol Rhinol Laryngol 75:553–558, 1966.

Leigh RJ, Zee DS (eds): The Neurology of Eye Movements, ed 3: New York: Oxford University Press, 1999.

LeLiever WC: Comparative repositioning maneuvers for benign paroxysmal positional vertigo. Proceedings of the Combined Otolaryngologic Spring Meeting, Palm Beach, FL; May 7–13, 1994.

LeLiever WC, Barber HO: Recurrent vestibulopathy. Laryngoscope 91:1–6, 1981.

Lempert T: Horizontal benign positional vertigo. Neurology 44:2213–2214, 1994.

Lempert T, Tiel-Wilck T: A positional maneuver for treatment of horizontal-canal benign positional vertigo. Laryngoscope 106:476–478, 1996.

Lepore FE: Disorders of ocular motility following head trauma. Arch Neurol 52:924–926, 1995.

Levenson MJ, Parisier SC, Jacobs M, Edelstein DR: The large vestibular aqueduct syndrome in children. Arch Otolaryngol Head Neck Surg 115:54–58, 1989.

Lilienfeld SO: Vestibular dysfunction followed by panic disorder with agoraphobia. J Nerv Ment Dis 177:700–701, 1989.

Lin J, Elidan J, Baloh RW, Honruba V: Direction-changing positional nystagmus: Incidence and meaning. Am J Otolaryngol 7:306–310, 1986.

Lobel E, Kleine J, Le Bihan D, Leroy-Willig A, Berthoz A: Functional MRI of galvanic vestibular stimulation. J Neurophysiol 80:2699–2709, 1998.

Longridge NS, Mallinson AI: A discussion of the dynamic illegible "E" test: A new method of screening for aminoglycoside vestibulotoxicity. Otolaryngol Head Neck Surg 92(6):671–677, 1984.

Luetje CM: Theoretical and practical implications for plasmapheresis in autoimmune inner ear disease. Laryngoscope 99:1137–1146, 1989.

Lundborg T: Diagnostic problems concerning acoustic tumors. Acta Otolaryngol (Suppl) 99:1–111, 1950.

Lunsford LD, Linskey ME, Flickinger JC: Stereotactic radiosurgery for acoustic nerve sheath tumors. In: Tos M, Thompson J (eds): Proceedings of the First International Conference on Acoustic Neuroma. Amsterdam: Kugler, 1992, 279–287.

Mackenzie M, Wolfenden N: Otosclerosis. J Laryngol Otol 69:437–456, 1955.

Manolidis LS, Balojannis SJ: Ultrastructural alterations of the vestibular nuclei in Jacob-Creutzfeld disease. Acta Otolaryngol 95:508–521, 1983.

Massoud EAS, Ireland DJ: Post-treatment instructions in the nonsurgical management of benign paroxysmal positional vertigo. J Otolaryngol 25:121–125, 1996.

McAlpine D: Symptoms and signs, brain-stem multiple sclerosis. In McAlpine D, Lumsden CE, Acheson ED (eds). Multiple Sclerosis: A Reappraisal. London: Churchill Livingstone, 1972, pp 164–196.

McCabe BF: Autoimmune inner ear disease: Therapy. Am J Otolaryngol 10:196–197, 1989.

McCabe BF: Otosclerosis and vertigo. Trans Pacific Coast Oto-Ophthalmol Soc annual meeting 47:37–42, 1966.

McClure JA: Horizontal canal BPV. J Otolaryngol 14:30–35, 1985.

McClure JA, Copp JC, Lycett P: Recovery nystagmus in Meniere's disease. Laryngoscope 91:1727–1737, 1981.

Mckiernan D, Jonathan D: Driving and vertigo. Clin Otolaryngol Allied Sci 26(1):1–3, 2001.

Meissner I, Wiebers DO, Swanson JW, O'Fallon WM: The natural history of drop attacks Neurology 36:1029–1034, 1986.

Melvill Jones G: Adaptive modulation of VOR parameters by vision. In: Berthoz A, Melvill Jones G (eds). Adaptive Mechanisms in Gaze Control: Reviews in Oculomotor Research. Amsterdam: Elsevier, 1985, pp 21–50.

Melvill Jones G, Berthoz A: Mental control of the adaptive process. In: Berthoz A, Melvill Jones G (eds). Adaptive Mechanisms in Gaze Control. Amsterdam: Elsevier, 1985, pp 203–212.

Merikangas KR, Angst J, Isler H: Migraine and psychopathology: Results of the Zurich cohort study of young adults. Arch Gen Psychiatry 47:849–853, 1990.

Merikanges KR, Stevens DE: Comorbidity of migraine and psychiatric disorders. Adv Headache 15(1):115–123, 1997.

Meyerhoff WL, Cass S, Schwaber MK, Sculerati N, Slattery WH: Progressive sensorineural hearing loss in children. Otolaryngol Head Neck Surg 110:569–579, 1994.

Meyerhoff WL, Kim CS, Paparella MM: Pathology of chronic otitis media. Ann Otol 87:749–760, 1978.

Meyerhoff WL, Paperella MM, Shea D: Meniere's disease in children. Laryngoscope 88:1504–1511, 1978.

Minor LB, Haslwanter T, Straumann D, Zee DS: Hyperventilation-induced nystagmus in patients with vestibular schwannoma. Neurology 53(9):2158–2168, 1999.

Minor LB, Solomon D, Zinreich J, Zee DS. Sound- and/or pressure-induced vertigo due to bone dehiscence of the superior semicircular canal. Arch Otolaryngol Head Neck Surg 124(3):249–258, 1998.

Moller AR: Audiotory neurophysiology. J Clin Neurophysiol 11(3):284–308, 1994.

Moller AR, Janetta PJ: Neural generators of the brainstem auditory evoked potentials. In: Nodar RH, Barber C (eds). Evoked Potentials II: The Second International Evoked Potentials Symposia. Boston: Butterworth, 1984, pp 137–144.

Moller MB, Moller AR, Jannetta PJ, Jho HD, Sekhar LN: Microvascular decompression of the eighth nerve in patients with disabling positional vertigo: Selection criteria and operative results in 207 patients. Acta Neurochir (Wien) 125:75–82, 1993.

Monday LA, Tetrault L: Hyperventilation and vertigo. Laryngoscope 109:1003–1010, 1988.

Money K, Johnson W, Corlett R: Role of semicircular canals in positional alcohol nystagmus. Am J Physiol 208:1065–1070, 1965.

Monsell EM, Brackmann DE, Linthicum FH: Why do vestibular destructive procedures sometimes fail? Otolaryngol Head Neck Surg 99:472–479, 1988.

Monsell EM, Cass SP, Rybak LP: Chemical labyrinthectomy: Methods and results. In: Brackmann DE (ed). Otologic Surgery. Philadelphia: WB Saunders, 1994, pp 509–518.

Monsell EM, Wiet RJ: Endolymphatic sac surgery: Methods of study and results. Am J Otol 9:396–402, 1988.

Monsell EM, Wiet JR, Young NM, Kazan RP: Surgical treatment of vertigo with retrolabyrinthine vestibular neurectomy. Laryngoscope 98:835–839, 1988.

Moore BE, Atkinson M: Psychogenic vertigo. Arch Otolaryngol 67:347–353, 1958.

Morales-Garcia C: Cochleo-vestibular involvement in otosclerosis. Acta Otolaryngol 73:484–492, 1972.

Moscatello AL, Worden DL, Nadelman RB, Wormser G, Lucente F: Otolaryngologic aspects of Lyme disease. Laryngoscope 101:592–595, 1991.

Moscicki RA, San Martin JE, Quintero CH, Rauch SD, Nadol JB Jr, Bloch KJ: Serum antibody to inner ear proteins in patients with progressive hearing loss. JAMA 272:611–616, 1994.

Moser M: An objective testing method to determine driving ability. Acta Otolaryngol (Stockh) 99:326–329, 1985.

Mossman S, Halmagyi GM: Partial ocular tilt reaction due to unilateral cerebellar lesion. Neurology 49(2):491–493, 1997.

Murakami S, Hato N, Horiuchi J, Honda N, Gyo K, Yanagihara N: Treatment of Ramsay Hunt syndrome with acyclovir-prednisone: Significance of early diagnosis and treatment. Ann Neurol 41(3):353–357, 1997.

Murphy TP: Mal de debarquement syndrome: A forgotten entity? Otolaryngol Head Neck Surg 109:10–13, 1993.

Nadol JB: Positive "fistula sign" with an intact tympanic membrane. Arch Otolaryngol 100:273–278, 1974.

Nakada T, Kwee I: Oculopalatal myoclonus. Brain 109:431–441, 1986.

National Institutes of Health, National Center for Complementary and Alternative Medicine: http://nccam.nih.gov Frequently Asked Questions, 10/27/01.

Nedzelski JM: Cerebellopontine angle tumors: Bilateral flocculus compression as cause of associated oculomotor abnormalities. Laryngoscope 93:1251–1260, 1983.

Nedzelski JM, Barber HO, McIlmoyl L: Diagnoses in a dizziness unit. J Otolaryngol 15(2):101–104, 1986.

Neuhauser H, Leopold M, von Brevern M, Arnold G, Lempert T: The interrelations of migraine, vertigo, and migrainous vertigo. Neurology 56(4):436–441, 2001.

Neuhuber WL, Zenker W: Central distribution of cervical primary afferents in the rat, with emphasis on proprioceptive projects to vestibular, perihypoglossal, and upper thoracic spinal nuclei. J Comp Neurol 280:231–253, 1989.

Nielsen JM: Tornado epilepsy simulating Meniere's syndrome. Neurology 9:794–796, 1959.

Niklasson M, Tham R, Larsby B, Eriksson B: Effects of toluene, styrene, trichloroethylene, and trichloromethane on the vestibulo- and opto-oculo motor system in rats. Neurotoxicol Teratol 15:327–334, 1993.

Nirankari VS, Hameroff SB: Spasm of the near reflex. Ann Ophthalmol 12:1050–1051, 1980.

Nunez RA, Cass SP, Furman JM: Short- and long-term outcomes of canalith repositioning for benign paroxysmal positional vertigo. Otolaryngol Head Neck Surg 122(5):647–653, 2000.

Nuti D, Agus G, Barbieri MT, Passali D: The management of horizontal-canal paroxysmal positional vertigo. Acta Otolaryngol (Stockh) 118(4):455–460, 1998.

Nuti D, Nati C, Passali D: Treatment of benign paroxysmal positional vertigo: No need for postmaneuver restrictions. Otolaryngol Head Neck Surg 122:440–444, 2000.

Oas JG, Baloh RW: Vertigo and the anterior inferior cerebellar artery syndrome. Neurology 42:2274–2279, 1992.

Odkvist LM, Larsby B, Fredrickson MF, Liedgren SR, Tham R: Vestibular and oculomotor disturbances caused by industrial solvents. J Otolaryngol 9:53–59, 1980.

Odkvist LM, Larsby B, Tham R, Ahlfeldt H, Andersson B, Eriksson B, Liedgren SR: Vestibulo-oculomotor disturbances in humans exposed to styrene. Acta Otolaryngol 94:487–493, 1982.

Odkvist LM, Moller C, Thuomas K-A: Otoneurologic disturbances caused by solvent pollution. Otolaryngol Head Neck Surg 106:687, 1992.

Olsson JE: Neurotologic findings in basilar migraine. Laryngoscope 101 (Suppl 52):1–41, 1991.

Onofrj M, Thomas A, Paci CF, D'Andreamatteo G: Gabapentin in orthostatic tremor: Results of a double-blind cross over with placebo in four patients. Neurology 51:880–882, 1998.

Oosterveld WJ, Kortschot HW, Kingma GG, de Jong HA, Saatci MR: Electronystagmographic findings following cervical whiplash injuries. Acta Otolaryngol (Stockh) 111:201–205, 1991.

Opal P, Zoghbi HY: The spinocerebellar ataxias. Up to Date Online 9.3, November 15, 2001.

Pagnini P, Nuti D, Vannucchi P: Benign paroxysmal vertigo of the horizontal canal. ORL J Otorhinolaryngol Relat Spec 51:161–170, 1989.

Paige GD: Senescence of human visual–vestibular interactions. J Vestib Res 2:133–151, 1992.

Paparella MM: The cause (multifactorial inheritance) and pathogenesis (endolymphatic malabsorption) of Meniere's disease and its symptoms (mechanical and chemical). Acta Otolaryngol (Stockh) 99:445–451, 1985.

Paparella MM, Chasen WD: Otosclerosis and vertigo. J Laryngol Otol 80:511–517, 1966.

Paparella MM, Mancini F, Liston SL: Otosclerosis and Meniere's syndrome: Diagnosis and treatment. Laryngoscope 94:1414–1417, 1984.

Paparella MM, Morizono T, Le CT, Mancini F, Sipila P, Choo YB, Liden G, Kim CS: Sensorineural hearing loss in otitis media. Ann Otol Rhinol Laryngol 93:623–629, 1984.

Paparella M, Sugiura S: The pathology of suppurative labyrinthitis. Ann Otol Rhinol Laryngol 76:554–586, 1967.

Parisier SC, Birken EA: Recurrent meningitis secondary to idiopathic oval window CSF leak. Laryngoscope 86:1503–1515, 1976.

Parnes LS, McClure JA: Free-floating endolymph particles: A new operative finding during posterior semicircular canal occlusion. Laryngoscope 102:988–992, 1992.

Parnes LS, McClure JA: Posterior semicircular canal occlusion for intractable benign paroxysmal positional vertigo. Ann Otol Rhinol Laryngol 99:330–334, 1990.

Parnes LS, McClure JA: Posterior semicircular canal occlusion in the normal hearing ear. Otolaryngol Head Neck Surg 104:52–57, 1991.

Parnes LS, Price-Jones R: Particle repositioning maneuver for benign paroxysmal positional vertigo. Ann Otol Rhinol Laryngol 102:325–331, 1993.

Peitersen E: Vestibulospinal reflexes. Arch Otolaryngol 79:481–486, 1976.

Peppard SB: Effect of drug therapy on compensation from vestibular injury. Laryngoscope 96:878–898, 1986.

Peterka R, Black F: Age-related changes in human posture control: Sensory organization tests. J Vestib Res 1:73–85, 1990.

Peterka R, Black F, Schoenhoff M: Age-related changes in human vestibulo-ocular reflexes: Sinusoidal rotation and caloric tests. J Vestib Res 1:49–59, 1990.

Platzer W (ed): PERNKOPF, Atlas der topographischen und angewandten Anatomie des Menschen, ed 3. Mauunchen, Wien, and Baltimore: Urban & Schwarzenberg, 1989.

Prusiner SB: Prions and neurodegenerative diseases. N Engl J Med 317:1571–1581, 1987.

Pullen FW: Perilymphatic fistula induced by barotrauma. Am J Otol 13:270–272, 1992.

Rabinowitz Dagi LR, Chrousos GA, Cogan DC: Spasm of the near reflex associated with organic disease. Am J Ophthalmol 103:582–585, 1987.

Rascol O, Hain TC, Brefel C, Benazet M, Clanet M, Montastruc JL: Antivertigo medications and drug-induced vertigo. Drugs 50:777–791, 1995.

Rassekh CH, Harker LA: The prevalence of migraine in Meniere's disease. Laryngoscope 102:135–138, 1992.

Rhoton AL: Microsurgical anatomy of posterior fossa cranial nerves. In: Barrow DL (ed). Surgery of the Cranial Nerves of the Posterior Fossa. Park Ridge: American Association of Neurological Surgeons, 1993, pp 1–103.

Richter E: Quantitative study of human Scarpa's ganglion and vestibular sensory epithelia. Acta Otolaryngol 90:199–208, 1980.

Richter E, Schuknecht HF: Loss of vestibular neurons in clinical otosclerosis. Arch Otorhinolaryngol 234:1–9, 1982.

Rintelmann WF (ed): Hearing Assessment. Perspectives in Audiology Series. Austin: Pro-Ed, 1991.

Rosenhall U, Rubin W: Degenerative changes in the human vestibular sensory epithelia. Acta Otolaryngol 79:67–80, 1975.

Ross MD, Peacor D, Johnsson LG, Allard LF: Observations on normal and degenerating human otoconia. Ann Otol 85:310–326, 1976.

Russell G, Abu-Arafeh I: Paroxysmal vertigo in children—an epidemiological study. Int J Pediatr Otorhinolaryngol 49(Suppl 1):S105–S107, 1999.

Rutka JA, Barber HO: Recurrent vestibulopathy: Third review. J Otolaryngol 15:105–107, 1986.

Ryan GMS, Cope S: Cervical vertigo. Lancet 2:1355–1358, 1955.

Rybak LP, Matz GJ: Auditory and vestibular effects of toxins. Manifestations of Systemic Disease. In: Cummings W (ed). Otolaryngology—Head and Neck Surgery, Vol 4. St Louis: CV Mosby, 1986, pp 3161–3172.

Ryu H, Yamamoto S, Sugiyama K, Nozue M: Neurovascular compression syndrome of the eighth cranial nerve. What are the most reliable diagnostic signs? Acta Neurochir (Wien) 140:1279–1286, 1998.

Sando I, Miller D, Hemenway WG, Black FO: Vestibular pathology in otosclerosis. Temporal bone histopathological report. Laryngoscope 84(4):593–605, 1974.

Sarkies NJC, Sanders MD: Convergence spasm. Trans Ophthalmol 104:782–786, 1985.

Schluederberg A, Struas SE, Peterson P, Blumenthal S, Komaroff AL, Spring SB, Landay A, Buchwald D: Chronic fatigue syndrome research. Ann Intern Med 117:325–331, 1992.

Schmid R, Jeannerod M: Vestibular habituation: An adaptive process? In: Berthoz, A, Melvill Jones G (eds). Adaptive Mechanisms in Gaze Control. Amsterdam: Elsevier, 1985, pp 113–122.

Schuknecht HF: A clinical study of auditory damage following blows to the head. Ann Otol Rhinol Laryngol 59:331–359, 1950.

Schuknecht HF: Cupulolithiasis. Arch Otolaryngol 90:113–126, 1969.

Schuknecht HF: Mondini dysplasia: A clinical and pathological study. Ann Otol Rhinol Laryngol 89(Suppl 65):3–23, 1980.

Schuknecht HF: Pathology of the Ear. Cambridge: Harvard University Press, 1974.

Schuknecht HF: Positional vertigo: Clinical and experimental observations. Trans Am Acad Ophthalmol Otolaryngol 166:319–332, 1962.

Schuknecht HF, Kitamura K: Vestibular neuritis. Ann Otol Rhinol Laryngol (Suppl) 78(90):1–19, 1981.

Schuknecht HF, Neff WD, Perlman HD: An experimental study of auditory damage following blows to the head. Ann Otol Rhinol Laryngol 60:273–289, 1951.

Schwaber MK, Whetsell WO: Cochleovestibular nerve compression syndrome. II. Vestibular nerve histopathology and theory of pathophysiology. Laryngoscope 102:1030–1036, 1992.

Scully RE, Mark E, McNeely W, McNeely B: Weekly clinicopathological exercises. N Engl J Med 329:1560, 1993.

Sekhar LN, Gormley WB, Wright DC: The best treatment for vestibular schwannoma (acoustic neuroma): Microsurgery or radiosurgery? Am J Otol 17(4):676–689, 1996.

Selesnick SH, Jackler RK: A typical hearing loss in acoustic neuroma patients. Laryngoscope 103:437–446, 1993.

Selters WA, Brackmann DE: Acoustic tumor detection with brain stem electric response audiometry. Arch Otolaryngol 103:181–187, 1977.

Semont A, Greyss G, Vitte E: Curing the BPPV with a liberatory maneuver. Adv Otorhinolaryngol 42:290–293, 1988.

Sharpe JA, Fletcher WA: Saccadic intrusions and oscillations. Can J Neurol Sci 11:426–433, 1984.

Shea JJ, Ge X, Orchik DJ: Endolymphatic hydrops associated with otosclerosis. Am J Otol 15:348–357, 1994.

Sheehy JL, Brackmann DE, Graham MD: Cholesteatoma surgery: Residual and recurrent disease. Ann Otol Rhinol Laryngol 86:1–12, 1977.

Sheehy JL, Hughes RL: The ABC's of impedance audiometry. Laryngoscope 134(11):1935–1949, 1974.

Shen WK, Gersh BJ: Syncope: mechanisms, approach, and management. In: Low PA (ed). Clinical Autonomic Disorders: Evaluation and Management. Boston: Litle, Brown and Company, 1993, 605–640.

Shumway-Cook A, Horak FB: Assessing the influence of sensory interaction on balance. J Am Phys Ther Assoc 66(10):1548–1550, 1986.

Shumway-Cook A, Horak FB: Rehabilitation strategies for patients with vestibular deficits. In: Arenberg, IK (ed). Dizziness and Balance Disorders. New York: Kugler, 1993, pp 667–691.

Silverstein H, Norell, H: Retrolabyrinthine vestibular neurectomy. Otolaryngol Head Neck Surg 90:778–782, 1982.

Silverstein H, Smouha E, Jones R: Natural history vs. surgery for Meniere's disease. Otolaryngol Head Neck Surg 100:6–16, 1989.

Silverstein H, Wolfson RJ, Rosenberg S: Diagnosis and management of hearing loss. Clin Symp 44(3):5, 1992.

Sindwani R, Parnes LS, Goebel JA, Cass SP: Approach to the vestibular patient and driving. A patient perspective. Otolaryngol Head Neck Surg 121:13–17, 1999.

Sinel M, Eisenberg MS: Two unusual gait disturbances: Astasia abasia and camptocormia. Arch Phys Med Rehab 71:1078–1080, 1990.

Skedros DG, Cass SP, Hirsch BE, Kelly RH: Sources of errors in use of beta 2 transferrin analysis for diagnosing perilymphatic and cerebral spinal fluid leaks. Otolaryngol Head Neck Surg 109:861–864, 1993.

Smith BH: Vestibular disturbances in epilepsy. Neurology 10:465–469, 1960.

Smith P, Curthoys I: Mechanisms of recovery following unilateral labyrinthectomy: A review. Brain Res Rev 14:155–180, 1989.

Smullen JL, Andrist EC, Gianoli GJ: Superior semicircular canal dehiscence: A new cause of vertigo. J LA State Med Soc 151:397–400, 1999.

Soliman AM: Experimental autoimmune inner ear disease. Laryngoscope 99:188–194, 1989.

Steele JC, Richardson JC, Olszewski J: Progressive supranuclear palsy. Arch Neurol 10:333–359, 1964.

Stewart WF, Linet MS, Celentano DD: Migraine headaches and panic attacks. Physcosom Med 51:559–569, 1989.

Stolz SE, Chatrian G-E, Spence A: Epileptic nystagmus. Epilepsia 32:910–918, 1991.

Strasnick B, Glasscock ME, Haynes D, McMenomey SO, Minor LB. The natural history of untreated acoustic neuromas. Laryngoscope 104:1115–1119, 1994.

Straus SE, Gluckman SJ: Clinical features of chronic fatigue syndrome. UptoDate Online 9.3, November 15, 2001.

Strupp M, Arbusow V, Dieterich M, Sautier W, Brandt T: Perceptual and oculomotor effects of neck muscle vibration in vestibular neuritis. Ipsilateral somatosensory substitution of vestibular function. Brain 121:677–685, 1998.

Strupp M, Arbusow V, Maag KP, Gall C, Brandt T: Vestibular exercises improve central vestibulospinal compensation after vestibular neuritis. Neurology 51(3):838–844, 1998.

Supance JS, Bluestone CD: Perilymph fistulas in infants and children. Otolaryngol Head Neck Surg 91:663–671, 1983.

The Alternative Medicine HomePage: http://www.pitt.edu/~cdw/altm.html, 10/27/01.

The Combined Health Information Database: http//child.nih.gov/subfile/contribs/am.html, 10/27/01.

Theunissen EJ, Huygen PL, Folgering HT: Vestibular hyperactivity and hyperventilation. Clin Otolaryngol 111:161–169, 1986.

Thompson PD: Orthostatic tremor. J Neurol Neurosurg Psychiatry 66:278, 1999.

Tinetti ME, Speechley M, Ginter SG: Risk factors for falls among elderly persons living in the community. N Engl J Med 319:1701–1707, 1988.

Toglia J, Thomas K, Kuritzky A: Common migraine and vestibular function electronystagmographic study and pathogenesis. Ann Otol 90:267–271, 1981.

Tusa RJ, Kaplan PW, Hain TC, Naidu S: Ipsiversive eye deviation and epileptic nystagmus. Neurology 40:662–665, 1990.

Uemura T, Suzuki J, Hozawa J, Highstein SM: Neuro-Otological Examination. Baltimore: University Park Press, 1977.

Uimonen S, Laitakari K, Kiukaanniemi H, Sorri M: Does posturography differentiate malingerers from vertiginous patients? J Vestib Res 5(2):117–124, 1995.

Veilleux M, Sharbrough FW, Kelly JJ, Westmoreland BF, Daube JR: Shaky-legs syndrome. J Clin Neurophysiol 4(3):304–305, 1987.

Veldman JE, Roord JJ, O'Connor AF, Shea JJ: Autoimmunity and inner ear disorders: An immune-complex mediated sensorineural hearing loss. Laryngoscope 94:501, 1984.

Vogel H, Thumler R, Von Baumgarten RJ: Ocular counterrolling. Acta Otolaryngol (Stockh) 102:457–462, 1986.

Von Baumgarten RJ: Plasticity in the nervous system at the unitary level. In: Schmitt FO (ed). The Neurosciences: Second Study Program. New York: Rockefeller University, 1970, pp 260–271.

Wackym PA: Molecular temporal bone pathology: II. Ramsay Hunt syndrome (herpes zoster oticus). Laryngoscope 107(9):1165–1175, 1997.

Wackym PA, Linthicum FH Jr, Ward PH, House WF, Micevych PE, Bagger-Sjoback D: Re-evaluation of the role of the human endolymphatic sac in Meniere's disease. Otolaryngol Head Neck Surg 102:732–744, 1990.

Waespe W, Cohen B, Raphan T: Dynamic modification of the vestibulo-ocular reflex by the nodulus and uvula. Science 288:199–202, 1985.

Walby PA, Barrerra A, Schuknecht HF: Cochlear pathology in chronic suppurative otitis media. Ann Otol Rhinol Laryngol 103(Suppl):3–19, 1983.

Walker JS, Barnes SB: Dizziness. Emerg Med Clin North Am 16(4):845–875, 1998.

Watson CP, Terbrugge K: Positional nystamus of the benign paroxysmal type with posterior fossa medullobastoma. Arch Neurol 39:601–602, 1982.

Watson P, Barber HO, Deck J, Terbrugge K: Positional vertigo and nystagmus of central origin. J Can Sci Neurol 8:133, 1981.

Watson SRD, Halmagyi M, Colebatch, JG: Vestibular hypersensitivity to sound (Tullio phenomenon). Neurology 54:722–728, 2000.

Weber PC, Cass SP: Clinical assessment of postural stability. Am J Otol 14(6):566–569, 1993.

Weber PC, Cass SP: Neurotologic manifestations of Chiari 1 malformation. Otolaryngol Head Neck Surg 109:853–860, 1993.

Weiser M, Strosser W, Klein P: Homeopathic vs conventional treatment of vertigo. A randomized double-blind controlled clinical study. Arch Otolaryngol Head Neck Surg 124:879–885, 1998.

Weller TH: Varicella and herpes zoster: Changing concepts of the natural history, control, and importance of a not-so-benign virus. N Engl J Med 309:1434–1440, 1983.

Wennmo K, Wennmo C: Drug-related dizziness. Acta Otolaryngol 455(Suppl):11–13, 1988.

Westheimer G, Blair S: The ocular tilt reaction—a brainstem oculomotor routine. Invest Ophthalmol 14:833–839, 1975.

Whitman GT, Tang T, Lin A, Baloh RW: A prospective study of cerebral white matter abnormalities in older people with gait dysfunction. Neurology 57(6):990–994, 2001.

Whitney SL, Wrisley DM, Brown KD, Furman JM: Physical therapy for migraine-related vestibulopathy and vestibular dysfunction with history of migraine. Laryngoscope 110(9):1528–1534, 2000.

Wiet RJ, Zappia JJ, Hecht CS, O'Connor CA: Conservative management of patients with small acoustic tumors. Laryngoscope 105:795–800, 1995.

Williams NP, Roland PS, Yellin W: Vestibular evaluation in patients with early multiple sclerosis. Am J Otol 18:93–100, 1997.

Williams DP, Troost BT, Rogers J: Lithium-induced downbeat nystagmus. Arch Neurol 45:1022–1023, 1988.

Wilson DF, Hodgson RS, Gustafson MF, Hogue S, Mills L: The sensitivity of auditory brainstem response testing in small acoustic neuromas. Laryngoscope 102:961–964, 1992.

Wist ER, Brandt T, Krafczyk S: Oscillopsia and retinal slip. Brain 106:153–168, 1983.

Wladislavosky-Waserman P, Facer GW, Mokri B, Kurland LT: Meniere's disease: A 30 year epidemiology and clinical study in Rochester, MN, 1951–1980. Laryngoscope 94:1098–1102, 1984.

Wrisley DM, Sparto PJ, Whitney SL, Furman JM: Cervicogenic dizziness. J Orthop Sports Phys Ther 30(12):755–766, 2000.

Yamanobe S, Harris JP: Inner ear-specific antibodies. Laryngoscope 103:319–326, 1993.

Yates BJ: Vestibular influences on the sympathetic nervous system. Brain Res Rev 17:51–59, 1992.

Yates BJ, Jakus J, Miller A: Vestibular effects on respiratory outflow in the decerebrate cat. Brain Res 629:209–217, 1993.

Yates BJ, Miller AD (eds): Vestibular Autonomic Regulation. Boca Raton: CRC Press, 1996.

Yazawa Y, Kitahara M: Bilateral endolymphatic hydrops in Meniere's disease: Review of temporal bone autopsies. Ann Otol Rhinol Laryngol 99:524–528, 1990.

Yee C, Baloh R, Honrubia V: Effect of Baclofen on congenital nystagmus. In: Lennerstrand G, Zee D, Keller E (eds), Functional Basis of Ocular Motility Disorders. Oxford: Pergamon Press, 1982, pp 151–158.

Yee RD, Farlow MR, Suzuki DA, Betelak KF, Ghetti B: Abnormal eye movements in Gerstmann-Straussler-Scheinker disease. Arch Ophthalmol 110:68–74, 1992.

Yoo TJ: Etiopathogenesis of Meniere's disease: A hypothesis. Ann Otol Rhinol Laryngol 93(Suppl 113):6–12, 1984.

Yoo TJ, Yazawa Y, Tomoda K, Floyd R: Type II collagen-induced autoimmune endolymphatic hydrops in guinea pig. Science 222:65–67, 1983.

Zee DS: Ophthalmoscopy in examination of patients with vestibular disorders. Ann Neurol 3(4):373–374, 1978.

Zee DS, Friendlich AL, Robinson DA: The mechanism of downbeat nystagmus. Arch Neurol 30:227–237, 1974.

Zee DS, Robinson DA: A hypothetical explanation of saccadic oscillations. Ann Neurol 5:405–414, 1979.

Zee D, Yee R, Robinson D: Optokinetic responses in labyrinthine-defective human beings. Brain Res 113:423–428, 1976.

Zilstorff-Pedersen K, Peitersen E: Vestibulospinal reflexes. Arch Otolaryngol 77:237–245, 1963.

Appendix of Diagnoses

Diagnosis/Condition	Case No.
Acoustic neuroma	2, 50
Anterior inferior cerebellar artery syndrome	30
Anxiety disorder	5, 22, 24
Autoimmune inner ear disease	27
Benign paroxysmal positional vertigo	7, 22, 25, 31,39
Benign paroxysmal vertigo of childhood	13
Bilateral vestibular loss	4
Brainstem infarction	29, 30, 38
Cerebellar degeneration	19
Cerebellar hemorrhage	6
Cerebellopontine angle lesion	2, 50
Cervicogenic dizziness	53
Chiari malformation	40
Chronic fatigue syndrome	54
Congenital nystagmus	42
Convergence spasm	36
Creutzfieldt-Jakob disease	48
Disequilibrium of aging	10
Drop attacks	34
Drug-induced dizziness	32
Endolymphatic hydrops (Meniere's disease)	9, 16, 21, 25, 34, 58
Enlarged vestibular aqueduct syndrome	37
Herpes zoster oticus	35
Horizontal semicircular canal benign positional vertigo	39

Impaired compensation	3
Labyrinthine concussion	11, 23, 42
Mal de débarquement syndrome	26
Malformation of the inner ear	37
Meniere's disease (endolymphatic hydrops)	9, 16, 21, 25, 34, 58
Migraine-associated dizziness	8, 13, 21, 24, 33
Multiple sclerosis	20
Multisensory disequilibrium	14
Nonspecific vestibulopathy	17
Ocular flutter	41
Orthostatic hypotension	28
Orthostatic tremor	49
Otitis media and cholesteatoma formation	18
Otosclerosis and otosclerotic inner ear disease	43
Ototoxicity	4
Perilymphatic fistula	18, 52
Posterior inferior cerebellar artery syndrome	29
Progressive supranuclear palsy	44
Psychiatric dizziness	5, 22, 24
Ramsay Hunt syndrome	35
Recurrent vestibulopathy	15
Solvent toxicity	45
Superior semicircular canal dehiscence syndrome	51
Syncope	33
Tullio's phenomenon	51
Vascular cross compression syndrome of the eighth cranial nerve	57
Vertebrobasilar insufficiency	12
Vestibular epilepsy	47
Vestibular neuritis	1,3
Wallenberg's syndrome	29
Wernicke's encephalopathy	46

INDEX

Acoustic neuroma, 74, 75, 223, 226, 341–346
Acoustic reflex testing, 43–44
Acyclovir, 69, 263, 264
Aging, 128–132
AICA. *See* Anterior-inferior cerebellar artery
Alcohol, 324, 325
Alexander's law, 65, 70, 322–323
Aminoglycoside ototoxicity, 83–84, 87
Amitriptyline, 94, 115, 118, 148, 220, 336, 377
Ampulla, 4–5, 109, 246
Anterior-inferior cerebellar artery (AICA), 75–76, 99, 142–143, 237–242
Antivert, 172
Anxiety disorders, 57, 91–96, 101, 145, 148
 benign paroxysmal positional vertigo and, 200–203
 migraine-related dizziness and, 208–212
Aspirin, 235, 240
Audiogram, 42–43, 164
Auditory-evoked potential testing. *See* Brain stem auditory-evoked potential testing
Auditory system. *See* Hearing
Autoimmune inner ear disease, 83, 124, 222–227
Autonomic nervous system
 vestibular projections to, 12

Balcofen, 318, 380–381
Basilar artery migraine, 253–255, 257
Benign paroxysmal positional vertigo (BPPV), 26–27, 48, 54, 105–114, 136–137, 282

anxiety disorder and, 200–203
endolymphatic hydrops and, 213–216
horizontal semicircular canal variant and. *See* Horizontal semicircular canal variant
Brandt-Daroff exercises and, 243–244
particle repositioning maneuver for. *See* Particle repositioning maneuver
surgical options and, 243–248
Benign paroxysmal vertigo of childhood. *See* Benign recurrent vertigo of childhood
Benign positional vertigo. *See* Benign paroxysmal positional vertigo
Benign recurrent vertigo of childhood, 145–148
Bilateral Meniere's disease, 382–387
Bilateral vestibular loss. *See* Vestibular loss, bilateral
Bony labyrinthine fistula, 175–176, 178
BPPV. *See* Benign paroxysmal positional vertigo
BPV. *See* Benign paroxysmal positional vertigo
Brainstem auditory-evoked potential (BAEP) testing, 44–45
Brainstem infarction, 97–98, 237, 244, 279–280
Brain stem concussion, 97–98, 133, 137, 204, 206, 301
Brandt-Daroff exercises, 110, 112
Bromocryptine, 315
Buspirone, 94

Caloric testing, 32–35
Canalithiasis, 107, 109, 245
Carbamazepine, 377, 380–381
Carbidopa-levodopa, 336
Carbonic anhydrase, 220
Central vestibular system, 13, 317, 321
Cerebellar degeneration. See Cerebellum,
    degeneration
Cerebellar hemorrhage, 97
Cerebellar infarction, 97–101, 237
Cerebellopontine angle neoplasm, 17, 41, 43,
    72–76, 87
Cerebellum, 7, 23, 73, 82, 92, 99, 142, 239, 294,
    314, 331
  degeneration, 180–185
  effect on vestibular system, 13
Cervical vertigo, 359–363
  cervico-ocular reflex, 12, 28, 87, 361–362
Cervicogenic dizziness, 204, 363, 559
Cervicogenic vertigo, 133, 137
Chiari malformation, 169–170, 173, 181, 184,
    253, 255, 267, 287–292
Chlordiazepoxide, 94
Cholesteatoma, 174–175, 177–178, 357
Chronic fatigue syndrome, 364–367
Chronic middle ear disease. See Chronic otitis
    media
Chronic otitis media, 174–179
Clonazepam, 94, 110, 118, 171–172, 198, 210,
    220, 336, 345, 390
Clorazepate, 336
Cogan's syndrome, 166–167, 223, 225, 227
Compazine, 126
Compensation, 13–14, 37, 63–71, 74, 136, 149,
    164, 205–207
Complementary and alternative therapies for
    dizziness, 388–392
Congenital inner ear malformations, 269–277,
    348, 351, 357–358
Congenital nystagmus, 24
Convergence spasm, 23, 265–268
Creutzfeldt-Jakob disease, 331–333
Cupula, 4
Cupuloithiasis, 107, 109, 245, 318
Cyclizine, 172
Cyclobenzaprine, 362

Dandy's syndrome, 83, 88
Demyelinating diseases. See Multiple sclerosis
Desipramine, 94
Diabetes mellitus, 228. See also Multisensory
    disequilibrium and, 149–153
Diazepam, 94, 110, 172, 200, 220, 366, 377
Dimenhydrinate, 172
Diphenhydramine, 172
Directional preponderance, 35–36
Disabling positional vertigo. See Vascular
    compression syndrome; Eighth cranial
    nerve
Disequilibrium of aging, 128–132, 332, 336

Dix-Hallpike maneuver, 21, 26, 32, 49, 106,
    108, 111, 113, 201
Dizziness. 16–20. See also Vertigo
Dizziness Handicap Inventory, 49
Dolls' eyes, 313
Downbeating nystagmus. See Nystagmus,
    downbeating
Driving and dizziness, 368–372
Drop attacks, 140, 141, 256–259
Drug-Induced dizziness. See Lithium-induced
    dizziness
Dysautonomia. See Othorstatic hypotension

Earth-vertical axis rotational testing, 36–37. See
    also Rotational testing
Eighth cranial nerve, 4, 6–9, 41–43, 241
  disorders of, 377–381
  root entry-zone lesions, 68
Electrocochleography, 45–46
Electronystagmography (ENG), 32, 117
Electro-oculography, 31–32
Endolymphatic hydrops, 45, 100, 121–127, 154,
    156, 158–168, 195–199, 213–216, 377
  Tumarkin's otolithic crisis and, 257, 259,
    370, 372
Endolymphatic sac
  surgery of, 159, 167
ENG. See Electronystagmography
Enlarged vestibular aqueduct syndrome, 274
Epstein-Barr virus
  chronic fatigue syndrome and, 365
Ethanol use, 324–325
Eye movement abnormalities. See Nystagmus;
    specific disorders

Fludrocortisone, 230
Frenzel glasses, 24, 26, 67, 71

Gabapentin, 150, 251, 336, 380–381
Gaze-evoked nystagmus. See Nystagmus,
    gaze-evoked
Gentamicin, 83, 85, 161

Hair cells, 4–7, 130–131, 161, 270
HCBPV. See Horizontal semicircular canal
    benign positional vertigo
Head-fixed body-turned maneuvers, 28,
    360–361
Head trauma, 204–207
  persistent dizziness, etiology of, 206
Hearing, 17, 23–24, 42
Hennebert's sign, 176, 178, 348, 351
Herpes zoster, 261–264
Histamine injection, 126
History of the dizzy patient, 16–20
Horizontal semicircular canal benign
    positional vertigo (HCBPV), 244,
    282–286
Hydrochlorothiazide, 126, 195, 213, 258, 377
Hydroxyzine, 94, 172
Hyperventilation, 93, 95, 100, 201, 254

Imipramine, 94, 210, 369
Impaired compensation, 79–80, 344
Industrial solvent exposure. *See* Solvent
  exposure
Internal auditory artery, 142–143, 238
Internuclear ophthalmoplegia, 23, 187, 189,
  191

Labyrinth. *See* Peripheral vestibular system
Labyrinthectomy
  chemical, 161, 167
  surgical, 159, 161, 167
Labyrinthine artery. *See* Internal auditory
  artery
Labyrinthine concussion, 107, 133–138,
  204–206, 265, 301, 354–355, 358, 374, 389
Labyrinthine infarction, 107
Lateral medullary syndrome. *See* Wallenberg's
  syndrome
Lateral vestibulospinal tract (LVST), 11
Lateropulsion, 233, 236
  saccadic, 234
Lithium, 249
Lithium-induced dizziness, 249–252
Lyme disease, 262–263

Macula, 4, 6
Mal debarquement syndrome, 219–221
Malformation of the inner ear. *See* Congenital
  inner ear malformation
Malingering, 373–376
Meclizine, 77–78, 82, 110, 126, 128, 133, 136,
  150, 152, 158, 169, 172, 190, 204, 219,
  220, 222, 265, 300, 341, 347, 353, 366, 377
Medial vestibulospinal tract (MVST), 11
Meniere's disease. See Endolymphatic
  hydrops
Midbrain, 314–315
Migraine, 100, 146–148, 154, 156, 257, 326, 388
  basilar artery, 195–199, 254
  dizziness and, 17–18, 115–120, 141, 170, 173,
    208–212, 249, 326–327, 368–369, 388
  vestibular laboratory abnormalities, 117
Mondini malformation. *See* Congenital inner
  ear malformations
Multiple sclerosis, 17–18, 97, 100, 170, 173,
  186–191, 267, 296
Multisensory disequilibrium, 180
  diabetes mellitus and 149–153

Neurotologic examination, 24–29
Nicotinic acid, 126
Nonspecific vestibulopathy, 169–173, 390, 367
Nystagmus, 23–25, 28, 31–33, 35, 37, 122–123
  Alexander's law, 65, 70
  Brun's, 72, 76
  caloric, 34
  cervical, 28
  congenital, 299–303
  downbeating, 249–251, 288, 290–291

epileptic, 328
gaze-evoked, 30, 73, 98, 290, 292
jerk, 23, 302–303
pendular, 23, 191, 302–303
periodic alternating, 220
positional, 26, 31, 129, 300, 317, 319, 379
  paroxysmal, 32, 283, 286, 391
  persistent, 26
spontaneous, 21, 34, 81, 223, 241, 290–291
upbeating, 201, 322
vestibular, 65, 67, 70, 98, 220, 241

Ocular flutter. *See* Saccadic fixation
  instabilities
Ocular motor testing, 29–31
Ocular tilt reaction, 278–281
Opsoclonus. *See* Saccadic fixation instabilities
Orthostatic hypotension, 228–232, 251, 254
Orthostatic tremor, 334–337
Oscillopsia, 83, 88
Otitis media, 174–179
  cholesteatoma formation and, 177
Otolith organs, 3–4, 12, 22, 215–216, 220, 280
Otologic examination, 21–22
Otosclerosis, 42, 223, 226
  otosclerotic inner ear disease and, 304–311
Ototoxicity, 82–90, 222, 226

Papaverine, 126
Particle repositioning maneuver, 110, 113, 202,
  215–216, 283–284, 286
Pendular nystagmus. *See* Nystagmus,
  pendular
Periactin, 147–148
Perilymphatic fistula, 43, 136–137, 175, 178,
  271, 276, 348, 351, 353–358
Peripheral vestibular system, 7, 12–15, 317
  aging effects, 130–131
Phenobarbital, 336
PICA. *See* Wallenberg's syndrome
Positional nystagmus. *See* Nystagmus,
  positional
Positional testing, 31–32
Positional vertigo. *See* Benign paroxysmal
  positional vertigo
Posterior-inferior cerebellar artery (PICA), 99,
  143–142, 233–236, 238, 242
Posterior semicircular canal occlusion, 246, 248
Postural sway, 21
Posturography, 27, 30, 38–40, 117
Prednisone, 69, 225, 227, 263–264, 275, 297
Presbyastasis, 130–131
Primidone, 336
Prion disease, 330–333
Prochlorperazine, 156, 172
Progressive supranuclear palsy, 312–315
Promethazine, 105, 126, 156, 171–172, 220, 309,
  377
Propranolol, 118, 147–148, 255, 336
Pseudoephedrine, 171–172

Psychiatric dizziness, 56, 58, 91–96
Psychogenic dizziness. *See* Psychiatric
　　dizziness
Psychosomatic mechanisms, 58

Ramsay Hunt syndrome, 260–264
Recurrent vestibulopathy, 154–157
Rheumatologic diseases, 225, 227
Rinne's test, 21, 24
Romberg's test, 21, 27, 50
Root entry-zone lesion, 187–188, 190
Rotational testing, 30–31, 35–38, 89, 117

Saccadic fixation instabilities, 23, 92, 201,
　　293–298, 313–314
Saccadic lateropulsion. *See* Lateropulsion,
　　saccadic
Saccule, 3–4, 6, 122
Scopolamine, 172, 219, 251
Semicircular canals, 3–5, 11–12, 32–34,
　　107–109, 113, 161, 175, 246, 284,
　　317–318, 347–352
Sensorineural hearing loss. *See* Hearing
Serous labyrinthitis, 175, 178
Singular neurectomy, 246, 248
Sjogren's syndrome, 83
Skew deviation, 22, 279–281
Solvent exposure, 316–320
Space and motion discomfort, 58, 92–93, 95,
　　118, 201, 210, 388
Square-wave jerks. *See* Saccadic fixation
　　instability
Stepping test, 21, 27–28
Superior semicircular canal dehiscence
　　syndrome, 347–352
Syncope, 231, 253–256

Thiamine, 324
Tinnitus, 17, 72, 137, 141, 210, 213, 237, 242,
　　254
　　congenital inner ear malformations and,
　　　269–270
　　endolymphatic hydrops or Meniere's
　　　disease and, 121, 126, 159, 163–164, 166,
　　　195–196
　　otosclerosis and, 306, 310
　　perilymphatic fistula and, 356, 358
　　Ramsay Hunt syndrome and, 260, 263
　　vascular compression syndrome of the
　　　eighth cranial nerve and, 378, 381
Tornado epilepsy. *See* Vestibular epilepsy
Trauma. *See* Head trauma

Triameterene, 126, 195, 213, 258, 377
Trimethobenzamine, 172
Tullio's phenomenon, 347–352
Tumarkin's otolithic crisis. *See* Endolymphatic
　　hydrops, Tumarkin's crisis
Tympanometry, 43–44

Unterberger stepping test, 28
Utricle, 3–4, 6, 107, 122

Valproic acid, 118, 251, 336
Vascular compression syndrome, 377–381
Verapamil, 118
Vertebrobasilar insufficiency, 17, 116, 139–144,
　　155, 253, 255, 257, 267, 326, 328
Vertigo, 16, 20, 32, 77, 97, 105–114, 121–122,
　　126, 139–140, 144–148, 154, 158, 161,
　　163–164, 166, 213–216, 241–248, 254,
　　260, 282–286, 326
　　defined, 16
Vestibular-autonomic projections, 12
Vestibular compensation. *See* Compensation
Vestibular epilepsy, 326–329
Vestibular laboratory testing, 30–40, 211
　　indications for, 30
　　types of, 31–40
Vestibular labyrinth. *See* Peripheral vestibular
　　system
Vestibular loss, 47
　　bilateral, 25, 34–35, 51, 82–90, 383
　　unilateral, 12–15, 25, 35, 63–71
Vestibular nerve, 7
Vestibular nerve section, 159, 161, 163, 167,
　　246, 248
Vestibular neuritis, 41, 63–71, 77–81
Vestibular nuclei, 7–11, 14, 45, 143, 235, 241,
　　324–325
Vestibular paroxysmia. *See* Vascular
　　compression syndrome of the eighth
　　cranial nerve
Vestibular rehabilitation, 47–53, 59, 118, 152,
　　210, 212, 336
Vestibulo-ocular reflex (VOR), 9–11, 14, 17, 21,
　　24, 30–31, 36, 48, 314, 324
Vestibulospinal reflexes, 12–13, 31
Video-oculography, 31–32
Visual-vestibular interaction testing, 37
VOR. *See* Vestibulo-ocular reflex

Wallenberg's syndrome, 143, 233–236, 238, 242
Weber's test, 21, 24
Wernicke's encephalopathy, 321–325